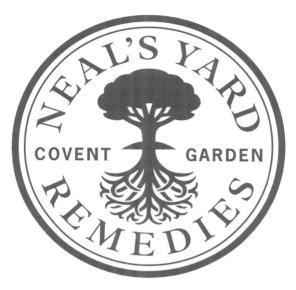

BEAUTY
BOOK

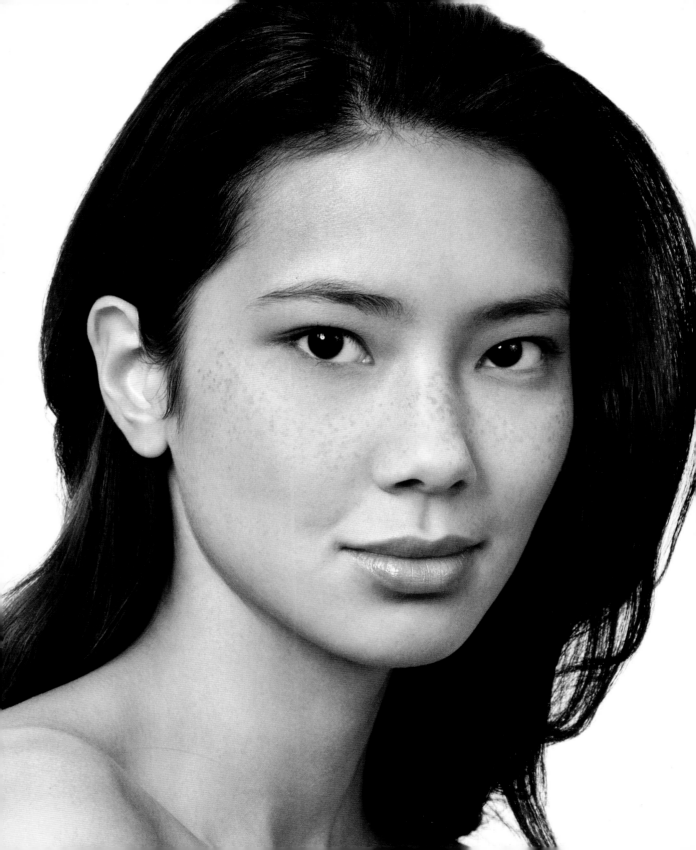

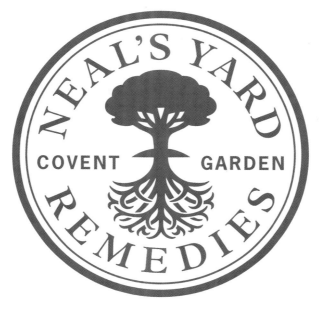

BEAUTY
BOOK

LONDON, NEW YORK, MELBOURNE, MUNICH, AND DELHI

DK LONDON
Project Editor Martha Burley
Senior Art Editor Tessa Bindloss
Design Assistant Laura Buscemi
Managing Editor Dawn Henderson
Managing Art Editor Christine Keilty
Jacket Art Editor Kathryn Wilding
Senior Jacket Creative Nicola Powling
Senior Producer, Pre-Production Tony Phipps
Senior Producer Jen Scothern
Art Director Peter Luff
Publisher Peggy Vance

DK INDIA
Senior Art Editor Balwant Singh
Editors Manasvi Vohra, Janashree Singha
Art Editor Vikas Sachdeva
Assistant Art Editor Pallavi Kapur
Managing Editor Alicia Ingty
Managing Art Editor Navidita Thapa
Pre-Production Manager Sunil Sharma
DTP Designer Satish Chandra Gaur

First published in Great Britain in 2015 by
Dorling Kindersley Limited
80 Strand, London, WC2R 0RL

2 4 6 8 10 9 7 5 3 1

001 – 256554 – Feb/2015

A CIP catalogue record for this book is available from
the British Library.

ISBN 978-0-2411-8391-5

Printed and bound in China by Hung Hing (DK)

Discover more at **www.dk.com**

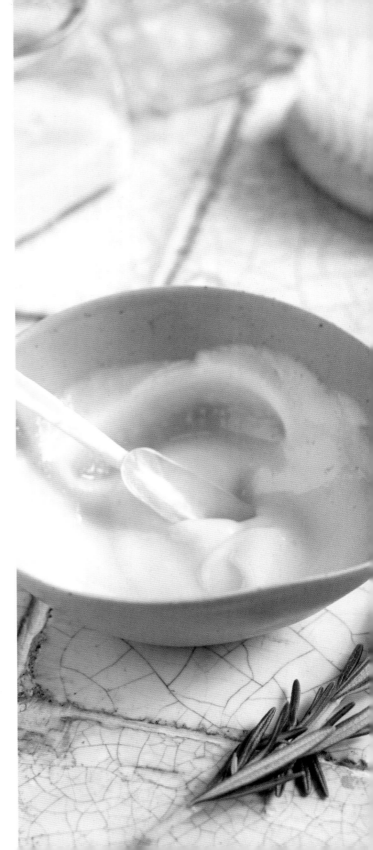

CONTENTS

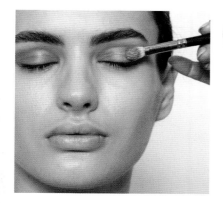

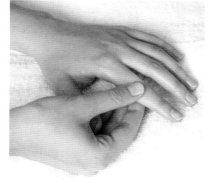

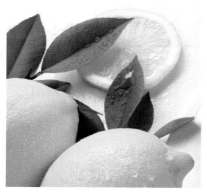

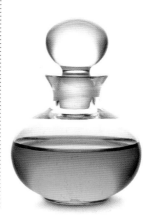

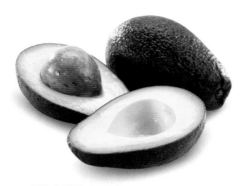

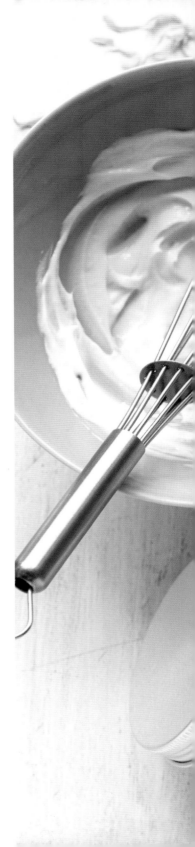

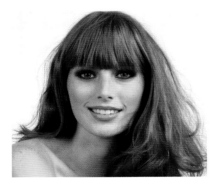

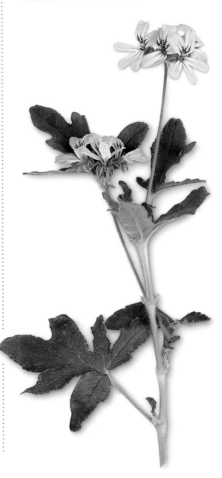

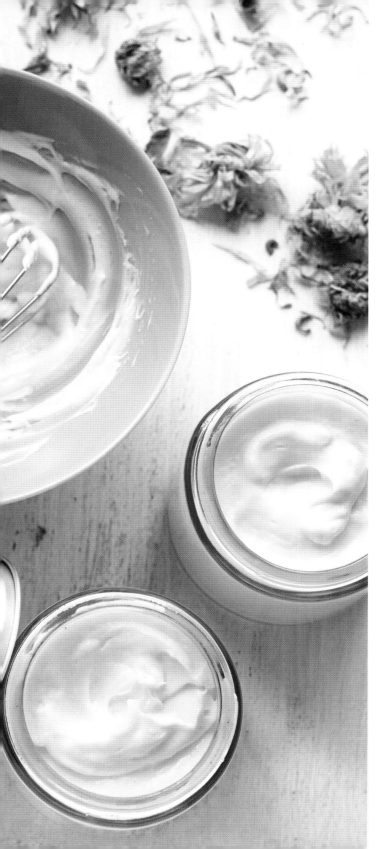

THE AUTHORS

Susan Curtis is a qualified homoeopath and naturopath and is the Director of Natural Health for Neal's Yard Remedies. She is the author of several books including *Looking Good and Feeling Younger* and *Essential Oils* and co-author of *Natural Healing for Women*. Susan has two grown-up children and is passionate about helping people to live a more natural and healthy lifestyle.

Fran Johnson is a passionate Cosmetic Scientist and has been the Formulator at Neal's Yard Remedies since 2006. She is a practising aromatherapist and plans and teaches a number of Neal's Yard Remedies courses that cover making cosmetic products, aromatherapy, and natural perfumery, including the best-selling course, Recipes for Natural Beauty.

Pat Thomas is a journalist, campaigner, and broadcaster. Her previous books include *Cleaning Yourself to Death*, *What's in this Stuff*, and *Skin Deep*. Through her work she has led the way in exposing the harmful chemicals in many everyday beauty products, as well as promoting natural alternatives that work. She is a former editor of *The Ecologist* magazine and currently sits on the Council of Trustees of the Soil Association – the UK's premier organic certification body – and is the editor of Neal's Yard Remedies' natural health website, *NYR Natural News*.

THE MAKE-UP ARTIST

Justine Jenkins is a renowned and influential celebrity make-up artist, cruelty-free cosmetics ambassador, broadcaster, and writer about natural beauty and make-up. Her work frequently appears in print and online.

INTRODUCTION

TAKING **CARE** OF OURSELVES ON THE INSIDE AND THE OUTSIDE ENABLES OUR TRUE BEAUTY TO SHINE THROUGH. **NATURE** PROVIDES ALL WE NEED TO **NOURISH** AND **LOOK AFTER** OUR BODIES, AND BRINGS OUT THE **NATURAL BEAUTY** IN EVERY ONE OF US.

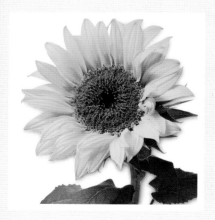
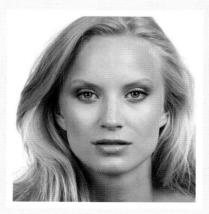
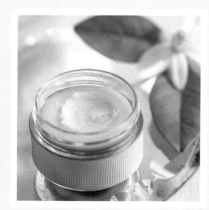

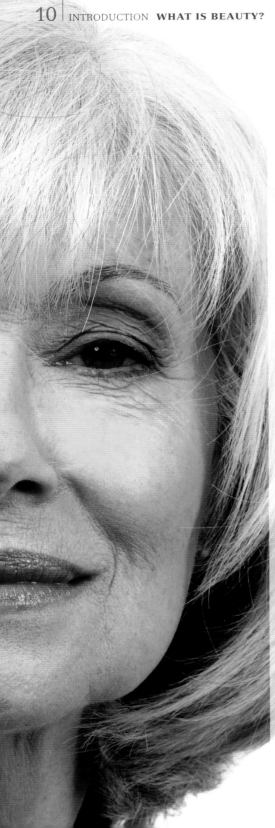

What Is Beauty?

Ask the question "what is beauty?", and you'll get a multitude of different answers. Everybody has a theory. In fact, mankind has been searching for the answer for a long time. The truth is, throughout your life, your own concept of beauty will change. What was appropriate for you at one age or stage of life may not be appropriate at another.

CHANGING PERCEPTIONS

Less than a century ago, the dictionary defined beauty as "properties pleasing the eye, the ear, the intellect, the aesthetic faculty, or the moral sense". Today, the default definition of beauty is narrow, focusing only on what is pleasing to the eye. This change has gained momentum because, for a long time, beauty, even natural beauty, has been defined by the media, Hollywood, and the globalized beauty industry. And yet, when we think of beauty as outwardly focused – a mask that we put on, or what we project in order to please others – we make a game for ourselves that is impossible to win.

Research shows that for most females, the inner beauty critic arrives at age 14 and continues to erode her self-esteem as she ages. This erosion has a profound effect on health and well-being. Research also shows that people who accept their looks are happier and healthier – the stress of fighting who you are can affect your health, which in turn affects physical beauty.

WORKING WITH NATURE

A revolution seeks to redefine beauty as natural and holistic, and more reflective of our needs, emotions, and perceptions. This leaves behind a static, one-size-fits-all philosophy and embraces a broader appreciation of diverse human beings

PRO-AGEING

The notion that youth equates to beauty is not sustainable in a world where the population is ageing. Research shows that interest in youth potions and invasive surgeries falls off after the age of 45. Older women, it seems, are more interested in looking good for their age than looking eternally young. They are also more likely to try therapeutic beauty treatments, such as massage or facials. These therapies don't just improve the appearance, they also embrace the inner self and promote a sense of well-being.

of all ages and cultures. It has also triggered a movement away from synthetic and mass-produced beauty products made from polluting and increasingly scarce petrochemical ingredients, to those made from safe and sustainable natural substances.

As many of us become environmentally aware, we know that there is no real beauty if the means to achieve it are ugly. Animal testing, toxic industrial chemicals, avoidable waste, science experiments such as GMO or nanotechnology that turn customers into lab rats, and lies on the labels are all ugly.

Our increasing interest in natural beauty, which mirrors an increased awareness of being environmentally friendly, is a positive and inspiring cultural shift, and a valuable alternative to plastic beauty.

Concern for what we put in our bodies, and a recent trend for natural and wholesome foods, extends into concern for what we are applying to our bodies. It is hard to feel healthy when one subsists on a diet of refined and highly processed junk food. It is just as hard to feel beautiful when one uses "junk" beauty products, made with petrochemicals or synthetic fragrances that some studies say disrupt the body's hormonal or nervous systems, cause cancer, provoke allergies, or cause harm to your unborn baby.

FROM THE INSIDE OUT

Wanting to be sure of what is actually in the products we use has started another revolution in beauty – an interest in making our own products from known and trusted ingredients. Nature provides much of what we need to stay beautiful in the form of healthy unadulterated foods but also in the form of ingredients such as luxurious oils and plant essences – and you may be surprised to find that some of the best beauty ingredients are already in your kitchen cupboards.

The recipes and tips in his book show how effective natural products are and how you can use them in your day-to-day life. Combining these in creative ways gives you total control over exactly what you are putting on your skin and hair, and is an art and a science that is within your grasp.

First and foremost, beauty should be something we do for ourselves, to feel better, to look better, to express what's inside us, to occasionally treat and indulge. Real beauty should promote a happier, healthier, more relaxed, more confident and comfortable "you". Studies show that our concepts of what is beautiful and what we think others find beautiful are often miles apart. Reclaiming the notion of natural beauty, then, could be seen as a process of narrowing that gap between who you are on the inside and what others see.

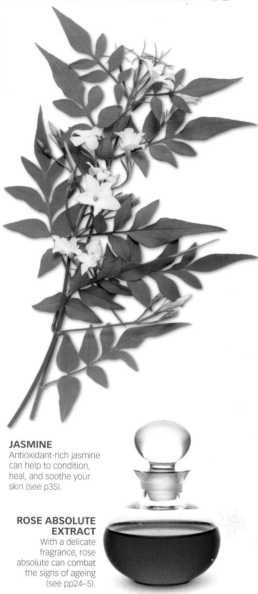

JASMINE
Antioxidant-rich jasmine can help to condition, heal, and soothe your skin (see p35).

ROSE ABSOLUTE EXTRACT
With a delicate fragrance, rose absolute can combat the signs of ageing (see pp24–5).

ECO CONCERNS

Many chemicals in conventional products, such as hormone-disrupting parabens, also harm the planet – either through unsustainable sourcing, during their manufacture, or when they are washed into drains and into our water supplies. As we become more aware of the damage that humankind has done to the planet, it is clear that trashing the planet in the name of vanity simply isn't beautiful.

THE SECRET LIFE OF YOUR SKIN

Your skin is alive and dynamic. It breathes, grows, and changes. It protects the body from bacteria, viruses, and pollutants, takes in nutrients and, through sweat, helps remove toxins. It regulates body temperature, manufactures vitamin D from sunlight, and provides information through touch and pain. Every day the skin reflects and reacts to what you eat and drink, your exposure to the elements, how you sleep, the stress you are under, and your general health.

UNDER YOUR SKIN

The skin consists of three layers: the epidermis, the dermis, and the subcutis. Each layer has particular functions that help skin to renew, react, and protect your body.

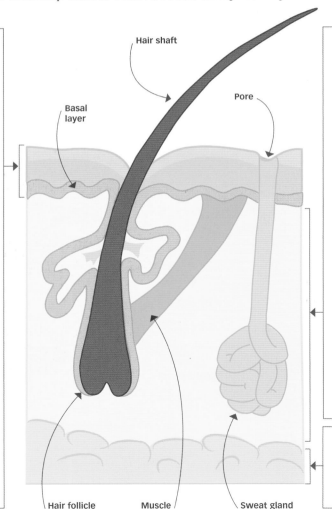

EPIDERMIS

An elastic layer on the outside, the epidermis is continually regenerating. It is made up of a number of different kinds of cells.

KERATINOCYTES
The main cells of the epidermis, keratinocytes are formed by cell division at its base. New cells continually move towards the surface. Gradually, as they move they die, are flattened, and are sloughed off. This process takes around 14 days (longer as we age).

CORNEOCYTES
Flattened dead keratinocytes, corneocytes make up a tough, protective, and virtually waterproof layer called the *stratum corneum* or horny layer. This layer continually renews and is sloughed off. In fact, each of us sloughs off millions of dead skin cells every day.

MELANOCYTES
These produce the pigment melanin that protects against UV radiation and gives skin its colour. Exposure to the sun stimulates increased melanin production, and this results in the skin becoming darker – or tanned. When melanin is unable to absorb all the ultra-violet rays, because of prolonged and unaccustomed exposure, the skin is damaged and it will burn.

DERMIS

The inner layer of the skin is composed of connective tissue, containing both elastin (the fibres that give the qualities of stretch and suppleness to the skin) and collagen (the fibres that provide strength). The dermis also contains numerous blood vessels, follicles, and glands.

HAIR FOLLICLES
These are pits where hair grows. Protective hair plays a role in temperature regulation.

SEBACEOUS GLANDS
These produce sebum (a natural oil), to keep hairs free from dust and bacteria. Sebum and sweat make up the surface "film" of the skin.

SWEAT GLANDS
Sweat is produced in the glands and travels via sweat ducts to openings in the epidermis called pores. They play a role in temperature regulation. Specific types of sweat glands called apocrine glands occur in hair parts of the body and only become active during puberty.

SUBCUTIS

Under the dermis lies the subcutis or subcutaneous layer, which is made up of connective tissue and fat. It is a good insulator.

Hair shaft

Pore

Basal layer

Hair follicle   Muscle   Sweat gland

WORK WITH YOUR SKIN

You should not see normal skin changes as problems that need to be fixed. Try to stop obsessing over minute and transient shifts in skin tone and colour, and adopt a sensible approach to skin care. Some things are beyond our control – how skin ages, for instance, is a complicated process involving a number of internal and external factors, some of which are within our control, many of which are not.

Ageing causes a decrease in collagen and elastin, the "scaffolding" of the skin, causing the skin to wrinkle and sag. Gravity can also make loose skin around eyes and jowls fall even more. Aged skin also appears more translucent because of the decrease in the number of pigment-containing cells (melanocytes). It is also thinner and more fragile, and at increased risk of injury and less able to repair itself.

Accepting the complex secret life of your skin and responding to it with a "from the inside out" approach is not only sensible and healthy, but can also make the difference between being at war or at peace with your skin.

MAKE PEACE WITH YOUR SKIN

If you want beautiful skin – whether it is youthful or mature – then you need to identify and work with the skin's natural rhythms (see pp14–15) and support them with healthy lifestyle choices.

Have a lot of good-quality sleep, which is vital for skin health. Don't only focus on the number of hours, but think about the quality of sleep. A chronic lack of good-quality sleep can age skin by as much as 10 years.

Relieve stress and see a miraculous effect on skin. Help your health and appearance by addressing stress and anxiety, perhaps by engaging in a hobby that absorbs you.

Drink at least 2 litres (3^1/$_2$ pints) of water a day to make a big difference to the radiance and moisture of your skin.

Avoid cigarettes and alcohol, which are highly damaging. Both can dehydrate the skin and interfere with its ability to utilize nutrients – just take a look at your skin after a heavy night out.

Use good-quality skin products that make use of gentle natural cleansing agents and natural oils and plant extracts instead of industrial petrochemical derivatives.

Eat healthily because your diet is influential on the health of your skin in both the short and the long term. For instance, studies show that diets that are high in sugar can make the skin look older. In contrast, diets rich in healthy omega-3 fats can protect against sun damage and even acne.

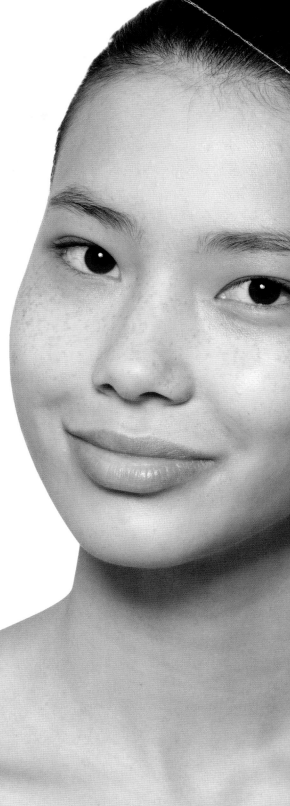

THE RHYTHMS OF YOUR SKIN

As the largest organ in the body, your skin has its own rhythms. It is tempting to try to tame and bully your skin into submission, but getting in touch with its natural rhythms is the most straightforward path to a healthier complexion.

THE DAILY CYCLE

Healthy, normal skin can change on almost an hourly basis. The clocks below show just how regularly your skin changes in the cycle of a day.

AM

You're much more likely to have an allergic skin reaction in the morning than in the afternoon.

AT 8am
Your skin is less likely to absorb products at 8am than in the afternoon, so it is not a good time to apply rich nourishing masks and serums.

PM

Skin is calmer in the late afternoon and evening. However, water loss is high at night, so apply moisturising creams and serums before you go to sleep.

9pm–MIDNIGHT
Skin is more sensitive to histamine late in the evening, which means itchy skin conditions such as dermatitis may be worse. If you need a skin-allergy test, schedule it for as late in the day as possible. Your skin is more acidic, and as a result oilier, when you sleep. Don't make the problem worse by using harsh acidic peels and scrubs before bedtime.

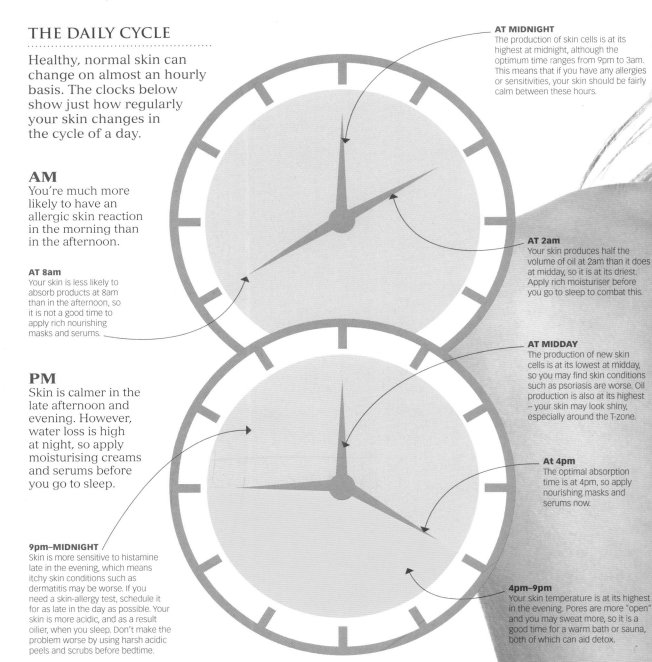

AT MIDNIGHT
The production of skin cells is at its highest at midnight, although the optimum time ranges from 9pm to 3am. This means that if you have any allergies or sensitivities, your skin should be fairly calm between these hours.

AT 2am
Your skin produces half the volume of oil at 2am than it does at midday, so it is at its driest. Apply rich moisturiser before you go to sleep to combat this.

AT MIDDAY
The production of new skin cells is at its lowest at midday, so you may find skin conditions such as psoriasis are worse. Oil production is also at its highest – your skin may look shiny, especially around the T-zone.

At 4pm
The optimal absorption time is at 4pm, so apply nourishing masks and serums now.

4pm–9pm
Your skin temperature is at its highest in the evening. Pores are more "open" and you may sweat more, so it is a good time for a warm bath or sauna, both of which can aid detox.

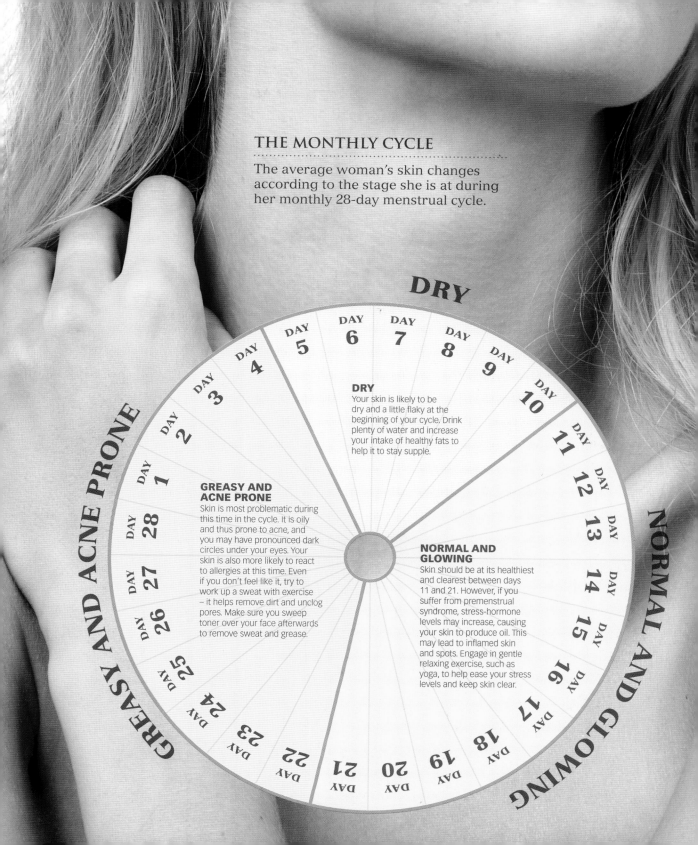

THE MONTHLY CYCLE

The average woman's skin changes according to the stage she is at during her monthly 28-day menstrual cycle.

DRY

DAY 1 · DAY 2 · DAY 3 · DAY 4 · DAY 5 · DAY 6 · DAY 7 · DAY 8 · DAY 9 · DAY 10 · DAY 11 · DAY 12 · DAY 13 · DAY 14 · DAY 15 · DAY 16 · DAY 17 · DAY 18 · DAY 19 · DAY 20 · DAY 21 · DAY 22 · DAY 23 · DAY 24 · DAY 25 · DAY 26 · DAY 27 · DAY 28

DRY
Your skin is likely to be dry and a little flaky at the beginning of your cycle. Drink plenty of water and increase your intake of healthy fats to help it to stay supple.

GREASY AND ACNE PRONE
Skin is most problematic during this time in the cycle. It is oily and thus prone to acne, and you may have pronounced dark circles under your eyes. Your skin is also more likely to react to allergies at this time. Even if you don't feel like it, try to work up a sweat with exercise – it helps remove dirt and unclog pores. Make sure you sweep toner over your face afterwards to remove sweat and grease.

NORMAL AND GLOWING
Skin should be at its healthiest and clearest between days 11 and 21. However, if you suffer from premenstrual syndrome, stress-hormone levels may increase, causing your skin to produce oil. This may lead to inflamed skin and spots. Engage in gentle relaxing exercise, such as yoga, to help ease your stress levels and keep skin clear.

GREASY AND ACNE PRONE

NORMAL AND GLOWING

WHAT'S IN THAT BOTTLE?

Cosmetics and toiletries offer the promise of magical transformation. They promise to refine and clarify skin, to give us manageable and shiny hair, and to melt away the years. We want to believe these promises – so much so, that sometimes we don't ask what's in the bottle. The truth is that most conventional beauty products contain exactly the same ingredients – moisturising agents, detergents, oils and waxes, silicones, emulsifiers, preservatives, colours, and perfumes – because there are only a limited number of chemicals that can clean, moisturise, and condition skin or hair.

CHEMICAL BEAUTY

We use products daily and in quantity, so you would think these ingredients would have been proven both safe and effective. But this is not necessarily the case – beyond proving that products do not produce immediate allergic reactions, cosmetic companies are not required to prove they are safe over the longer term; and as for effectiveness, almost any claim goes.

If you regularly use conventional products, then you are exposing yourself to a staggering range of harmful industrial chemicals. Look at a label on a typical shampoo bottle – you may see as many as 20 ingredients, many of which have been synthesized in the lab. To the average person, the list is an incomprehensible alphabet soup that makes most of us switch off. We open the bottle, cross our fingers, and pray that the companies have our beauty and welfare at heart.

Laboratory tests have shown many ingredients to be harmful and capable of producing not only short-term health issues, such as contact allergies, but also more serious long-term health problems, such as cancer, birth defects, and central nervous system damage. Some of the chemicals found in modern beauty products are also considered hazardous waste by many governments.

Cosmetics manufacturers may claim that they use only a little of these chemicals, but apart from this notion being disingenuous, it ignores the fact that we use them every day (as opposed to once, during a laboratory test). It also ignores that individual chemicals can combine in the bottle to produce unexpected toxins – that manufacturers don't always test for.

Your skin can't protect you from these chemicals. Most can easily penetrate the protective barrier of the skin and build up in your body. Is any promised transformation really worth this risk?

On average we each use nine different products, with a total of 126 unique chemical ingredients, daily. Yet 90 per cent of these chemicals have never been fully evaluated for safety.

A Better Way

If more of us refuse to buy toxic products and transform our beauty routine, manufacturers will quickly get the message that using industrial chemicals in beauty products is not acceptable.

1 SIMPLIFY YOUR ROUTINE

Use fewer products daily and be choosy about what you use.

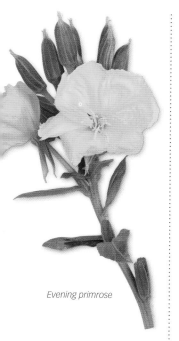

Evening primrose

2 CHOOSE CERTIFIED ORGANIC COSMETICS

These help you to avoid the worst cosmetic offenders, which are simply not allowed under organic rules. But watch out for the organic "pretenders" – those products that have a small percentage of organic ingredients in an otherwise toxic mix of synthetic chemicals. Only a product carrying a certified organic stamp is guaranteed to be free of these.

Chamomile Roman essential oil

3 TRY NATURAL FRAGRANCES

Look for products that are fragranced with essential oils rather than those that use generic "parfum", which is usually synthetic (see pp18–19).

4 MAKE YOUR OWN

A satisfying and creative pastime, making your own products may also be good for your health. Not only can you tailor the ingredients to your personal needs, but you can also be absolutely sure of what goes into them.

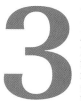
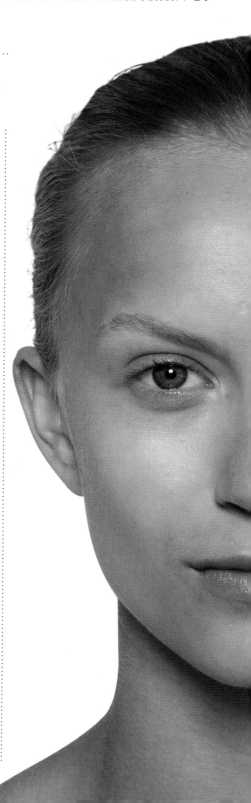

THE SCIENCE OF THE LABEL

It may surprise you to find out what goes into your toiletries and cosmetics. Natural and organic brands avoid the worst chemical offenders, and you can, too, if you learn to read ingredient labels. The more you do it, the easier it gets. Certain ingredients should always

INGREDIENT	WHAT IS IT?
BHA AND BHT PRESERVATIVES	These artificial preservatives are commonly found in cosmetics to extend shelf life, such as in make-up, body lotions, and soaps.
FORMALDEHYDE-RELEASING PRESERVATIVES Such as MDM hydantoin, diazolidinyl urea, imidazolidinyl urea, methenamine, quaternium-15, and sodium hydroxymethylglycinate	These artificial preservatives are used to help prolong the shelf life of products and cosmetics.
PARABENS Such as Methyl-, Propyl-, Butyl-, and Ethyl-Paraben	These are the most widely used preservatives in the cosmetic industry. Parabens are found in shampoos, shower gels, make-up, body lotions, scrubs, and facial toners.
ISOPROPANOL	A solvent and penetration enhancer that drives other ingredients deeper into the skin. Isopropanol is found in make-up, shampoos, moisturisers, and nail polish.
PARAFFINUM LIQUIDUM (Mineral oil)	A cheap and abundant ingredient, paraffinum liquidum is found in face creams, make-up, body lotions, and baby oils. It makes the products easy to apply and forms a film on the skin to prevent water loss.
PETROLATUM (Petroleum jelly)	This mineral-oil derivative is used for its emollient (film-forming) properties. It is found in lipsticks and balms, hair-care products, moisturisers, depilatories, and deodorants.
PROPYLENE GLYCOL, PEG (POLYETHYLENE GLYCOL), AND PPG (POLYPROPYLENE GLYCOL)	These combinations of synthetic petrochemicals are found in moisturisers, deodorants, make-up, depilatories, and soaps to keep the product moist and drive other ingredients deeper into the skin.
PVP/VA COPOLYMER	A plastic-like substance that helps the product to stick to the skin or to hold the hair in place. It is found in hairsprays, styling aids, make-up, tanning products, toothpastes, and skin creams.
SODIUM LAURYL OR SODIUM LAURETH SULFATE DETERGENTS	These are detergents and foaming agents found in shampoos, body washes, and toothpastes.
SYNTHETIC COLOURS (Numbers with the prefix CI)	These add colour to most toiletries and cosmetics but add nothing to the effectiveness of some products, such as shampoos, and cleansers.
PARFUM	Around 95 per cent of the fragrances used in toiletries and cosmetics are petrochemically based, made of dozens of separate ingredients.
DIBUTYL PHTHALATE	A solvent and plasticizer, dibutyl phthalate is often found in perfumes and nail polishes.
SILOXANES Such as cyclotetrasiloxane, cyclopentasiloxane, cyclohexasiloxane, and cyclomethicone	These silicone-based compounds are used to make products, such as lotions and creams, feel better on your skin. The siloxanes make products easy to apply and form a film that temporarily makes the skin feel smoother.
TRICLOSAN	An antibacterial agent that absorbs easily into the skin, it is commonly found in antiperspirants, facial cleansers, hand sanitizers, and toothpastes.
BENZOYL PEROXIDE	A harsh antibacterial agent used mainly in products to treat oily skin and acne.
MIT (METHYLISOCHLOROTHIAZOLINONE)	A preservative added to prolong the shelf life of a product. It is found in most types of toiletries and cosmetics.

ring alarm bells – especially those that are carcinogenic, which means they are linked to cancer; or neurotoxic, meaning that they are capable of causing damage to the body's nervous system. Check all labels against this helpful table.

WHAT CAN IT DO TO YOUR HEALTH?

BHA and BHT can cause allergic skin reactions. BHA is also a hormone disrupter – it mimics the natural action of hormones in the body (in this case oestrogen). This can raise the risk of oestrogen-dependent cancers, such as breast and ovarian cancer. As such BHA and BHT are potential carcinogens.

In low doses, these preservatives can cause eye and skin irritations and can trigger allergies. In larger doses, formaldehyde fumes are carcinogenic.

Parabens can cause allergic reactions and skin rashes. Parabens easily absorb into the skin; studies show they are oestrogen mimics that have been found in samples of breast tumours.

Studies show it is neurotoxic, skin drying or irritating, and potentially toxic for the liver.

Research suggests that it can interfere with the body's own natural moisturising mechanism, which over time leads to dryness and chapping.

Studies show that, like paraffinum liquidum, it can interfere with the body's own natural moisturising mechanism, which over time leads to dryness and chapping.

Studies have linked these to allergic reactions, hives, and eczema. Propylene glycol can be derived from natural sources (see box, opposite). PEG compounds may be contaminated with the carcinogen 1,4-dioxane.

If sensitive people inhale particles of this plastic-like substance, it can damage their lungs. Used topically, it can prevent the skin from "breathing".

These detergents can cause eye irritation, scalp "scurf" (similar to dandruff), skin rashes, and allergic reactions. Sodium laureth sulphate may be contaminated with the carcinogen 1,4-dioxane.

Many synthetic colours are carcinogenic. Exceptions are mineral-based colours (see box, opposite).

Perfumes are neurotoxic and can cause headaches, mood swings, depression, dizziness, and skin irritation. They are also very common triggers of asthma attacks.

Studies show it can cause developmental and reproductive abnormalities. It is toxic to the liver and kidneys.

Some siloxanes can disrupt hormones, which means they are potential carcinogens as well as reproductive toxins.

Research shows that triclosan is a hormone disrupter. It is also implicated in causing resistance to commonly used antibiotics.

This chemical can dry the skin and cause redness, itching, and swelling. In sensitive individuals, it can cause blistering.

MIT has caused an epidemic of skin reactions, which has provoked dermatologists to demand that it be removed from toiletries and cosmetics. It is also a neurotoxin and potential carcinogen.

GREEN SCIENCE

There is no excuse for any manufacturer to use toxic chemicals when viable natural alternatives exist. Leading natural brands prove that you don't have to compromise your health in order to be beautiful.

TOXIC COMPONENT	NATURAL ALTERNATIVE
Parabens	Vitamins E (alpha tocopherol) and C (L ascorbic acid), citric acid, propolis, and rosemary (*Rosmarinus officinalis*).
Paraffinum liquidum, petrolatum, and siloxanes	Coconut oil (*Cocos nucifera*), apricot seed oil (*Prunus armeniaca*), almond oil (*Prunus amygdalus dulcis*). Plant oils and butters, such as jojoba (*Simmondsia chinensis*), avocado (*Persea gratissima*), rosehip seed (*Rosa canina*), and shea butter (*Shea Butyrospermum parkii*).
Propylene glycol, PEG (polyethylene glycol), and PPG (polypropylene glycol)	Vegetable glycerine, lecithin, and panthenol (pro-vitamin B5).
Emulsifiers, such as PEG compounds	Xanthan gum, *Cetearyl oliva*, quince seed (*Pyrus cydonia*), rice bran, and plant waxes, such as candelilla (*Euphorbia antisyphillitica*), carnauba (*Copernica cerifera*), jojoba (*Simmondsia chinensis*).
Synthetic colours	Mineral-based colours (denoted on the label as CI 75 or CI 77, indicating mineral or other naturally derived colours).
Parfum	Essential oils or herbal and floral extracts.
Triclosan	Tea tree essential oil (*Melaleuca alternifolia*), thyme essential oil (*Thymus vulgaris*), grapefruit seed extract (*Citrus grandis*), bitter orange extract (*Citrus aurantium amara*).
Benzoyl peroxide	Tea tree essential oil (*Melaleuca alternifolia*), lemongrass essential oil (*Cymbopogon*), grapefruit essential oil (*Citrus paradisi*), sugar compounds.

THE KIT YOU NEED

Discover everything you need to create and apply natural beauty products like a professional. It is so easy to make a vast array of fantastic products with very little specialized equipment. You could also simplify your beauty kit, leaving yourself with basic, versatile tools that help to give perfect results.

MAKE YOUR OWN PRODUCTS

It is hugely satisfying, cheap, and fun to make your own products. You have full control over the ingredients that you use and the source, quality, and quantity. Much of the equipment you need is probably already in your kitchen cupboards. It is fine to use the same tools for food preparation and cosmetics, provided everything is completely clean.

KEEPING PRODUCTS

Use all products within a short period of time as they will perish more quickly than conventional products. Make only enough for personal use or for gifts.

Fresh ingredient-based products should be used on the same day, but you could use them throughout the day and keep them in the fridge between uses.

Oil-based products, such as balms, keep for up to 6 months. Store in an airtight container in a cool, dry, and dark place.

Recipes containing water, such as emulsion-based creams, perish quickly. Store them in airtight containers and keep them in the fridge.

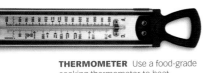

THERMOMETER Use a food-grade cooking thermometer to heat mineral water to 80℃ (175°F) – the optimum temperature to create water-based emulsions.

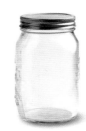

LIDS, DROPPERS, ATOMIZERS, AND PUMPS Finding the right dispenser for your product is key – think about how much of the product you need for application and match that with the appropriate closure.

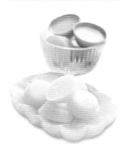

MOULDS Try specialized silicone moulds for soaps, bath bombs, or melts. These are very durable. Ice-cube trays or baking trays are also suitable.

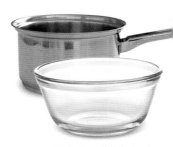

BAIN-MARIE Essentially just a glass bowl that sits inside a saucepan, a bain-marie is necessary for most balm, cream, and lotion recipes. Make sure that the bottom of the glass bowl never touches the boiling water.

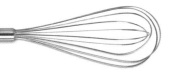

HAND-HELD WHISK Use a balloon whisk to mix emulsions to the right consistency.

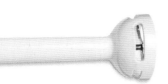

STICK BLENDER Save time and energy by using a plastic or metal stick blender – these are cheap and easy to clean. They are useful for making emulsions and soaps.

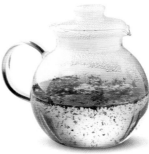

TEA POT Use a tea pot with a filter inside or use a tea strainer to make healthy herbal infusions to drink or use in products.

STERILIZED JARS, BOTTLES, AND CONTAINERS Use specialized vessels or sterilize whatever you have to hand. All products keep for longer in containers with airtight lids.

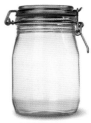

KILNER JARS These are especially useful for scrubs and powders, as they are airtight and keep contents fresh for longer.

APPLY YOUR BEAUTY PRODUCTS

You can use your fingers or hands to apply many products – this allows you to control the pressure and movement. However, you do need some simple and cheap beauty tools for certain tasks. Use organic and non-animal derived cotton and brushes where possible, and always make sure that wooden tools have been sustainably sourced. You may also need an easy-to-wash hairband to keep products out of your hair.

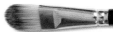

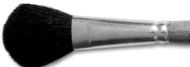

FOUNDATION BRUSH
This is a multi-purpose brush that you can use to apply make-up and clay-based masks.

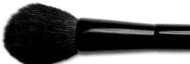

BLUSHER BRUSH Use this brush to apply powder and/or mineral blusher to the cheek area.

POWDER BRUSH Use this brush to apply loose, pressed, or mineral powder to the face and décolleté (the neck, shoulders, chest, and upper back).

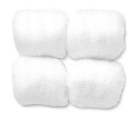

COTTON WOOL PADS AND BALLS
Versatile cotton wool pads and balls are useful for removing make-up and applying cleansing products. Always buy organic.

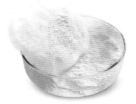

POWDER PUFF After bathing, smooth body powders over dry skin with a powder puff.

EYESHADOW BRUSH Apply eyeshadow and contour the eye area using a variety of eyeshadow brushes.

EYESHADOW BLENDING BRUSH Create a refined finish by using this brush to blend your eyeshadow.

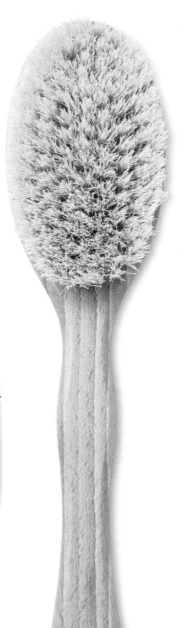

FLANNEL OR MUSLIN CLOTH Use to remove products from the skin. Always wash flannels and muslin cloths thoroughly every time they have been in contact with the skin.

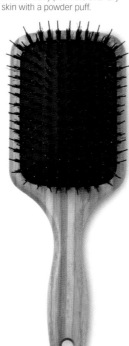

SMUDGE BRUSH Soften and blend eyeliner and apply eyeshadow to the lower lash line with this brush.

EYELINER BRUSH Use this brush to apply eyeliner to both the upper and lower lash lines.

ANGLED BRUSH Use a small angled brush to apply brow powder and eyeliner, and a large brush to add contour to the face.

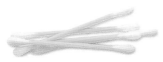

COTTON BUDS The perfect tool to erase mistakes and blend eyeliner and eyeshadow. You can even use cotton buds to apply lip colour.

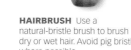

HAIRBRUSH Use a natural-bristle brush to brush dry or wet hair. Avoid pig bristles where possible.

DRY BODY BRUSH Once a week, invigorate the skin all over the body before you bathe. Use a long-handled brush for difficult-to-reach parts.

LIP BRUSH Apply lipstick, lip gloss, and lip stains with this brush.

DIRECTORY OF INGREDIENTS

INGREDIENTS DERIVED FROM NATURE, WITH
NO HIDDEN NASTIES, ARE REVOLUTIONIZING
THE BEAUTY INDUSTRY. MAKE AND USE PRODUCTS
THAT COMBINE THESE **CARING** HERBS, FLOWERS,
AND FRUITS WITH **RICH** OILS AND WAXES.

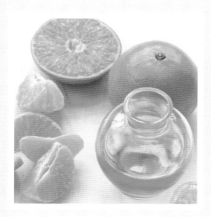
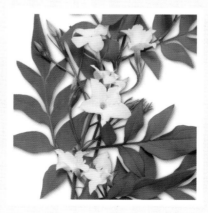
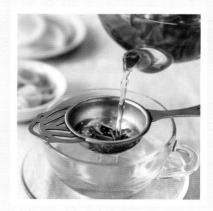

ROSE *Rosa damascena*

Rose petals produce an exquisite essential oil with a delicate, uplifting scent and a **healing**, **rejuvenating** effect on the skin. There are two main types of rose essential oil – rose absolute, which is solvent-extracted; and rose otto, which is steam-distilled and more costly. Rose also yields a **nourishing** oil pressed from its seeds, as well as **skin-toning** floral water.

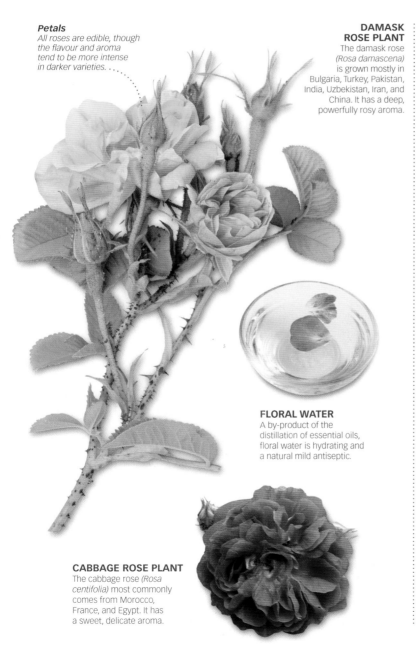

Petals
All roses are edible, though the flavour and aroma tend to be more intense in darker varieties.

DAMASK ROSE PLANT
The damask rose *(Rosa damascena)* is grown mostly in Bulgaria, Turkey, Pakistan, India, Uzbekistan, Iran, and China. It has a deep, powerfully rosy aroma.

FLORAL WATER
A by-product of the distillation of essential oils, floral water is hydrating and a natural mild antiseptic.

CABBAGE ROSE PLANT
The cabbage rose *(Rosa centifolia)* most commonly comes from Morocco, France, and Egypt. It has a sweet, delicate aroma.

WHAT IS IT GOOD FOR?

REPAIRS AND PROTECTS SKIN Rosehip seed oil is great for treating broken capillaries, sun damage, skin redness, scars, and stretch marks. Rub a small amount directly into the problem areas, or dilute a little rose essential oil and apply to the skin.

CONDITIONS AND SOOTHES SKIN Anti-inflammatory, cooling, and soothing, rosehip seed oil or diluted essential oil absorbs quickly and easily and is beneficial for dry, hot, inflamed, itchy, or even broken skin.

TONES SKIN Good-quality rose floral water (also known as hydrosol) is an excellent skin toner, especially for combination and mature skins. You can use it in place of harsher synthetic products to refresh and balance all types of skin. Rosehip seed oil also tones skin and minimizes the appearance of pores.

TREATS ACNE Rosehip seed oil is a source of trans-retinoic acid, which the body turns into vitamin A. This makes it useful for treating acne-prone skine and acne rosacea.

COMBATS SIGNS OF AGEING Rose essential oil supports cell and tissue regeneration, maintains the elasticity of the skin, and reduces the appearance of fine lines around the eyes – making it perfect for both youthful and mature skins.

Valuable for dry, normal, and mature skin, rose essential oil supports cell and tissue regeneration.

NOURISHING MASSAGE You can use rosehip seed oil neat on your skin, but as good-quality oil is expensive, blend it with other good-quality base oils and essential oils to make a skin-nourishing massage oil. Add rose essential oil to massage blends to act as a general tonic for heart and lungs, to aid detox, and also to relieve menstrual pains.

PROVIDES GOOD FATS Rosehip seed oil is among the best vegetable oil sources of omega 3 and is also a good source of omega 6, both of which are involved in cellular membrane and tissue regeneration.

FIGHTS BACTERIA Rose essential oil is often added to cosmetics, due to its antimicrobial properties. In one laboratory study, damask essential oil demonstrated antibacterial activity against 15 strains of bacteria.

ENHANCES SENSE OF WELL-BEING Rose essential oil has been valued for centuries for its ability to lift the spirit.

RELIEVES STRESS Use rose essential oil for aromatherapy when you feel stressed or low, have headaches, or are grieving. Studies show it can calm breathing and lower heart rate.

EAT YOURSELF BEAUTIFUL

Petals Often dried and used only for decoration, rose petals are actually edible, so long as they are organic. Recent research shows they are high in beneficial antioxidants, which help to fight the signs of premature ageing. Remove the white base, which can be bitter, and float the petals in summer drinks, scatter on desserts or salads, or add to jams and vinegars. Rose petal syrup is delicious over a fresh fruit salad.

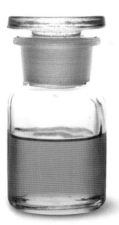

ROSEHIP SEED OIL
A rich source of omega 3 and omega 6, rosehip seed oil can help regenerate cellular membrane and tissue, and provides natural vitamin A.

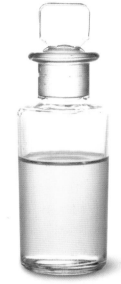

ROSE OTTO ESSENTIAL OIL
This oil is rich and intense – better quality and more expensive than rose absolute as it is produced by steam extraction. You only need a few drops to reap the benefits.

CREATE A SCENT

Make a **romantic floral scent** by combining rose oil with geranium, palmarosa, cedarwood, and patchouli oils. You can also blend it with sage or lavender oil.

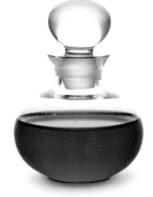

ROSE ABSOLUTE EXTRACT
A thick, concentrated extract, rose absolute is produced by solvent extraction. It has a light fragrance.

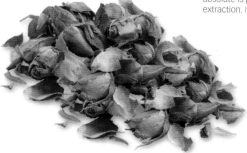

DRIED PETALS
Use dried rose petals and buds in herbal tea to add fragrance. They have a calming and mildly diuretic action.

ARNICA *Arnica montana*

Arnica flowers contain caffeine-like substances with **anti-inflammatory** and **toning** properties, and are a remedy for bruising and wounds. In cosmetic formulations they help to reduce puffiness, for instance around the eyes. The extract can **stimulate blood flow** and **boost circulation** beneath the skin, helping to **revitalize** the complexion. Do not consume arnica in any form, as it may be toxic.

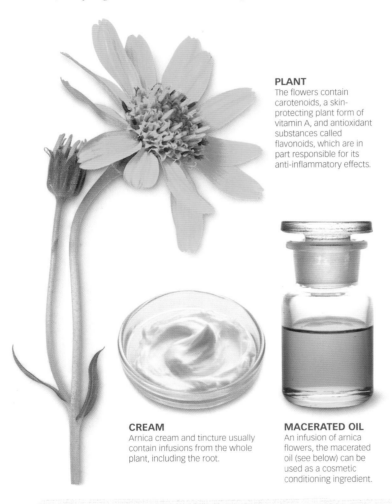

PLANT
The flowers contain carotenoids, a skin-protecting plant form of vitamin A, and antioxidant substances called flavonoids, which are in part responsible for its anti-inflammatory effects.

CREAM
Arnica cream and tincture usually contain infusions from the whole plant, including the root.

MACERATED OIL
An infusion of arnica flowers, the macerated oil (see below) can be used as a cosmetic conditioning ingredient.

MAKE YOUR OWN

Macerated oil Pack a clean, sterile jar with your choice of herbs. Top up with a base oil such as olive, grapeseed, or sunflower. Store at room temperature and shake vigorously each day for 2–6 weeks to help infuse the oil. The oil will take on a dark golden colour and have a distinctive "woody" aroma when it is fully infused. Strain the oil through a muslin cloth into a clean, sterile bottle and cap tightly. Store in a cool, dark place.

WHAT IS IT GOOD FOR?

HEALS CUTS, SCRAPES, AND BRUISES
By improving circulation, arnica flowers support fast, effective healing. Arnica flowers can be distilled into a macerated oil, tincture, or cream. These preparations have healing properties and are traditional treatments for burns, bruising, and wounds. Use them neat on the skin to heal cuts, grazes, and bruises – but avoid using them on broken skin.

CONDITIONS AND SOOTHES SKIN Arnica oil and cream help to soften rough patches of skin. Applied neat, it is a great remedy for preventing chapped lips.

HEALS SCARS Massage arnica oil onto the skin, in gentle circular motions, to help reduce the appearance of stretch marks.

IMPROVES SKIN TONE Massaging with arnica oil improves blood circulation and also has a mild skin-lightening effect. With damp hands, apply a few drops on the face in a light, circular motion.

TONES SKIN Arnica oil can help diminish the appearance of spider veins. To use it, apply a few drops of the oil to the area in a light, circular motion. Or use it in massage to help to reduce the swelling and pain of varicose veins.

ACTS AS AN ANTI-INFLAMMATORY Keep arnica tincture to hand to reduce redness and inflammation caused by insect stings.

CONDITIONS HAIR AND SCALP Arnica oil can condition your hair and scalp – use it just as you would a normal conditioner. Alternatively, dilute arnica tincture in water and use it as a hair rinse to treat dandruff. In Ayurvedic medicine it is also used as a treatment for hair loss.

RELIEVES ACHES AND PAINS Use arnica oil during massage to relieve backache and the pain caused by arthritis and rheumatism.

SUNFLOWER *Helianthus annuus*

Sunflower seeds produce a light-coloured oil with a delicate, nutty scent, ideal for use as a base oil in massage or as a carrier for essential oil blends. Sunflower oil is rich in vitamin E, omega-6 linoleic acid, and carotenoids, which can help **repair** and **protect skin**. It can be **soothing** and **nourishing** if you have dry, rough skin, or are suffering from eczema and other inflammatory skin conditions.

WHAT IS IT GOOD FOR?

REPAIRS AND PROTECTS SKIN Rich in vitamin E, sunflower oil can help prevent scarring, smooth the appearance of existing wrinkles, and generally improve the health and appearance of your skin. Studies show that sunflower oil can help to protect the skin of premature babies, who are more susceptible to infection and disease. It also helps to prevent and repair sun-damaged skin. Apply with damp hands to skin – it will soak in easily and does not need to be washed off.

CLEANSES AND TONES SKIN The oil is a good all-rounder for removing dirt and make-up. The presence of light waxes help form a protective emollient barrier on the skin to keep moisture in. It is a light, dry oil and can be used on all skin types, even oily skin. Its linoleic acid has a toning quality on the skin that can help reduce inflammation and minimize the appearance of large pores. Apply using damp cotton wool or even damp fingers. Remove any excess oil with a damp muslin or microfibre cloth and rinse with warm, not hot, water.

TREATS ACNE An excellent oil for cleansing and moisturising acne-prone skin. It contains carotenoids, a plant-based form of vitamin A. Beta-carotene in skincare products can help lighten the appearance of red, inflamed spots and blemishes and can even out skin tone.

CONDITIONS HAIR AND SCALP The oil can tame flyaway hair and reduce the appearance of split ends. Use as a conditioning treatment before shampooing or rub 1 or 2 drops onto damp hands and run through the ends of your hair to control frizz. It is also a good treatment to massage into the scalp to treat dandruff or seborrhoeic dermatitis.

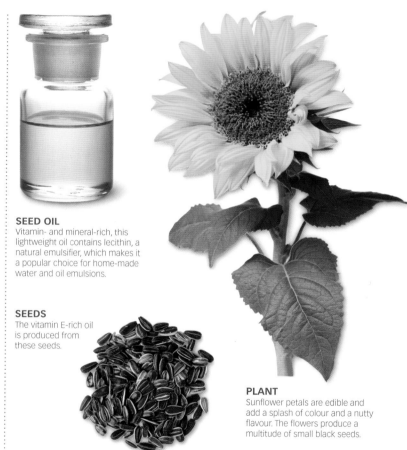

SEED OIL
Vitamin- and mineral-rich, this lightweight oil contains lecithin, a natural emulsifier, which makes it a popular choice for home-made water and oil emulsions.

SEEDS
The vitamin E-rich oil is produced from these seeds.

PLANT
Sunflower petals are edible and add a splash of colour and a nutty flavour. The flowers produce a multitude of small black seeds.

EAT YOURSELF BEAUTIFUL

Seeds The seeds are edible and have diuretic and antioxidant properties. They are a tasty source of protein and vitamins B, D, E, and K.

Salad dressing Phytonutrients are destroyed by heat, so the best way to get the best from sunflower oil is to use it cold as a salad dressing. Use unrefined sunflower oil, which retains more of the original nutritional content of the seeds and has a more pronounced flavour.

CALENDULA *Calendula officinalis*

Calendula has a **healing** action on the skin and can be used in a variety of infusions, tinctures, liquid extracts, creams, or ointments. It has **rejuvenating** properties and is often incorporated into moisturisers, sun, hair, and baby-care products. Its popularity – especially for sensitive and dry skins – is due to its ability to quickly **soothe** irritated skin and **repair** skin tissue.

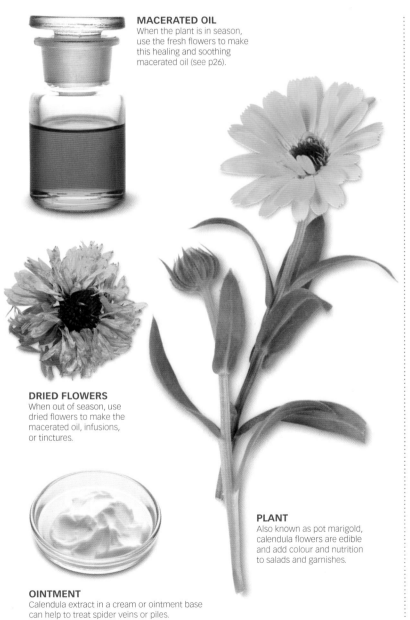

MACERATED OIL
When the plant is in season, use the fresh flowers to make this healing and soothing macerated oil (see p26).

DRIED FLOWERS
When out of season, use dried flowers to make the macerated oil, infusions, or tinctures.

PLANT
Also known as pot marigold, calendula flowers are edible and add colour and nutrition to salads and garnishes.

OINTMENT
Calendula extract in a cream or ointment base can help to treat spider veins or piles.

WHAT IS IT GOOD FOR?

CONDITIONS AND SOOTHES SKIN Along with potent natural resins and volatile oils, calendula oil is bursting with antioxidants that help to fight inflammation. Herbalists combine calendula, comfrey, echinacea, and St John's wort to make an all-purpose skin salve.

REPAIRS AND PROTECTS SKIN Calendula oil or cream is a good choice for healing cuts and skin ulcers and soothing dermatitis. It is mildly antiseptic so also helps to prevent infection. Hypercal cream, which is a staple of most natural first-aid kits, is a mixture of hypericum (St John's wort) and calendula. Calendula ointment is also a good remedy for perineal tears after childbirth. You can also apply calendula oil or cream after sun exposure to keep skin in good condition.

TEETH AND GUM CARE Toothpaste with calendula extract can significantly reduce plaque, gingivitis, and bleeding gums. Use a calendula infusion or tincture as a mouthwash or gargle.

FOOT CARE Calendula oil is a traditional remedy for bunions, verrucae, and foot ulcers. Modern studies show that combined with a protective dressing, a cream made from a variant of calendula, *Tagetes patula* (French marigold), reduced the size and pain of bunions. The flowers of this variety should never be consumed.

Calendula oil is bursting with antioxidants that help to fight inflammation.

CHAMOMILE *Matricaria recutita*

As a skin and beauty treatment, chamomile is mildly **astringent** and **antibacterial**. The essential oil penetrates below the skin surface into the deeper layers, where its **anti-inflammatory** action can **repair** and **soothe** irritated skin and **heal** mouth ulcers, eczema, burns, bruises, and more. Buy organic to ensure that you get all the benefits minus the harmful chemicals or pesticides.

WHAT IS IT GOOD FOR?

SOOTHES SENSITIVE SKIN Chamomile oil's anti-inflammatory, soothing action makes it useful for problem, allergic, or sensitive skin. Chamomile in creams and ointments helps to relieve itchy and inflamed skin conditions such as rashes, including nappy rash, cracked nipples, and chicken pox. For eczema, the creams or ointments have been found to be as effective as hydrocortisone.

TONES SKIN The astringent properties of chamomile make it a useful pore-cleansing treatment, applied with cotton wool. You could try mixing a little tincture with water, infusing a strong chamomile tea, or simply adding the oil to your own home-made cleanser (see recipes, pp103–05).

HEALS CUTS, SCRAPES, AND BRUISES Use the tincture or oil to help heal scratches and treat wounds – chamomile has been shown to promote faster healing than corticosteroids. Add 4–5 drops of the essential oil to a bath to heal wounds or soothe the skin.

CONDITIONS HAIR AND SCALP Although it will not change your hair colour, rinsing blonde hair in a chamomile infusion brings shine and can enhance highlights. Add chamomile oil to hair treatments to calm a sensitive or allergic scalp.

EASES ACHES AND PAINS Research has shown that chamomile contains two powerful anti-inflammatories – bisabolol and apigenin. Both substances work to reduce inflammation in a similar way to NSAIDS like paracetamol. Bisabolol, which is often added to cosmetics, can reduce inflammation, fever, and even arthritic pain.

SOOTHES EYES Apply a tepid, moist chamomile teabag to tired eyes to soothe them. This remedy can also alleviate eye infections such as conjunctivitis.

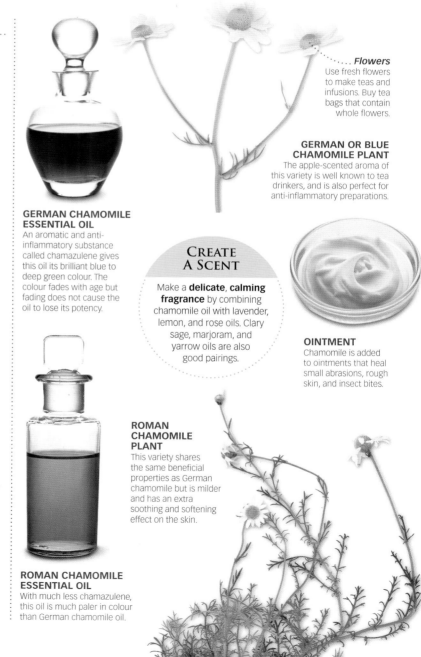

Flowers
Use fresh flowers to make teas and infusions. Buy tea bags that contain whole flowers.

GERMAN OR BLUE CHAMOMILE PLANT
The apple-scented aroma of this variety is well known to tea drinkers, and is also perfect for anti-inflammatory preparations.

GERMAN CHAMOMILE ESSENTIAL OIL
An aromatic and anti-inflammatory substance called chamazulene gives this oil its brilliant blue to deep green colour. The colour fades with age but fading does not cause the oil to lose its potency.

CREATE A SCENT

Make a **delicate**, **calming fragrance** by combining chamomile oil with lavender, lemon, and rose oils. Clary sage, marjoram, and yarrow oils are also good pairings.

OINTMENT
Chamomile is added to ointments that heal small abrasions, rough skin, and insect bites.

ROMAN CHAMOMILE PLANT
This variety shares the same beneficial properties as German chamomile but is milder and has an extra soothing and softening effect on the skin.

ROMAN CHAMOMILE ESSENTIAL OIL
With much less chamazulene, this oil is much paler in colour than German chamomile oil.

BEAUTIFUL BEE INGREDIENTS

Bees are remarkable creatures. They are responsible for pollinating around 85 per cent of the world's food crops. They also make honey, wax, and propolis, all of which have been regarded as skin healers for thousands of years. All three ingredients are valued for their **moisturising**, **antiseptic**, and **skin-conditioning** properties. You can use honey for everything, from a face mask to a wound healer.

HONEY *Mel mellis* ▶

HEALS CUTS, SCRAPES, AND BRUISES
Honey is a natural antibacterial, antifungal, and antiseptic. It contains hydrogen peroxide, which is partly responsible for its healing properties. Medical-grade honey is used widely to treat wounds of all kinds – from minor cuts and scalds to skin ulcers.

ACTS AS AN ANTISEPTIC Honey is a traditional remedy for infected acne spots. The benefits of honey are also being researched in the fight against a strain of bacteria called MRSA.

REPAIRS AND PROTECTS SKIN A natural humectant (a substance that attracts and retains moisture), honey makes a good addition to skin-care products, especially those meant for sensitive skin.

IMPROVES SKIN TONE Honey is a natural and traditional way to lighten skin and hair, an effect that is the result of its hydrogen peroxide content. You can apply it neat to the skin, but it is widely used as an ingredient in products.

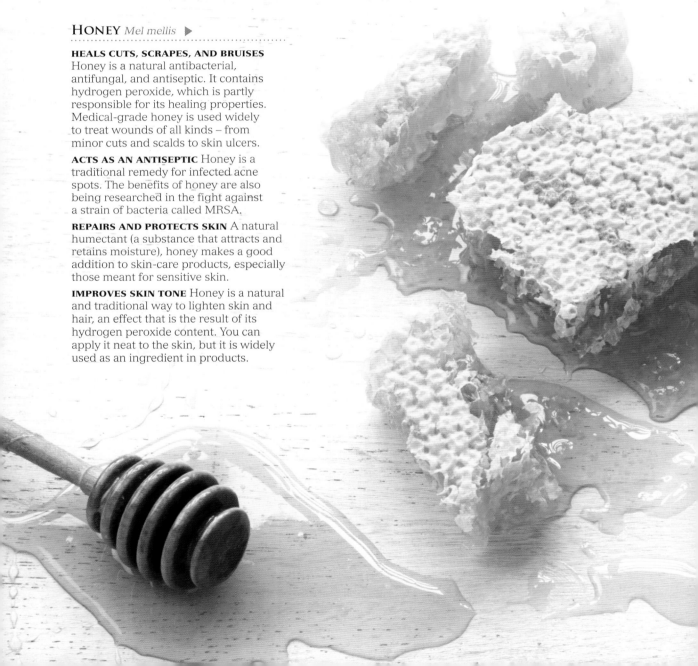

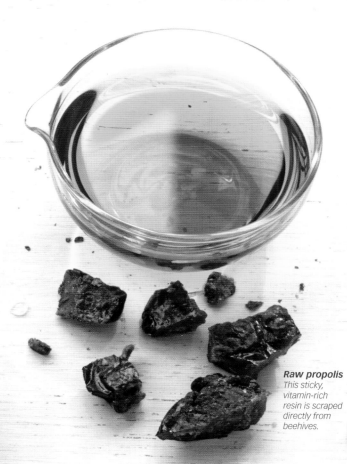

Raw propolis
This sticky, vitamin-rich resin is scraped directly from beehives.

◄ PROPOLIS

ACTS AS AN ANTISEPTIC Skin creams containing propolis have been shown to have beneficial effects on burns, wounds, inflammation of the skin, and other skin lesions and leg ulcers.

TREATS ACNE Many natural acne treatments make use of the antibacterial properties of propolis. It helps remove acne-causing bacteria from the skin.

REPAIRS AND PROTECTS SKIN The phenolic compounds in propolis, particularly its caffeic-acid content, are more potent than both vitamins C and E. This gives propolis antioxidant and anti-inflammatory properties, making it a good addition to creams for sunburn and scalds. It may also help to enhance skin-cell growth, increase circulation, and prevent scars.

BEESWAX *Cera alba* ►

HEALS CUTS, SCRAPES, AND BRUISES A good base for ointments and salves, beeswax is also used to heal burns, bruises, and inflammation. This makes it an ideal ingredient for skin creams and salves.

CONDITIONS AND SOOTHES SKIN Beeswax adds a rich, emollient quality to creams, which is very useful for dry skin. Deeply moisturising, it also creates a waterproof barrier on the skin, which makes it ideal for skin conditions such as psoriasis and dermatitis.

REPAIRS AND PROTECTS SKIN A natural hydrating agent, beeswax moisturises the skin. It is great for chapped or weather-damaged lips and hands.

ACTS AS AN ANTIBACTERIAL Studies suggest that beeswax has an antibacterial action against the bacteria staphylococcus, and may help heal fungal infections such as candida.

LAVENDER *Lavendula angustifolia*

Lavender has a sweet, **calming** fragrance and is the most versatile and widely used of all the essential oils. Its **regenerative** effect on the skin **stimulates** the growth of healthy new cells, promotes rapid **healing**, and helps to prevent scarring. The essential oil and the floral water have **soothing** and **balancing** properties when used on burns, wounds, bites, and inflammatory skin conditions.

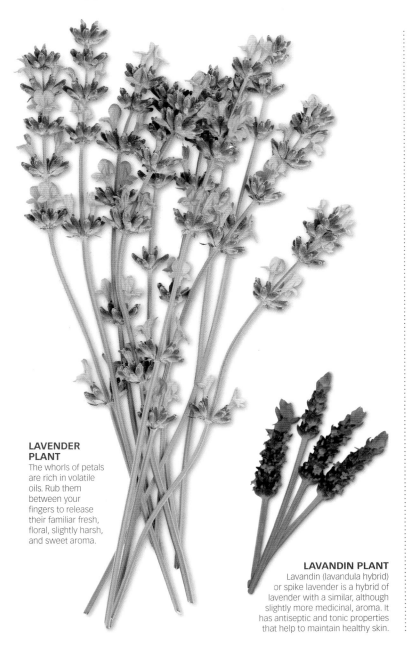

LAVENDER PLANT
The whorls of petals are rich in volatile oils. Rub them between your fingers to release their familiar fresh, floral, slightly harsh, and sweet aroma.

LAVANDIN PLANT
Lavandin (lavandula hybrid) or spike lavender is a hybrid of lavender with a similar, although slightly more medicinal, aroma. It has antiseptic and tonic properties that help to maintain healthy skin.

WHAT IS IT GOOD FOR?

HEALS CUTS, SCRAPES, AND BRUISES Lavender essential oil is extremely useful for treating wounds, ulcers, and sores of all kinds. Its antiseptic properties prevent infection setting in, while at the same time promoting healing and minimizing scarring. Unlike most essential oils, you can use it neat on the skin. As a first-aid remedy it can be used neat on abrasions, wounds, burns, insect bites, and stings.

TONES SKIN After cleansing, use lavender floral water (also known as hydrosol) as an effective skin toner, or decant it into a spray bottle and use it as a toning facial spritz. It revitalizes and refreshes, and its antiseptic properties make it a good choice for oily or acne-prone skin.

CONDITIONS AND SOOTHES SKIN Lavender floral water has regenerative effects on inflamed or damaged skin. Lavender oil helps calm inflammatory skin conditions such as dermatitis, eczema, and psoriasis. Added to lotions, massage oils, and bath preparations, it helps to soften and condition skin. Some commercial products can be adulterated with synthetic linalool and linalyl acetate – be sure to check under the ingredients label for the Latin name, *Lavendula angustifolia*.

REPAIRS AND PROTECTS SKIN If you have sunburn, a spritz of lavender floral water can help to cool and repair skin.

Lavender oil encourages restful sleep and can reduce stress levels and anxiety.

COMBATS OILY HAIR AND DANDRUFF Rinse hair with the essential oil mixed in warm water or with a strong infusion of lavender flowers to help combat oiliness and dandruff. Also useful for treating nits and lice.

STIMULATES HAIR GROWTH Research has shown that massaging lavender oil into the scalp can significantly improve hair growth.

FOOT CARE Lavender oil has an antiseptic and deodorizing action that makes it an ideal addition to a foot soak or a massage for tired feet – especially at the end of a long day.

RELIEVES STRESS Lavender oil encourages restful sleep. It can reduce stress levels and anxiety to a degree that can be measured scientifically via brainwave activity. Used as a massage oil, it can calm breathing and your heart rate. It also treats upset stomachs caused by anxiety and nervous exhaustion.

CLEARS THE AIR The soothing aroma and antiseptic properties make lavender essential oil an ideal choice as a room spray, especially for sick rooms. Add 5 drops of the essential oil to 120ml (4fl oz) water, or a mixture of half water half vodka, and decant into an atomizer. The fragrance will grow stronger if you allow the mixture to sit for a few hours before use.

EAT YOURSELF BEAUTIFUL

Flowers Although edible, the flowers are most often used to make a relaxing tea. Drink the tea before bed to help with insomnia and get a restful night's sleep, or after a meal to aid digestion.

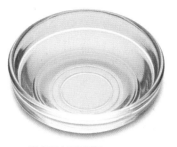

FLORAL WATER
This water, also known as hydrosol, is a by-product of the distillation of the essential oil. It has a milder aroma than the oil but retains the plant's beneficial properties.

CREATE A SCENT

Make your own **refreshing eau de Cologne** by blending lavender oil with rosemary oil and citrus oils such as bergamot, petitgrain, lemon, neroli, and orange.

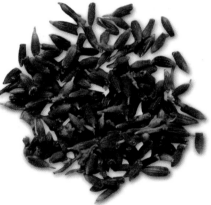

DRIED LAVENDER
Brew dried lavender flowers into an infusion that can be used as a skin toner or hair rinse.

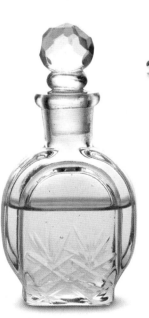

ESSENTIAL OIL
A colourless or pale yellow liquid, lavender oil is steam-distilled from the fresh flowers.

QUICK FIX

Headache remedy
Lavender oil is one of the few essential oils you can use neat on the skin. Rub it into the temples to relieve tension headaches, or try combining 2 drops of it with 2 drops of peppermint oil.

YLANG YLANG *Cananga odorata*

The exotic, floral scent of ylang ylang has an **uplifting** effect, dispelling stress and anxiety, while at the same time being arousing. The oil is highly prized by perfumiers and is used in many popular luxury perfumes. It is a **stimulating** and **balancing** essential oil that is suitable for all skin types. It was a key ingredient in a hair preparation called macassar oil, which was popular in the 19th century.

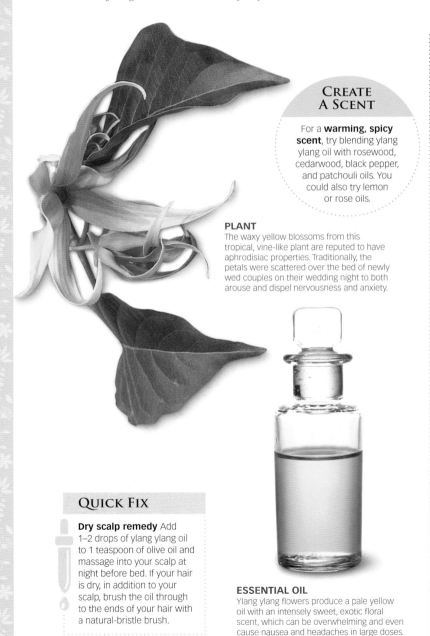

CREATE A SCENT

For a **warming, spicy scent**, try blending ylang ylang oil with rosewood, cedarwood, black pepper, and patchouli oils. You could also try lemon or rose oils.

PLANT
The waxy yellow blossoms from this tropical, vine-like plant are reputed to have aphrodisiac properties. Traditionally, the petals were scattered over the bed of newly wed couples on their wedding night to both arouse and dispel nervousness and anxiety.

ESSENTIAL OIL
Ylang ylang flowers produce a pale yellow oil with an intensely sweet, exotic floral scent, which can be overwhelming and even cause nausea and headaches in large doses.

QUICK FIX

Dry scalp remedy Add 1–2 drops of ylang ylang oil to 1 teaspoon of olive oil and massage into your scalp at night before bed. If your hair is dry, in addition to your scalp, brush the oil through to the ends of your hair with a natural-bristle brush.

WHAT IS IT GOOD FOR?

TREATS ACNE Ylang ylang oil has a balancing action on the secretion of sebum, which makes it ideal for both oily and dry skin types. As an ingredient in skin-care products, ylang ylang can have a good balancing effect on oily or problem skin.

TONES SKIN The oil adds a toning and firming effect to skin-care products. Its stimulating effect on circulation can also help to brighten the complexion.

COMBATS SIGNS OF AGEING When diluted in a good-quality base oil or in natural skin-care products, ylang ylang can improve the appearance of mature skin.

STIMULATES HAIR GROWTH The oil nourishes and stimulates the scalp and is a traditional treatment to promote hair growth. Mix a small amount of the oil with a base oil, such as sunflower, and rub it into the scalp.

ACTS AS AN ANTIDEPRESSANT Ylang ylang has a sedative and antidepressant action and acts as a tonic for the entire nervous system.

RELIEVES STRESS Mix 1 or 2 drops of ylang ylang oil in a teaspoon of base oil, such as apricot kernel or sunflower. It makes a simple perfume that is at once arousing but also has the aromatherapeutic benefits of increasing well-being, reducing anxiety, and lowering heart and breathing rates.

The oil nourishes and stimulates the scalp and is a traditional treatment to promote hair growth.

JASMINE *Jasminum officinale*

Although there are more than 200 species of jasmine, only about a dozen can be used to produce the heady, sensual essential oil so valued by perfumiers. In skin care, it is used as much for its **uplifting** aroma as its **skin-cooling** and **soothing** properties. Jasmine essential oil can be applied neat as a delightful perfume, which can relax and help to relieve stress.

WHAT IS IT GOOD FOR?

CONDITIONS AND SOOTHES SKIN Diluted jasmine oil is beneficial for treating hot, dry, sensitive, and inflamed skin, especially if the irritation is triggered by emotional stress.

HEALS SCARS The oil is often a key ingredient in stretch-mark formulas, due to its ability to help to reduce redness and minimize the appearance of scars. You can also apply diluted jasmine oil directly onto scars.

RELIEVES STRESS Inhaling jasmine oil has been shown to produce measurable change in brain waves, consistent with reduction in stress and listlessness, and an increase in feelings of alertness and well-being. Linalool, a natural constituent of jasmine essential oil, is responsible for its stress-busting properties. Research has shown that inhaling linalool reduced the activity of a number of genes that tend to be over-activated in moments of stress.

ACTS AS AN ANTIDEPRESSANT Added to a base massage or bath oil, jasmine essential oil has a strong antidepressant effect and can quickly help to promote a sense of well-being and optimism.

EAT YOURSELF BEAUTIFUL

Tea Brew jasmine flowers and green tea together to produce a tea that is subtly sweet, rich in antioxidants, and has an aroma that aids relaxation.

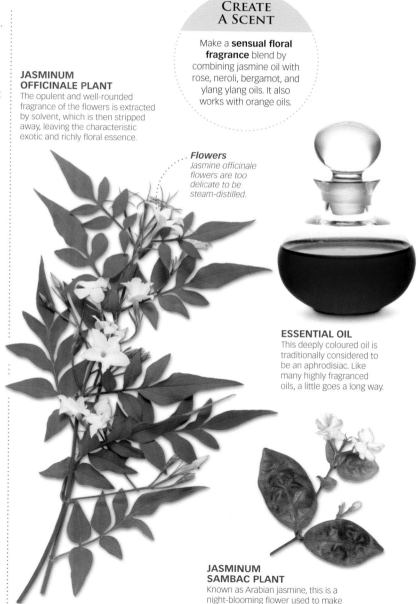

CREATE A SCENT

Make a **sensual floral fragrance** blend by combining jasmine oil with rose, neroli, bergamot, and ylang ylang oils. It also works with orange oils.

JASMINUM OFFICINALE PLANT
The opulent and well-rounded fragrance of the flowers is extracted by solvent, which is then stripped away, leaving the characteristic exotic and richly floral essence.

Flowers
Jasmine officinale flowers are too delicate to be steam-distilled.

ESSENTIAL OIL
This deeply coloured oil is traditionally considered to be an aphrodisiac. Like many highly fragranced oils, a little goes a long way.

JASMINUM SAMBAC PLANT
Known as Arabian jasmine, this is a night-blooming flower used to make most commercial Chinese jasmine teas.

GERANIUM *Pelargonium graveolens*

Surprisingly, geranium essential oil is produced from the leaf rather than the flower of this cheerful plant. The variety *P. graveolens*, or rose geranium, is the most widely cultivated for its oil. The oil has a **cooling** and **balancing** effect on the skin, making it suitable for dry or oily skin, or skin prone to acne. Its **regenerative** properties help to revive tired-looking skin.

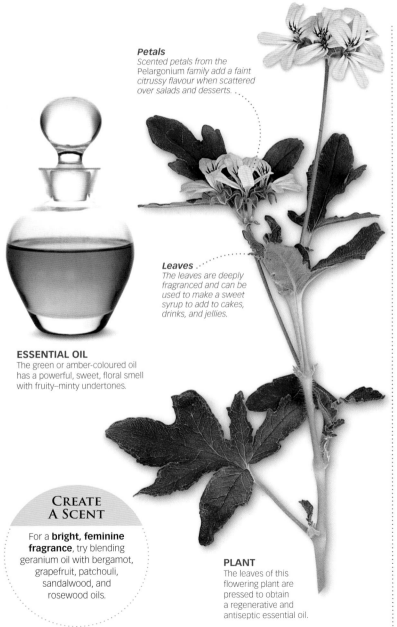

Petals
Scented petals from the Pelargonium *family add a faint citrussy flavour when scattered over salads and desserts.*

Leaves
The leaves are deeply fragranced and can be used to make a sweet syrup to add to cakes, drinks, and jellies.

ESSENTIAL OIL
The green or amber-coloured oil has a powerful, sweet, floral smell with fruity–minty undertones.

PLANT
The leaves of this flowering plant are pressed to obtain a regenerative and antiseptic essential oil.

CREATE A SCENT

For a **bright, feminine fragrance**, try blending geranium oil with bergamot, grapefruit, patchouli, sandalwood, and rosewood oils.

WHAT IS IT GOOD FOR?

CONDITIONS AND SOOTHES SKIN Suitable for all skin types, geranium oil has a balancing effect on the skin. It cools and moistens dry, irritated skin. Apply diluted essential oil to problem areas, but avoid on broken skin.

REPAIRS AND PROTECTS SKIN Diluted geranium oil is great for sunburnt skin and scars. It also helps to heal wounds and ulcers.

COMBATS SIGNS OF AGEING The cellular regenerative properties of geranium oil are ideal for rejuvenating mature or wrinkled skin.

COMBATS OILY SKIN AND DANDRUFF Geranium oil, as part of a skin toner or another facial product, can clean and revive sluggish or oily skin. Mix with a base oil and apply to your scalp to fight dandruff and balance the secretion of sebum. Leave for an hour, then wash as normal.

TREATS ACNE The antiseptic and anti-inflammatory properties of geranium oil help to control acne. Apply diluted essential oil to affected areas.

COMBATS HEAD LICE Try diluting 1–2 drops of geranium oil with unscented shampoo to help eliminate head lice.

ENHANCES SENSE OF WELL-BEING A very pleasant oil to use in the bath or as a massage oil. It has a balancing effect on body and mind, which makes it a good antidepressant.

AIDS DETOX Use geranium oil in massage – it has a general diuretic effect on the body, boosting the elimination of water and waste material, and reducing puffiness.

EVENING PRIMROSE *Oenothera biennis*

The beautiful flowers of the evening primrose may be the pretty face, but the soul of the plant is in the seeds, which produce a **rich**, **nourishing** oil with multiple skin benefits. It is naturally rich in essential fatty acids such as omega-6 linoleic acid, which **strengthen** the membranes surrounding the skin. It also contains omega-3 gamma linolenic acid (GLA), which has **anti-ageing** effects.

WHAT IS IT GOOD FOR?

COMBATS SIGNS OF AGEING The GLA in evening primrose oil possesses natural anti-inflammatory and skin-rejuvenating properties and reactivates certain cells into life after age or sun-related damage.

TREATS ACNE Acne-prone skin needs moisture too. This is a "dry" oil that is quickly and easily absorbed by the skin and does not clog pores. This is a great oil to use on its own to treat small localized areas, such as spots. Apply it neat to the skin.

CONDITIONS AND SOOTHES SKIN Although evening primrose provides a light, dry oil, it can penetrate into the skin and maintain its softness and suppleness. Its moisture-retaining properties keep skin from drying out, making it less prone to eczema and acne. It supports the optimum function of skin cells by increasing the cells' ability to absorb oxygen and to withstand infection. As well as applying the oil neat, you can use it to make your own products or massage oils. The oil should make up at least 5–10 per cent of the total recipe to ensure there is enough of it to bring benefits to your skin.

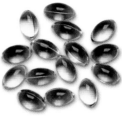

SUPPLEMENTS
These usually come in the form of gel-based capsules that contain the oil in concentrated form. Taking them regularly produces similar skin benefits to the topical application of the oil.

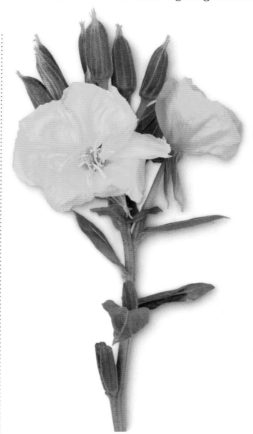

PLANT
The delicate yellow flowers are edible and add colour and nutrition to salads and garnishes. Never eat flowers that have been treated with pesticides.

EAT YOURSELF BEAUTIFUL

Supplements A daily evening primrose oil supplement can markedly improve skin tone and increase cellular respiration – skin cells' abilty to absorb and utilize oxygen, a key feature of healthy skin. It makes the skin more resilient to sun and environmental damage that cause premature ageing. It also increases levels of hormones called prostaglandins, an imbalance of which can cause loss of elasticity, wrinkles, and inflammation.

QUICK FIX

Healthy nails Give your nails a daily treat by rubbing 1–2 drops of the seed oil into them thoroughly. This helps to condition cuticles and soften and improve resilience of brittle and easily breakable nails.

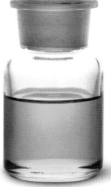

SEED OIL
The oil is pressed from the seeds of the plant. It does not keep well, so it is better to use the oil from capsules, rather than open bottles.

PEPPERMINT *Mentha piperita*

When applied to the skin, peppermint **stimulates** the circulation in a way that feels initially **cooling** and **refreshing,** then gently **warming**. Its **analgesic** properties mean it can be used to treat neuralgia, muscular pains, and headaches. It is also a first-class **antiseptic**. It is used in many beauty products. Always dilute the essential oil – it should constitute no more than 1 per cent of the final mixture.

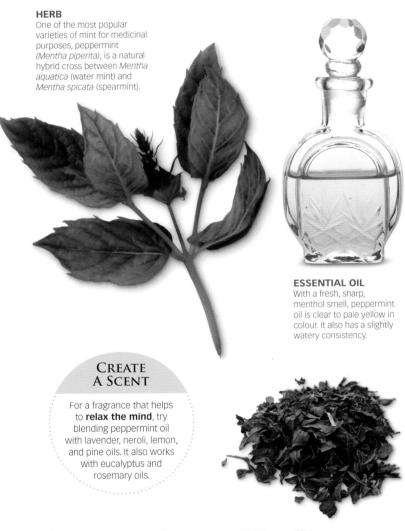

HERB
One of the most popular varieties of mint for medicinal purposes, peppermint *(Mentha piperita)*, is a natural hybrid cross between *Mentha aquatica* (water mint) and *Mentha spicata* (spearmint).

ESSENTIAL OIL
With a fresh, sharp, menthol smell, peppermint oil is clear to pale yellow in colour. It also has a slightly watery consistency.

CREATE A SCENT
For a fragrance that helps to **relax the mind**, try blending peppermint oil with lavender, neroli, lemon, and pine oils. It also works with eucalyptus and rosemary oils.

TEA
The astringent qualities of brewed mint tea make it suitable for external use as a skin toner.

EAT YOURSELF BEAUTIFUL

Tea As a drink, peppermint tea aids digestion, which results in better skin.

WHAT IS IT GOOD FOR?

CLEANSES AND TONES SKIN Peppermint oil and extracts are added to cleansers and toners meant for greasy and acne-prone skin. To make a quick toner, brew some peppermint tea, allow to cool, and use to cleanse and refresh tired skin.

CONDITIONS AND SOOTHES SKIN Added to lotions and body oils, peppermint oil cools and soothes skin after exposure to the elements. It is particularly soothing for tired feet or irritated skin – for a refreshing foot soak, try mixing some brewed mint tea or a few drops of the oil in a bowl of warm water.

ACTS AS AN ANTIVIRAL Peppermint oil has viricidal properties that make enable it to treat cold sores or even more resistant strains of the herpes simplex virus. Dab on a small amount of diluted oil to the area.

ACTS AS AN ANTISEPTIC The oil makes a useful antiseptic when added to products such as lip balms and hand creams.

SOOTHES BITES AND STINGS Peppermint oil is a natural insect repellent. It also soothes mosquito bites and other irritations, such as hives, poison ivy, and poison oak. Dilute in a base oil and dab on the affected area.

COMBATS BODY ODOUR Peppermint oil is a useful ingredient in deodorants and foot washes. It is also used in dental preparations, as its antiseptic and deodorizing properties can help to combat bad breath.

CONDITIONS HAIR AND SCALP Strong peppermint tea, allowed to cool, can act as a hair rinse to add shine and combat dandruff.

EASES HEADACHES The oil helps to refresh the mind and aid focus. It has long been recognized as a safe and effective treatment for tension headaches and has an action that is similar to conventional drugs, such as acetaminophen and paracetamol. Add a drop of eucalyptus oil to a diluted peppermint solution to enhance its effectiveness.

LEMON BALM *Melissa officinalis*

Lemon balm is also known as melissa. The essential oil is popular in skin-care products because of its **uplifting** lemony scent and its **calming**, **anti-inflammatory** action on irritated skin and allergic skin conditions. It exerts a **healing** action on skin complaints, such as eczema and ulcers. Always dilute the essential oil well – it should constitute no more than 1 per cent of the final mixture.

WHAT IS IT GOOD FOR?

CONDITIONS AND SOOTHES SKIN Inflamed skin and allergic skin conditions can be calmed with well-diluted melissa oil. You can also use it to treat ulceration on the body and eczema, especially when it is stress related. It can reduce redness and irritation from insect bites and stings, as well as sunburn, but never apply it neat to the skin.

IMPROVES SKIN TONE Melissa oil is a perfect ingredient for a home-made toner. It stimulates the circulation for a brighter complexion and has a tightening effect that helps to improve skin tone.

COMBATS SIGNS OF AGEING The oil has exceptionally high antioxidant properties, which can help fight skin ageing caused by free-radical damage.

REPAIRS AND PROTECTS SKIN Two of the compounds in lemon balm – caffeic acid and ferulic acid – have been shown to penetrate deeply into the cutaneous layers of the skin and provide protection against UV radiation-induced skin damage.

ANTISEPTIC AND ANTIVIRAL The oil has an antibacterial action that can be useful in treating acne and other skin eruptions. It is also effective at combatting the herpes virus and so can treat cold sores – dab on the tincture or diluted essential oil.

EASES HEADACHES AND MIGRAINES The scent of melissa oil is uplifting and can treat migraines and headaches, especially those associated with tension in the neck and shoulders.

EAT YOURSELF BEAUTIFUL

Tea Drink lemon balm tea to uplift the spirit and calm nervous exhaustion. In addition, it can treat stress headaches and migraines.

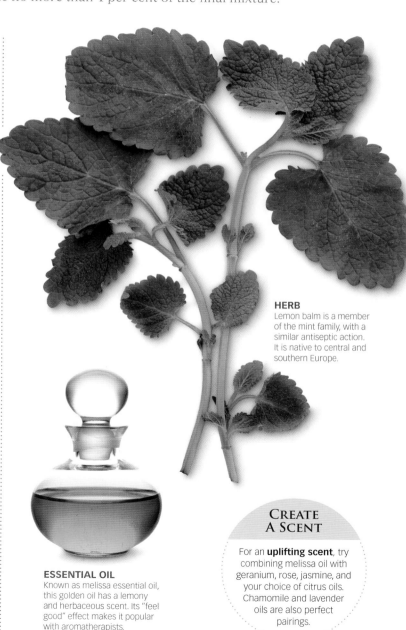

HERB
Lemon balm is a member of the mint family, with a similar antiseptic action. It is native to central and southern Europe.

ESSENTIAL OIL
Known as melissa essential oil, this golden oil has a lemony and herbaceous scent. Its "feel good" effect makes it popular with aromatherapists.

CREATE A SCENT

For an **uplifting scent**, try combining melissa oil with geranium, rose, jasmine, and your choice of citrus oils. Chamomile and lavender oils are also perfect pairings.

PATCHOULI *Pogostemon cablin*

The leaves of this herb produce an oil with **stimulating** and **strengthening** properties, which can help skin tissue to **regenerate** and can improve scar tissue and stretch marks. It may also **revitalize** ageing skin and reduce wrinkles. It has **antiseptic** properties that can be used to treat problem skin, such as acne, and a heady scent that helps to dispel stress and anxiety.

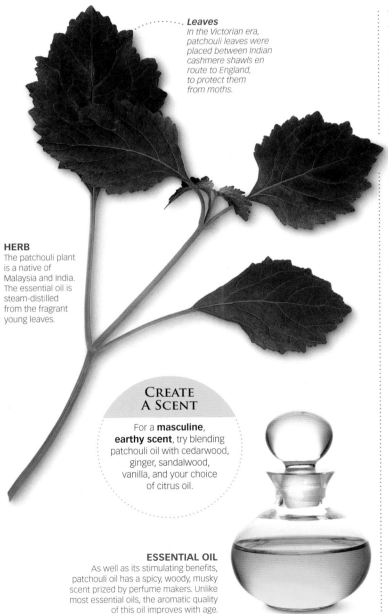

Leaves
In the Victorian era, patchouli leaves were placed between Indian cashmere shawls en route to England, to protect them from moths.

HERB
The patchouli plant is a native of Malaysia and India. The essential oil is steam-distilled from the fragrant young leaves.

CREATE A SCENT

For a **masculine, earthy scent**, try blending patchouli oil with cedarwood, ginger, sandalwood, vanilla, and your choice of citrus oil.

ESSENTIAL OIL
As well as its stimulating benefits, patchouli oil has a spicy, woody, musky scent prized by perfume makers. Unlike most essential oils, the aromatic quality of this oil improves with age.

WHAT IS IT GOOD FOR?

REPAIRS AND PROTECTS SKIN Patchouli oil has regenerative properties that can reduce the appearance of wrinkles, scars, and stretch marks. It is added to serums, lotions, and creams that are traditional remedies for spider veins, and superb moisturisers for rough, cracked, or dehydrated skin.

ACTS AS AN ANTISEPTIC Patchouli oil aids the treatment of acne, oily skin, weeping sores, and impetigo. It's antifungal action helps treat athlete's foot and other fungal infections.

TONES SKIN A good astringent, patchouli oil can help balance sebum secretions and normalize oily and acne-prone skin.

ACTS AS AN INSECT REPELLENT Patchouli oil makes an excellent insect repellant and it can be applied neat to the skin as an emergency treatment to help soothe insect bites and stings.

RELIEVES STRESS Use patchouli oil in the aromatherapy treatment of nervous exhaustion, stress, and anxiety.

AIDS DETOX Add patchouli oil to a massage oil blend to make the most of its diuretic properties – they can help to fight water retention and cellulite.

ACTS AS AN APHRODISIAC Stimulating patchouli oil is a traditional aphrodisiac, said to banish feelings of nervousness and lethargy.

Patchouli oil makes an excellent insect repellent.

ROSEMARY *Rosmarinus officinalis*

This Mediterranean native has a **cleansing** action. Its active constituents are carnosic acid, which is a **preservative** and **antioxidant**, and the **anti-inflammatory** rosmarinic acid. It **stimulates** the circulation of blood and lymphatic fluid, and makes a fine treatment for sluggish complexions or scalp problems. Always dilute the oil well – it should constitute no more than 1 per cent of the final mixture.

WHAT IS IT GOOD FOR?

ACTS AS A SKIN AND HAIR TONIC The astringent properties of rosemary oil make it an excellent skin toner and balancing hair rinse, which can treat hair loss and dandruff. Simply dilute it in a base oil.

COMBATS SIGNS OF AGEING Whether you drink rosemary tea or use the oil or tincture in massage, abundant antioxidants help to reduce inflammation and prevent oxidative damage that lead to premature ageing.

NOURISHING MASSAGE In massage, rosemary oil can stimulate the lymphatic system, aiding detox and the treatment of cellulite and water retention. Its warming effect is great for loosening up sore muscles, before or after exercise.

ACTS AS AN INSECT REPELLENT Rosemary oil can help remove lice and scabies. Dab the tincture neat on sores and insect bites to reduce inflammation and speed healing.

ACTS AS AN ANTIOXIDANT The carnosic acid in rosemary is a powerful antioxidant, making it useful as a natural preservative in products. Recent studies have shown it can prevent UVA damage to skin cells, meaning it has potential as a sunscreen ingredient.

ENHANCES FOCUS AND MEMORY Rosemary oil has a strengthening effect on the mind, aiding focus and memory. It has a reviving effect when tired, debilitated, or lethargic. Keep some on hand to relieve jet lag.

MAKE YOUR OWN

Tincture Fill a large jar three-quarters full with fresh or dried herbs. Cover with 500ml (16fl oz) vodka, brandy, or apple cider vinegar, and stir. Seal and store the jar in a cool, dark place for at least 3 weeks, shaking 3 times a week. Strain through muslin into a dark glass bottle.

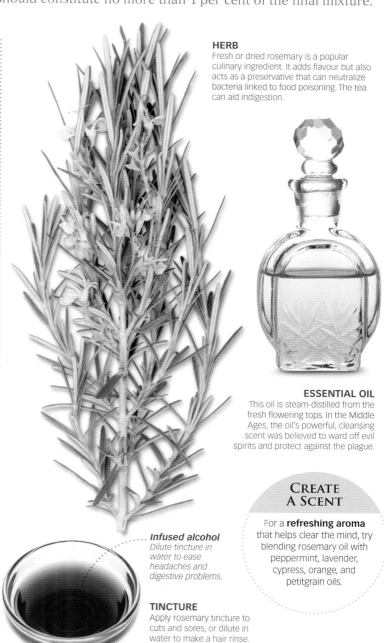

HERB
Fresh or dried rosemary is a popular culinary ingredient. It adds flavour but also acts as a preservative that can neutralize bacteria linked to food poisoning. The tea can aid indigestion.

ESSENTIAL OIL
This oil is steam-distilled from the fresh flowering tops. In the Middle Ages, the oil's powerful, cleansing scent was believed to ward off evil spirits and protect against the plague.

CREATE A SCENT

For a **refreshing aroma** that helps clear the mind, try blending rosemary oil with peppermint, lavender, cypress, orange, and petitgrain oils.

Infused alcohol
Dilute tincture in water to ease headaches and digestive problems.

TINCTURE
Apply rosemary tincture to cuts and sores, or dilute in water to make a hair rinse.

SAGE *Salvia officinalis*

Sage has an **astringent, anti-inflammatory** quality that helps **tone** the skin. It contains rosmarinic acid, which makes it a powerful **antiseptic** and **deodorizer**. It is also a mild diuretic that aids **detoxification**. It has a **stimulating** effect on circulation and a focusing effect on the mind and emotions. Use the oil well diluted, do not consume it, and *avoid during pregnancy* or if you are prone to seizures.

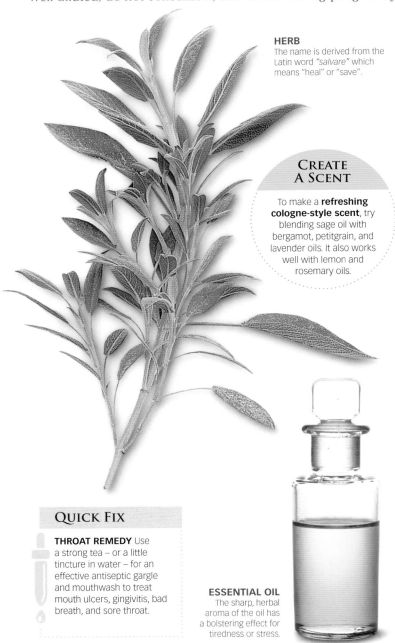

HERB
The name is derived from the Latin word "*salvare*" which means "heal" or "save".

CREATE A SCENT

To make a **refreshing cologne-style scent**, try blending sage oil with bergamot, petitgrain, and lavender oils. It also works well with lemon and rosemary oils.

WHAT IS IT GOOD FOR?

CONDITIONS AND SOOTHES SKIN Add sage oil to ointments and washes to treat cuts and grazes. The diluted oil can also help to dry up cold sores and soothe eczema and psoriasis.

IMPROVES SKIN TONE Sage oil or herbal infusion improves skin tone by increasing blood flow and diminishing the size of pores.

COMBATS SIGNS OF AGEING The antioxidant properties in sage oil help to delay the ageing process and reduce the harmful effects of free radicals.

NOURISHES HAIR Sage oil can be used as a hair rinse to control dandruff and restore shine and colour to greying hair – simply dilute it in water or vinegar. You can also make a hair treatment by diluting the oil in olive oil. Apply it to your hair and leave it on for a few hours, then shampoo as normal. You could leave it on your hair overnight for a more intensive treatment.

RELIEVES STRESS The oil acts as a tonic to the nervous system, enhancing its strength and vitality. It helps calm those under any kind of stress.

COMBATS BODY ODOUR Add the essential oil or tincture to natural deodorants to help to kill the bacteria that causes body odour and provide a refreshing, long-lasting natural fragrance. Add it to a foot bath to soothe and refresh tired feet.

QUICK FIX

THROAT REMEDY Use a strong tea – or a little tincture in water – for an effective antiseptic gargle and mouthwash to treat mouth ulcers, gingivitis, bad breath, and sore throat.

ESSENTIAL OIL
The sharp, herbal aroma of the oil has a bolstering effect for tiredness or stress.

EAT YOURSELF BEAUTIFUL

Tea Studies show that if you drink sage as a tea or take a supplement regularly, you can reduce excessive sweating, particularly during the menopause.

THYME *Thymus vulgaris*

Do not let the tiny leaves fool you – this aromatic, resinous herb packs a big punch. Since ancient times, thyme has been added to bath water to **relieve** aches and pains. Thymol, the active ingredient in thyme, is strongly **antiseptic**. Its aroma is **stimulating** and clears and **refreshes** the mind. The oil has a **warming**, **toning** effect on the skin which helps to improve circulation.

WHAT IS IT GOOD FOR?

CONDITIONS AND SOOTHES SKIN Thyme essential oil and tincture are effective healers for eczema, but always use them diluted. Do not use on hypersensitive or damaged skin, or on infants under 2 years of age.

IMPROVES SKIN TONE Diluted thyme oil or tincture has a stimulating and toning effect on the circulatory system and can help brighten the complexion. Antioxidant phenols and flavonoids help protect against free-radical damage.

TREATS ACNE Laboratory tests have shown that thyme tincture is more effective than benzoyl peroxide, the active ingredient in most anti-acne creams or washes, at killing Propionibacterium acnes – the bacterium that causes acne by infecting skin pores and forming spots, whiteheads, and pimples.

ACTS AS AN ANTISEPTIC Use well-diluted thyme oil in a compress to heal infections, boils, and sores. It also helps to eliminate body and head lice and scabies, and can be effective against *Candida albicans* as well as fungal nail infections and athlete's foot.

CONDITIONS HAIR AND SCALP Added to hair rinses and scalp treatments, thyme oil or tincture can help clear conditions like dandruff and seborrheic dermatitis.

EASES ACHES AND PAINS The oil, mixed into a warming liniment and lotion, is wonderful for rubbing into aching joints and muscles.

RELIEVES STRESS A massage blend made with thyme oil brings relief when you are anxious, stressed, or feeling low. It helps to promote restful sleep.

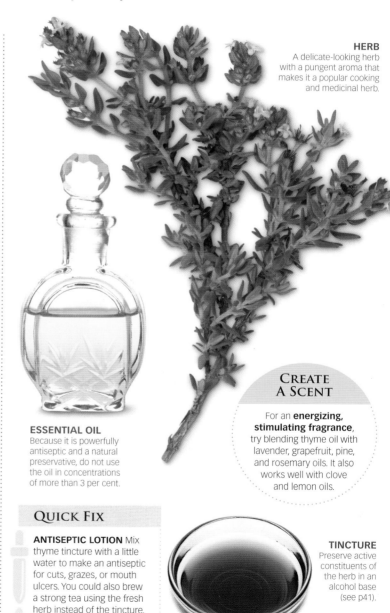

HERB
A delicate-looking herb with a pungent aroma that makes it a popular cooking and medicinal herb.

ESSENTIAL OIL
Because it is powerfully antiseptic and a natural preservative, do not use the oil in concentrations of more than 3 per cent.

CREATE A SCENT

For an **energizing, stimulating fragrance**, try blending thyme oil with lavender, grapefruit, pine, and rosemary oils. It also works well with clove and lemon oils.

QUICK FIX

ANTISEPTIC LOTION Mix thyme tincture with a little water to make an antiseptic for cuts, grazes, or mouth ulcers. You could also brew a strong tea using the fresh herb instead of the tincture.

TINCTURE
Preserve active constituents of the herb in an alcohol base (see p41).

TEA *Camellia sinensis*

Tea, particularly green and white tea extracts, are common cosmetic ingredients. Tea extracts possess **anti-inflammatory** and **anticarcinogenic** properties that help **protect** against sun and environmental damage and therefore impart **anti-ageing** effects. As tea is treated with a vast number of pesticides, choose organic varieties to get the most beneficial nutrients.

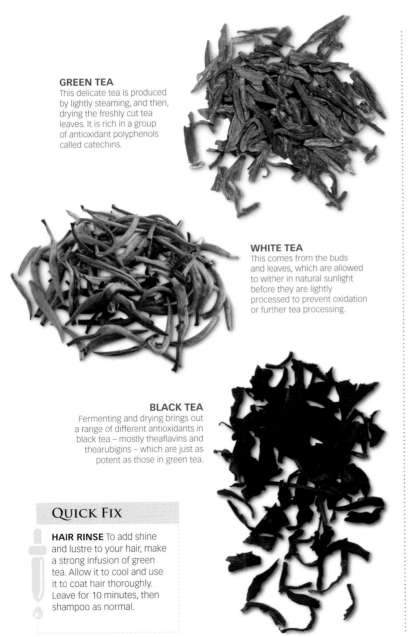

GREEN TEA
This delicate tea is produced by lightly steaming, and then, drying the freshly cut tea leaves. It is rich in a group of antioxidant polyphenols called catechins.

WHITE TEA
This comes from the buds and leaves, which are allowed to wither in natural sunlight before they are lightly processed to prevent oxidation or further tea processing.

BLACK TEA
Fermenting and drying brings out a range of different antioxidants in black tea – mostly theaflavins and thearubigins – which are just as potent as those in green tea.

WHAT IS IT GOOD FOR?

COMBATS SIGNS OF AGEING Tea extracts are rich in antioxidants. When added to cosmetics, they can help delay premature ageing caused by inflammation and oxidative stress. Antioxidant catechins in green tea, whether applied externally or consumed as a drink, can help make your skin more resistant to ultraviolet radiation and therefore premature skin ageing.

TONES SKIN Because tea leaves contain caffeine constituents, nutrients such as beta-carotene, vitamin C, and antioxidant polyphenols, extracts can boost circulation, improving the tone and structure of the skin.

PROTECTS FROM THE SUN Black, green, and white teas all have UV-absorbing properties, which when applied topically, can provide sun protection. Never use tea extracts as your only protection from the sun.

AIDS DETOX Tea has a mild astringent and diuretic effect that can help reduce puffiness and excess water.

QUICK FIX

HAIR RINSE To add shine and lustre to your hair, make a strong infusion of green tea. Allow it to cool and use it to coat hair thoroughly. Leave for 10 minutes, then shampoo as normal.

EAT YOURSELF BEAUTIFUL

Green tea A cup of green tea may have anti-allergy properties, for instance against hay fever, and can help reduce symptoms of eczema.

White tea Drinking a cup of white tea a day could help reduce your risk of cancer, rheumatoid arthritis, or even just age-associated wrinkles.

ST JOHN'S WORT *Hypericum perforatum*

It is well known that St John's wort is effective as a **sedative** and can help lift mild to moderate depression. Less well known are its benefits when used externally as a tincture or macerated oil. These include an **anti-inflammatory** action on the skin, a **calming** effect on nerve pain, and a **healing** action for minor cuts and abrasions.

WHAT IS IT GOOD FOR?

CONDITIONS AND SOOTHES SKIN St John's wort's macerated oil is particularly soothing for inflammatory skin conditions caused by eczema, psoriasis, and lupus. The oil, tincture, or strong tea can be used topically to treat cold sores and viral skin lesions. Apply the oil neat, but do not apply before sun exposure as it may increase the photosensitivity of the skin.

HEALS CUTS, SCRAPES, AND BRUISES St John's wort's oil or tincture is excellent at treating nerve pain, inflamed joints, and tendonitis, as well as soothing the pain and inflammation of sore skin, minor scalds, sunburns, cuts, and grazes. You can also dab the tincture on cuts and wounds.

RELIEVES MUSCLE PAIN St John's wort's oil helps alleviate muscle pain. Use as a massage oil to get the best from it.

ACTS AS AN ANTIDEPRESSANT The herb is soothing to the nervous system and has been used to good effect in treating mild to moderate depression and menopausal anxiety. The relaxing and antidepressant effect of St John's wort can also induce restful sleep, which in turn provides healthy skin and hair.

The relaxing and antidepressant effect of St John's wort can induce a restful night's sleep.

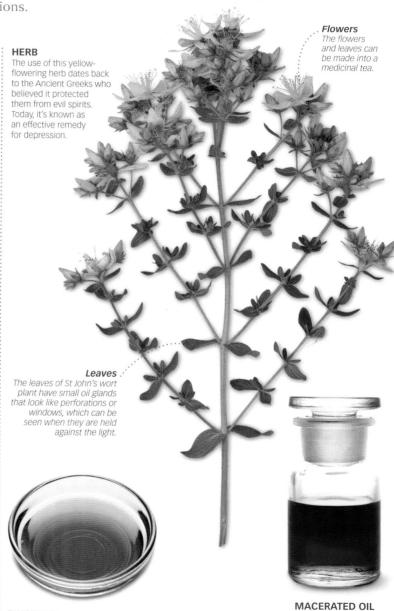

HERB
The use of this yellow-flowering herb dates back to the Ancient Greeks who believed it protected them from evil spirits. Today, it's known as an effective remedy for depression.

Flowers
The flowers and leaves can be made into a medicinal tea.

Leaves
The leaves of St John's wort plant have small oil glands that look like perforations or windows, which can be seen when they are held against the light.

TINCTURE
Taking St John's wort as a tincture (see p41) helps the herb get into your bloodstream quickly.

MACERATED OIL
Made by infusing the fresh flowers into an oil such as olive oil (see p26), this deeply coloured oil has anti-inflammatory and analgesic properties.

WITCH HAZEL *Hamamelia virginiana*

Astringent, **cooling,** and **refreshing**, witch hazel is usually used as an infusion or herbal water (also known as hydrosol) to **cleanse**, **tone**, and **refresh** the skin. It is rich in antioxidant phenols and tannins that can **calm** inflamed skin conditions, **soothe** irritation, roughness, and soreness and is also used to wash wounds and **heal** bruises and sores.

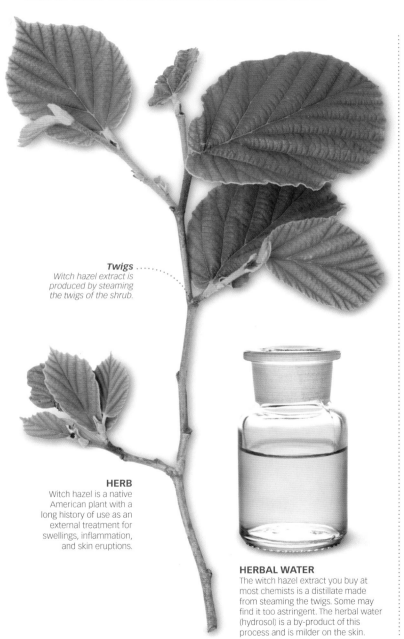

Twigs
Witch hazel extract is produced by steaming the twigs of the shrub.

HERB
Witch hazel is a native American plant with a long history of use as an external treatment for swellings, inflammation, and skin eruptions.

HERBAL WATER
The witch hazel extract you buy at most chemists is a distillate made from steaming the twigs. Some may find it too astringent. The herbal water (hydrosol) is a by-product of this process and is milder on the skin.

WHAT IS IT GOOD FOR?

COMBATS OILY SKIN Distilled witch hazel can be used on most skin types – though it may be too strong for very dry skin. It is especially beneficial for balancing oily skin and drying up spots – dab it neat on the face or use it to make products.

CONDITIONS AND SOOTHES SKIN Witch hazel has traditionally been used to calm skin conditions such as eczema, psoriasis, and allergic skin reactions. You can use it directly on problem areas.

ACTS AS AN ASTRINGENT Its astringent properties are also useful for easing varicose veins and shrinking spider veins.

HEALS CUTS, SCRAPES, AND BRUISES For minor skin injuries, use witch hazel to wash and disinfect the wound and stem bleeding. It helps heal bruises, insect bites, and makes a useful compress for sprains.

SOOTHING AFTERSHAVE Forget expensive and over-fragranced products and splash on distilled witch hazel or the herbal water to tone skin after shaving.

SOOTHES EYES To refresh tired eyes and reduce bags and puffiness, use witch hazel herbal water. Dip a cotton pad or facecloth into a little herbal water and place it over closed eyes. Rest for 20 minutes.

Witch hazel is especially benefical for balancing oily skin and drying spots.

BORAGE *Borago officinalis*

Borage yields a conditioning oil that is rich in gamma linolenic acid (GLA), an **anti-inflammatory** essential fatty acid. It can **rejuvenate** the skin, particularly if it is sun-damaged or ageing. Add a small amount of oil – roughly 2–10 per cent – to blends to reap benefits.

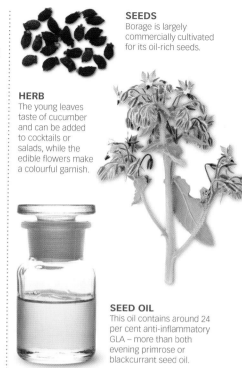

SEEDS
Borage is largely commercially cultivated for its oil-rich seeds.

HERB
The young leaves taste of cucumber and can be added to cocktails or salads, while the edible flowers make a colourful garnish.

SEED OIL
This oil contains around 24 per cent anti-inflammatory GLA – more than both evening primrose or blackcurrant seed oil.

WHAT IS IT GOOD FOR?

CONDITIONS AND SOOTHES SKIN
Oleic, palmitic, and stearic fatty acids give borage oil an emollient quality. GLA has an anti-inflammatory action known to ease eczema, psoriasis, and seborrheic dermatitis. Whether you choose to take supplements or apply it directly to your skin, the beauty benefits are very similar. Since this oil does not keep well, use capsules rather than open bottles in home-made cosmetics. The dried herb can be brewed as a tea and dabbed on the affected areas of the skin with cotton balls.

COMBATS SIGNS OF AGEING Borage oil soothes, hydrates, heals, and boosts the elasticity of skin. Its regenerative quality makes it a particularly good choice for mature skin. It can also help prevent water loss and increase skin-cell strength.

STRENGTHENS NAILS The GLA in borage oil can help strengthen nails and maintain healthy cuticles – simply rub the oil into them.

COMFREY *Symphytum officinale*

Comfrey is a traditional remedy for **healing** cuts, scratches, and even bones. It also has **anti-inflammatory** and skin **rejuvenating** properties. The leaves are rich in tannins and allantoin, which help prevent moisture loss and **stimulate** cell growth and repair.

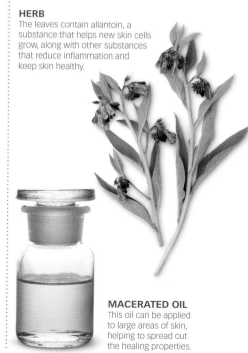

HERB
The leaves contain allantoin, a substance that helps new skin cells grow, along with other substances that reduce inflammation and keep skin healthy.

MACERATED OIL
This oil can be applied to large areas of skin, helping to spread out the healing properties.

WHAT IS IT GOOD FOR?

CONDITIONS AND SOOTHES SKIN
Comfrey contains allantoin, which provides healing and anti-inflammatory properties. Good for all skin types, it is particularly helpful for irritated, dry, and cracked skin.

PROTECTS FROM THE SUN Comfrey contains rosmarinic acid, which has anti-inflammatory and antioxidant properties. This helps to protect the skin from UV damage.

HEALS CUTS, SCRAPES, AND BRUISES Comfrey tincture, ointment, cream, or macerated oil has been used since ancient times for healing wounds, ulcers, insect bites, and other skin irritations. Its antibacterial properties help keep wounds from becoming infected. Do not use comfrey oils and ointments on deep wounds or infected skin, as it may promote surface healing before the wound is healed underneath.

NOURISHES HAIR Steep comfrey leaves in hot vinegar. Allow to cool, then rinse through your hair, leaving it soft and manageable.

LEMONGRASS *Cymbopogon citratus*

Lemongrass is a powerful tonic. It **refreshes** and **stimulates** body and mind and has an **astringent** effect that suits oily or acne-prone skin. It is also a **pain reliever** and a strong **antiseptic**, making it useful for treating cuts, grazes, and stings, and, in addition, it can also act as an **insect repellent**. Always dilute the essential oil – it should constitute no more than 1 per cent of the final mixture.

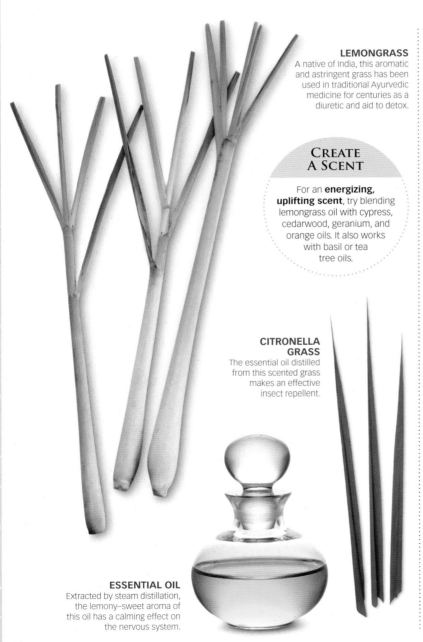

LEMONGRASS
A native of India, this aromatic and astringent grass has been used in traditional Ayurvedic medicine for centuries as a diuretic and aid to detox.

CREATE A SCENT

For an **energizing, uplifting scent**, try blending lemongrass oil with cypress, cedarwood, geranium, and orange oils. It also works with basil or tea tree oils.

CITRONELLA GRASS
The essential oil distilled from this scented grass makes an effective insect repellent.

ESSENTIAL OIL
Extracted by steam distillation, the lemony–sweet aroma of this oil has a calming effect on the nervous system.

WHAT IS IT GOOD FOR?

ACTS AS AN ASTRINGENT Lemongrass oil has an astringent and antiseptic effect on the skin. Add to a facial steam to deep-cleanse the skin and treat open or blocked pores.

REPAIRS AND PROTECTS SKIN The oil is useful for treating skin problems such as acne, eczema, and athlete's foot.

TONES SKIN The herbal water (also known as hydrosol), is a by-product of the production of the essential oil, which retains the essence of the plant. Use in skin-care lotions and creams, or as a facial toner.

COMBATS BODY ODOUR The fresh scent and antiseptic properties of lemongrass oil can help combat excessive perspiration. It is deodorizing due to active ingredients such as citral and myrcene, which are antibacterial.

ACTS AS AN INSECT REPELLENT Lemongrass oil is the key ingredient in natural insect repellents that fight mosquitoes and fleas. The oil can also be used against lice, scabies, and ticks. Another variety, Citronella (*Cymbopogon winterianus*), is an even more powerful insect repellent and a key ingredient in natural insecticides.

ACTS AS AN ANTIDEPRESSANT The oil is also a mild antidepressant. Inhaling lemongrass oil can relieve stress and nervous exhaustion.

EASES HEADACHES Lemongrass oil can soothe headaches and symptoms of jet lag.

EAT YOURSELF BEAUTIFUL

Tea This delicious herbal tea (see opposite) can help to lift your mood and aid focus. It also supports digestion and detox.

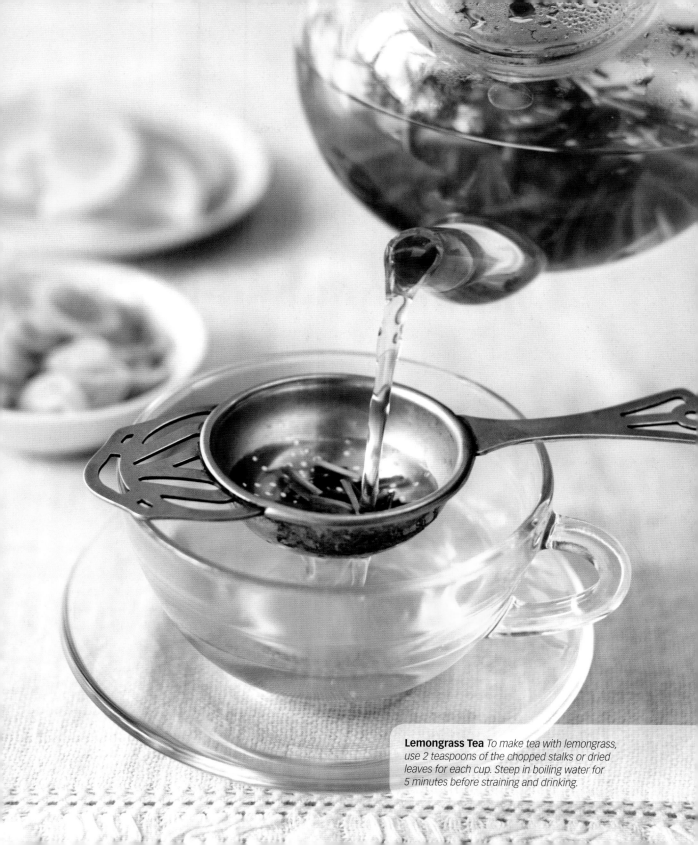

Lemongrass Tea *To make tea with lemongrass, use 2 teaspoons of the chopped stalks or dried leaves for each cup. Steep in boiling water for 5 minutes before straining and drinking.*

PALMAROSA *Cymbopogon martini*

Palmarosa essential oil is distilled from the scented grass, which is a relative of lemongrass. It grows wild in India. The essential oil has a pleasant, sweet, floral–rosy smell. It is best known for its skin-care properties, including a **balancing** action. It can help to **hydrate** dry skin or normalize the sebum secretions of oily skin. It also **tones** and **revitalizes** the appearance of tired or ageing skin.

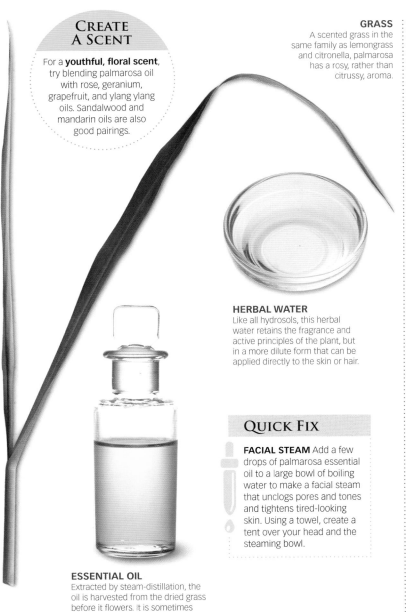

CREATE A SCENT

For a **youthful, floral scent**, try blending palmarosa oil with rose, geranium, grapefruit, and ylang ylang oils. Sandalwood and mandarin oils are also good pairings.

GRASS
A scented grass in the same family as lemongrass and citronella, palmarosa has a rosy, rather than citrussy, aroma.

HERBAL WATER
Like all hydrosols, this herbal water retains the fragrance and active principles of the plant, but in a more dilute form that can be applied directly to the skin or hair.

QUICK FIX

FACIAL STEAM Add a few drops of palmarosa essential oil to a large bowl of boiling water to make a facial steam that unclogs pores and tones and tightens tired-looking skin. Using a towel, create a tent over your head and the steaming bowl.

ESSENTIAL OIL
Extracted by steam-distillation, the oil is harvested from the dried grass before it flowers. It is sometimes called Indian or Turkish geranium.

WHAT IS IT GOOD FOR?

REPAIRS AND PROTECTS SKIN Palmarosa oil has a balancing and hydrating effect on all skin types. It helps minimize the appearance of scar tissue and stretch marks. Apply palmarosa oil, diluted in a light base oil, such as almond oil, to the problem areas.

IMPROVES SKIN TONE Add palmarosa oil to products for the face and body to improve skin tone all over.

COMBATS SIGNS OF AGEING Palmarosa oil stimulates cellular regeneration and reduces the appearance of wrinkles and fine lines. As an ingredient in skin-care products, it helps to brighten tired or ageing skin.

ACTS AS AN ANTISEPTIC Helpful ingredients in products for controlling oily skin, the oil and floral water also heal acne, dermatitis, athlete's foot, and minor skin infections.

RELIEVES STRESS Add palmarosa oil to massage oils to lift the spirits and soothe and strengthen mind and body. It is good for relieving stress, nervous tension, and anxiety.

ACTS AS AN APHRODISIAC The oil has a calming effect on the nerves as well as an ability to uplift – thought to contribute to its reputation as an aphrodisiac.

Palmarosa oil stimulates cellular regeneration and reduces the appearance of wrinkles and fine lines.

ALOE VERA *Aloe barbadensis*

Aloe vera gel can be found in hundreds of beauty products. It is a **cooling** remedy for burns, helps **repair** and **heal** wounds, and has a **soothing** effect on skin conditions such as eczema and psoriasis. Aloe is most effective if minimally processed. If you cannot source it fresh, direct from the leaves, look for 100 per cent aloe juice products and pure gels, not extracts from the macerated leaves.

WHAT IS IT GOOD FOR?

HEALS BURNS AND WOUNDS Aloe vera is often referred to as the "burn plant" because of the remarkable way the gel and herbal water, when applied externally, can heal a wide variety of burns – from sunburn to more serious scalds and burns. Aloe vera can help soften skin around minor wounds and prevent dryness as they heal.

CONDITIONS AND SOOTHES SKIN Anti-inflammatory properties of aloe vera gel and herbal water can help soothe skin that has had too much sun exposure. It also blocks the formation of histamine, so is useful for allergic conditions such as contact dermatitis. It has also been shown to help psoriasis.

IMPROVES SKIN TONE The gel and water can help lighten the appearance of blemishes.

TONES SKIN Use aloe vera juice as a skin-toning treatment or to treat oily skin. Apply as you would with an everyday toner.

TREATS ACNE The antimicrobial properties in aloe ingredients help to kill the bacteria that cause acne.

COMBATS SIGNS OF AGEING The gel or juice, added to beauty products, keeps the skin hydrated and moisturised. It can also plump up wrinkles and fine lines.

CONDITIONS HAIR AND SCALP The natural salicylic acid in aloe vera extracts can help remove dandruff build-up from the scalp. For seborrheic dermatitis, aloe has been shown to decrease scaliness and itching significantly.

TEETH AND GUM CARE You can dilute fresh aloe gel into a juice and use it as a mouthwash or toothpaste ingredient. When gargled, it is also a beneficial treatment for gingivitis, an inflammatory condition of the gums, relief for cold sores, and mouth ulcers. Apply fresh aloe gel to the gums to help pain and inflammation.

CARING AFTERSHAVE Men can use aloe vera gel as an aftershave. It reduces the irritation and inflammation of the skin and heals cuts and nicks.

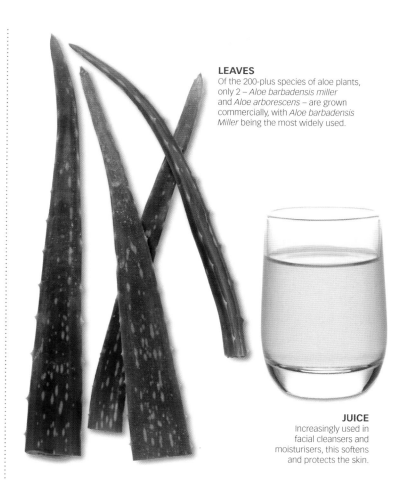

LEAVES
Of the 200-plus species of aloe plants, only 2 – *Aloe barbadensis miller* and *Aloe arborescens* – are grown commercially, with *Aloe barbadensis Miller* being the most widely used.

JUICE
Increasingly used in facial cleansers and moisturisers, this softens and protects the skin.

GEL
The fresh gel is obtained from the leaves, without any additives. If you wish to use gel made from the thickened juice, make sure aloe vera (*Aloe barbadensis miller*) is the first ingredient, not water or a sugary filler.

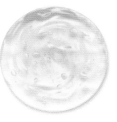

Fresh gel

Gel from the juice

AVOCADO *Persea gratissima*

Avocados are rich in vitamins and minerals, healthy fats, lecithin, and phytosterols (plant hormones), all of which can have a healing effect on the body, inside and out. The oil is highly **moisturising** and **revitalizing** for the skin. Whether you eat it or use it topically, avocado is deeply **nourishing** and can help to fight free radicals linked with illness and premature skin ageing.

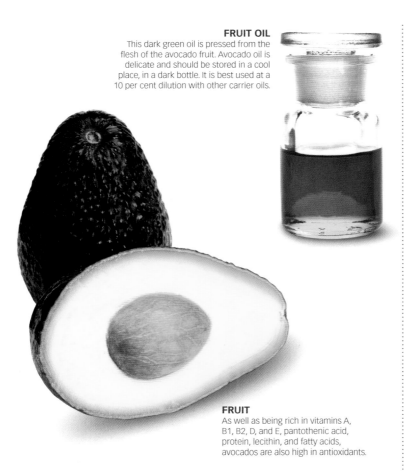

FRUIT OIL
This dark green oil is pressed from the flesh of the avocado fruit. Avocado oil is delicate and should be stored in a cool place, in a dark bottle. It is best used at a 10 per cent dilution with other carrier oils.

FRUIT
As well as being rich in vitamins A, B1, B2, D, and E, pantothenic acid, protein, lecithin, and fatty acids, avocados are also high in antioxidants.

WHAT IS IT GOOD FOR?

CONDITIONS SKIN AND HAIR Avocado oil helps to hydrate parched skin and aids the regeneration of skin cells. A high fatty-acid content means the oil is great for conditioning rough skin on feet, knees, or elbows and repairing hair damaged by styling, sun, or harsh winter weather. It can be applied neat to small areas of very dry skin, but for everyday use try it as a 10–25 per cent blend with lighter oils as it has a high viscosity. Mash fresh avocado into a smooth paste for a deeply nourishing and soothing facial mask for all skin types. Leave it on the skin for 20 minutes, then wash off to reveal glowing skin.

REPAIRS AND PROTECTS SKIN Used regularly, avocado oil can help prevent or minimize the appearance of stretch marks. Apply with damp hands straight after your bath or shower.

COMBATS SIGNS OF AGEING Avocado oil adds lustre and shine to a tired or dull complexion. Fatty acids and phytosterols (plant hormones) help replenish and revitalize mature skin.

PROTECTS FROM THE SUN While avocado oil cannot be used as a sunscreen on its own, it can boost protection to both skin and hair during sun exposure. The oil also helps to alleviate the pain of sunburn.

EAT YOURSELF BEAUTIFUL

Avocado Eat avocados for a good source of biotin, a deficiency of which can lead to dry skin and brittle hair and nails. The fruit is full of nourishing nutrients and helps fight the free radicals that cause disease and age skin prematurely.

Oil Add the oil to a salad to significantly increase the absorption of two skin-protecting antioxidants – lycopene and beta-carotene – by 200–400 per cent.

Avocado oil adds lustre and shine to a tired or dull complexion.

OLIVE *Olea europaea*

A rich, heavy oil, full of healthy fats, **skin-regenerating** phenolic antioxidants, vitamin E, squalene, and omega-9 oleic acids, olive oil is **moisturising** and **healing**. It has multiple uses in a natural beauty routine.

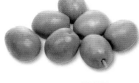

FRUIT
The skin is a rich source of anti-inflammatory antioxidant punicalagins.

FRUIT OIL
The whole fruit is ground into a fine paste from which olive oil can be extracted.

WHAT IS IT GOOD FOR?

CLEANSES AND CONDITIONS SKIN Olive oil will penetrate deep into the skin and provide long-lasting hydration to keep the skin smooth and supple. A drop or two of extra-virgin olive oil on a cotton wool pad gently and effectively removes even waterproof eye make-up without irritating delicate skin.

COMBATS SIGNS OF AGEING The antioxidants and vitamin E in olive oil help to prevent cell degeneration, thus preventing premature ageing. Squalene provides an effective barrier against water loss.

STRENGTHENS NAILS Rub a few drops of olive oil into the nails and cuticles to condition and protect, as well as add shine.

CONDITIONS HAIR AND SCALP Olive oil is great for treating dry hair and a sensitive scalp. Use as a pre-treatment before shampooing or as an overnight hair mask.

ACTS AS AN ANTIFUNGAL Olive oil is also an antifungal and the extract of the olive leaf has been shown to heal cold sores and fungal infections, such as candida, thrush, and athlete's foot.

EAT YOURSELF BEAUTIFUL

Oil Helps absorb vital fat-soluble vitamins from food, promoting healthy skin. Store away from heat and light.

POMEGRANATE *Punica granatum*

Extracted from the seeds, pomegranate oil has **anti-ageing**, **toning**, and **moisturising** effects. Extracts from the rind and pith are also rich in the antioxidant punicalagins, which **reduces inflammation** and helps to maintain collagen production.

SEEDS
Rich in skin-protecting nutrients and a good source of fibre. Enjoy them as part of a healthy diet.

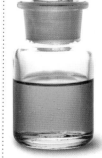

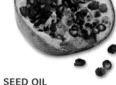

SEED OIL
A golden, clear oil produced from the seed and pith. It contains collagen-boosting isoflavones (plant hormones) similar to those found in soya.

WHAT IS IT GOOD FOR?

REPAIRS AND PROTECTS SKIN The rind contains ellagic acid, a strong anti-inflammatory that can aid the healing of burns and skin ulcers. It also helps to strengthen the membrane around skin cells, making them less susceptible to free-radical damage and preventing water loss.

CONDITIONS AND SOOTHES SKIN The oil nourishes and repairs dry skin, eczema, psoriasis, and sunburned skin. Its pucinic acid content reduces inflammation and swelling.

COMBATS SIGNS OF AGEING Topical application of products containing

the oil or extracts has been shown to improve skin elasticity by reducing inflammation. Research indicates that peel extracts, when used with the oil, boost collagen production and promote skin cell growth, thus effectively delaying skin ageing.

PROTECTS FROM THE SUN The extract, oil, and juice are added to sun-care preparations. The bioactive compounds of all these can protect skin cells from damage caused by UV radiation.

TEETH AND GUM CARE Gargle powdered pomegranate with water to fight bad breath.

EAT YOURSELF BEAUTIFUL

Juice Drink juice made from the pith and seeds, which contains high levels of beneficial antioxidants that can improve circulation and skin tone.

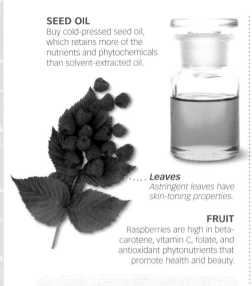

SEED OIL
Buy cold-pressed seed oil, which retains more of the nutrients and phytochemicals than solvent-extracted oil.

Leaves
Astringent leaves have skin-toning properties.

FRUIT
Raspberries are high in beta-carotene, vitamin C, folate, and antioxidant phytonutrients that promote health and beauty.

EAT YOURSELF BEAUTIFUL

Raspberries The fruits contain a variety of phytonutrients that have anti-cancer properties and can aid weight control.

RASPBERRIES *Rubus idaeus*

Recent studies show that raspberries and raspberry seed oil contain a vast array of antioxidants. One of these is the **anti-inflammatory** compound, ellagic acid. Raspberry leaf extract is **toning**, **antiseptic**, and helps to **soothe** and **calm** irritated skin.

WHAT IS IT GOOD FOR?

REPAIRS AND PROTECTS SKIN
The seed oil is exceptionally rich in the antioxidants alpha and gamma tocopherols (vitamin E). It also contains alpha linoleac acid, an anti-inflammatory essential omega-3 fatty acid.

TONES SKIN The leaf extract is mildly astringent and helps to tighten the surface of the skin. If you have oily skin, use a strong infusion made from dried raspberry leaves as a toner.

CONDITIONS AND SOOTHES SKIN The seed oil is gentle enough for use on sensitive skin. It is moisturising, softening, and helps to improve skin elasticity and moisture retention. The ellagic acid content makes the seed oil beneficial for skin conditions like psoriasis and eczema. You can pulp raw, ripe raspberries to make a quick facial mask to revive tired-looking skin.

PROTECTS FROM THE SUN Sun-protection research has shown that raspberry seed oil helps absorb UVB and UVC rays, suggesting that it may be a useful addition to sun cream.

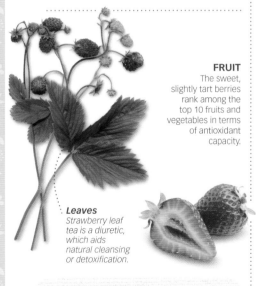

FRUIT
The sweet, slightly tart berries rank among the top 10 fruits and vegetables in terms of antioxidant capacity.

Leaves
Strawberry leaf tea is a diuretic, which aids natural cleansing or detoxification.

EAT YOURSELF BEAUTIFUL

Strawberries Salicylic acid, vitamin C, and alpha hydroxy acids (AHAs) in strawberry fruit and tea can help clear acne and balance oily skin.

STRAWBERRIES *Fragaria vesca*

Apart from being delicious, fresh strawberries are rich in vital nutrients, vitamins, minerals, and antioxidants, and are therefore beneficial for your health, skin, and hair. They are popular in fresh beauty preparations to help **cleanse**, **tone**, and **nourish** the skin.

WHAT IS IT GOOD FOR?

TONES SKIN Strawberries contain salicylic acid, which helps remove dead cells and impurities while tightening the pores.

PROTECTS AND REPAIRS SKIN
Ellagic acid helps fight inflammation associated with environmental damage, irritants, and pollution. To treat sunburn, fix a strong cup of strawberry leaf tea and then let it cool down. Dab the cooled tea on the skin to cool and soothe.

IMPROVES SKIN TONE Strawberry juice applied to the skin has skin-lightening properties and is a traditional treatment for removing age spots and freckles.

TEETH AND GUM CARE Strawberry extract is a gentle dentifrice, often used in toothpastes for children.

COMBATS SIGNS OF AGEING The extract acts as a photoprotective against skin ageing. In addition, it also increases cell survival and viability, and decreases the DNA damage caused by UV exposure.

BLUEBERRIES *Cyanococcus*

Native to North America, blueberries have long been valued for their nutritional and medicinal properties. They are one of the richest plant sources of key **antioxidants**, which have **anti-ageing** properties and are high in **skin-toning** vitamins A and C.

WHAT IS IT GOOD FOR?

BOOSTS CIRCULATION High in vitamin C and a good source of fibre, blueberries aid detox and help keep arteries and veins healthy. This contributes to healthier skin and fewer problems like spider veins and blotchiness.

COMBATS SIGNS OF AGEING The vitamin C in fresh blueberries also supports the production of collagen – which maintains the skin's elasticity and tone. Blueberries contain antioxidant polyphenols, which combat the effects of free radicals, a key cause of wrinkles. This is the reason why blueberry extracts are being used more and more in commercial products. Anthocyanins in blueberries reduce the production of substances in the body that accelerate the breakdown of collagen. Research on women aged 45–61 years has shown that diluted blueberry extract, applied daily for 3 months, significantly improves the quality of mature skin.

COMBATS OILY SKIN Nutrients in fresh blueberries help normalize oil levels in your skin, making clogged pores and acne breakouts less likely.

FRUIT
Studies show that blueberries have some of the highest levels of active antioxidants per serving of any food.

PLANT
All parts of the plant are high in antioxidants, but the extracts from the stems have the highest antioxidant activity of all.

EAT YOURSELF BEAUTIFUL

Blueberries 100g (3½oz) of the fruit contain the same amount of antioxidants as 5 servings of other fruits and vegetables.

SEA BUCKTHORN *Hippophae*

Sea buckthorn is highly prized for its ability to **hydrate** and **repair** dry, damaged, and ageing skin. Both the seed and pulp oils are rich in antioxidant carotenoids, vitamin E, and plant sterols that help to **tone** skin and **protect** it from day-to-day damage.

WHAT IS IT GOOD FOR?

TONES SKIN Antioxidants such as vitamins A, C, E, and beta-carotene in sea buckthorn oil help tone skin.

REPAIRS AND PROTECTS SKIN The oil is great for skin, hair, and nails. In addition to nourishing omega-3 (alpha linolenic acid), omega-6 (linoleic acid), and omega-9 (oleic acid), it is also the richest source of omega-7 (palmitoleic acid), which helps combat dryness and loss of elasticity, supports collagen production, and promotes cell-tissue regeneration.

CONDITIONS AND SOOTHES SKIN A high fatty acid content makes the oil emollient and nourishing. Especially good for dry, sun-damaged skin. When taken orally in supplements or applied neat on the skin, it softens and smoothes dry, cracked skin.

EAT YOURSELF BEAUTIFUL

Sea buckthorn The berries contain more vitamin C than strawberries, kiwis, and even oranges. Their tart juice is often added to fruit juice blends.

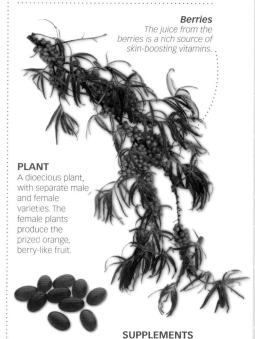

Berries
The juice from the berries is a rich source of skin-boosting vitamins.

PLANT
A dioecious plant, with separate male and female varieties. The female plants produce the prized orange, berry-like fruit.

SUPPLEMENTS
You can get the skin benefits of sea buckthorn by taking it in supplement form. You only need a little as the oil is highly concentrated.

COCONUT *Cocos nucifera*

Coconut fruit yields a light, **moisturising**, and **nourishing** oil. It is suitable for all skin and hair types but is especially beneficial for **soothing** and **softening** dry skin and hair. It also has an **anti-inflammatory** effect, which can help to **heal** wounds, blisters, and rashes. Coconut milk and water can also **nourish** and **condition** skin and hair.

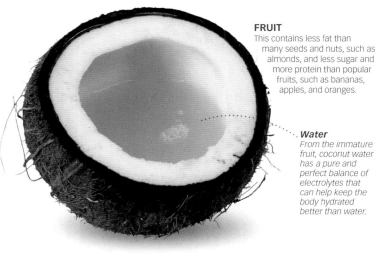

FRUIT
This contains less fat than many seeds and nuts, such as almonds, and less sugar and more protein than popular fruits, such as bananas, apples, and oranges.

Water
From the immature fruit, coconut water has a pure and perfect balance of electrolytes that can help keep the body hydrated better than water.

Organic oil
Avoid the odourless, flavourless, "pure" refined types, and opt instead for the organic, cold-pressed, virgin oil.

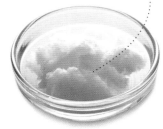

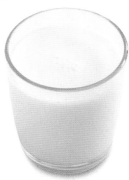

FRUIT OIL
Cooking coconut oil smells strongly of coconut and is solid at room temperature but melts easily when rubbed between the palms. Fractionated coconut oil has no odour, making it a good base for essential oils.

MILK
Obtained primarily by extracting the juice from the white kernel, the milk is rich in beneficial fats.

WHAT IS IT GOOD FOR?

CONDITIONS AND SOOTHES SKIN Coconut oil absorbs quickly and leaves the skin feeling silky smooth. Use it in place of a mineral oil for chapped lips, eczema and dermatitis, and as a shaving oil. Try applying it to damp skin or with damp hands to help spread it quickly and evenly over large areas of your body.

CLEANSES AND TONES SKIN A great make-up remover, coconut oil cleanses and moisturises all in one. You can use coconut water as a light skin cleanser and toner to help remove dirt, grease, and blemishes.

NOURISHES HAIR Use the oil as an overnight hair mask or pre-shampooing treatment. It helps combat dandruff and restores lustre and shine to dry or damaged hair.

ACTS AS AN ANTIFUNGAL The fatty acids in coconut oil help to prevent fungal and bacterial infections, making it an excellent all-purpose salve for healthy nails and feet.

TEETH AND GUM CARE Swish a small amount of coconut oil around in your mouth for 20 minutes – known as "oil pulling". Spit out when finished. There is no need to rinse afterwards. Oil pulling can help to reduce bacteria, control plaque, as well as fight tooth decay and gum infection. Studies have shown that this is as effective as the mouthwash ingredient chlorohexadine, for controlling bad breath.

EAT YOURSELF BEAUTIFUL

Oil Use in cooking as a nourishing substitute for butter and other cooking oils. It is very heat stable so is a better choice for cooking with than many other vegetable oils.

Water Coconut water is a superior drink for aiding hydration and maintaining the pH balance of the body.

VANILLA POD *Vanilla planifolia*

The vanilla pod is the fruit from the vanilla orchid. Vanilla pod extract has **soothing** and **softening** qualities and is rich in antioxidants, making it ideal for **repairing** rough or damaged skin. Its **antiseptic** properties can help to clear acne. Vanilla has long been popular with perfumiers; more recently it has become a favourite with cosmetic manufacturers due to its **rejuvenating** properties.

WHAT IS IT GOOD FOR?

REPAIRS AND PROTECTS SKIN The extract is perfect for use in face creams because it is rich in antioxidant properties that protect your skin from damage caused by environmental pollutants and toxins.

TREATS ACNE The antibacterial properties of vanilla make it an excellent ingredient in acne treatments. Vanillin, a constituent of vanilla, is antibacterial and helps cleanse your skin, reducing the occurrence of pimples and acne.

CONDITIONS HAIR Vanilla extract can help soften hair and minimize the appearance of split ends. It is reputed to aid hair growth.

RELIEVES PAIN The vanillin in vanilla extract has similar properties to capsaicin in chilli peppers and euganols in spices such as cinnamon. Used topically, it has a mild analgesic effect that provides temporary local relief from pain. In Ayurvedic medicine vanilla extract is used to relieve toothache.

RELIEVES STRESS Vanilla extract, when added to aromatherapy blends, helps to lift feelings of anxiety.

ACTS AS AN APHRODISIAC Vanilla extract has a euphoric effect on the emotions. This is thought to be responsible for its reputation as an aphrodisiac.

Vanilla extract can help to soften hair and minimize the appearance of split ends.

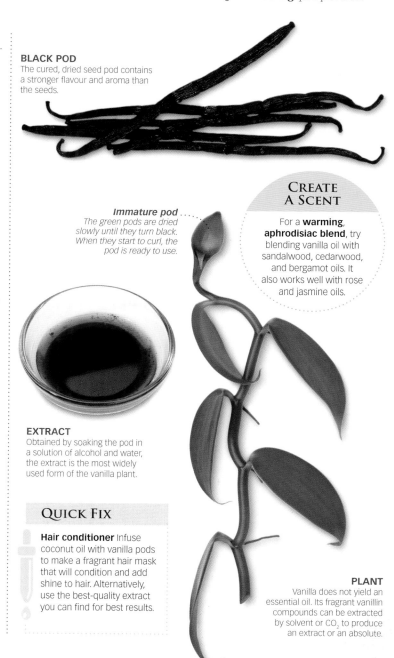

BLACK POD
The cured, dried seed pod contains a stronger flavour and aroma than the seeds.

Immature pod
The green pods are dried slowly until they turn black. When they start to curl, the pod is ready to use.

CREATE A SCENT

For a **warming**, **aphrodisiac blend**, try blending vanilla oil with sandalwood, cedarwood, and bergamot oils. It also works well with rose and jasmine oils.

EXTRACT
Obtained by soaking the pod in a solution of alcohol and water, the extract is the most widely used form of the vanilla plant.

QUICK FIX

Hair conditioner Infuse coconut oil with vanilla pods to make a fragrant hair mask that will condition and add shine to hair. Alternatively, use the best-quality extract you can find for best results.

PLANT
Vanilla does not yield an essential oil. Its fragrant vanillin compounds can be extracted by solvent or CO_2 to produce an extract or an absolute.

UPLIFTING CITRUS

The smell of citrus fruits is now so recognizable in commercial products that we don't always think of it as therapeutic. Yet the citrus family provides delightfully **refreshing** and **invigorating** aromas. The rinds of citrus fruits are rich in essential oils which means that oils from this family are plentiful and affordable. Used on the skin, the essential oils **balance**, **tone**, and **detoxify** all skin types.

LEMON *Citrus limonum* ▶

TONES SKIN When diluted and applied topically, lemon essential oil can boost circulation, making it good for toning varicose veins and preventing chilblains. It has a clarifying effect on greasy skin as well as toning properties that help to combat wrinkles and spider veins.

ACTS AS AN ANTISEPTIC Like most citrus oils, lemon essential oil also has antiseptic properties. As an ingredient in skin-care preparations, it helps to treat problem skin, such as acne.

AIDS DETOX The essential oil's diuretic action can reduce cellulite and fluid retention. Drinking hot water with a slice of lemon is good for detox as it supports the liver and aids lymphatic cleansing.

CONDITIONS HAIR Lemon juice, neat or mixed with water, makes a great, quick hair rinse that can lighten and condition the hair.

RELIEVES HEADACHES Lemon oil has a pleasing scent, which is good for treating headaches and supplying a dose of mental clarity and positivity.

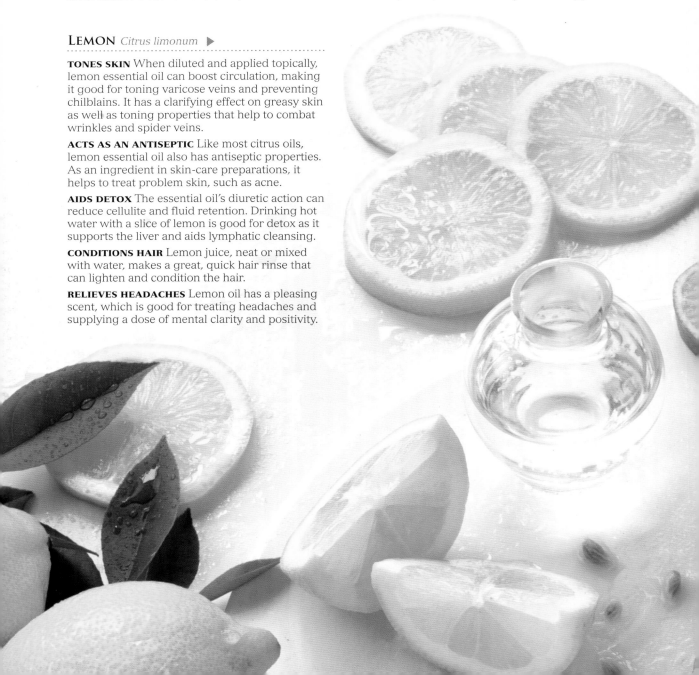

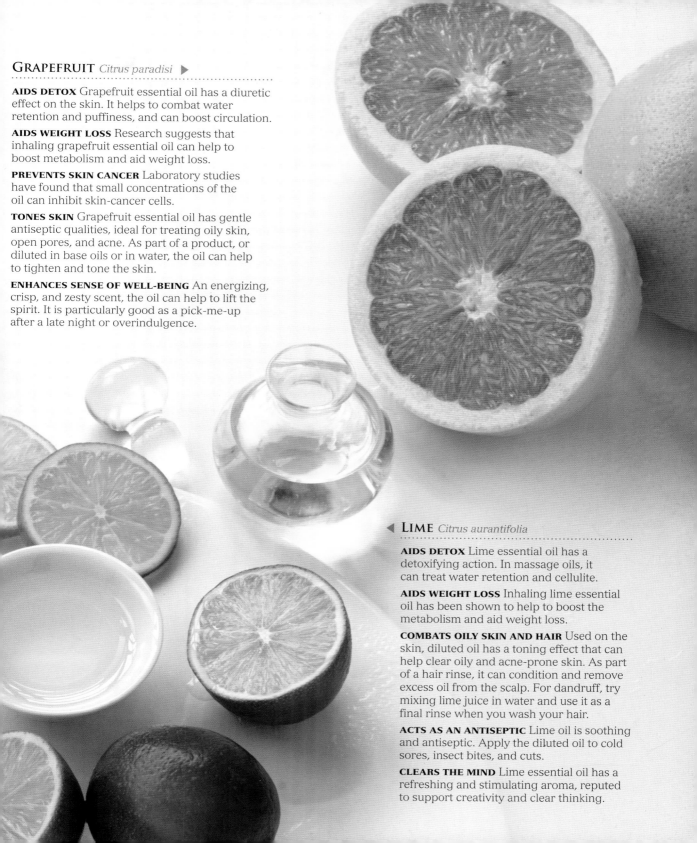

GRAPEFRUIT *Citrus paradisi* ▶

AIDS DETOX Grapefruit essential oil has a diuretic effect on the skin. It helps to combat water retention and puffiness, and can boost circulation.

AIDS WEIGHT LOSS Research suggests that inhaling grapefruit essential oil can help to boost metabolism and aid weight loss.

PREVENTS SKIN CANCER Laboratory studies have found that small concentrations of the oil can inhibit skin-cancer cells.

TONES SKIN Grapefruit essential oil has gentle antiseptic qualities, ideal for treating oily skin, open pores, and acne. As part of a product, or diluted in base oils or in water, the oil can help to tighten and tone the skin.

ENHANCES SENSE OF WELL-BEING An energizing, crisp, and zesty scent, the oil can help to lift the spirit. It is particularly good as a pick-me-up after a late night or overindulgence.

◀ LIME *Citrus aurantifolia*

AIDS DETOX Lime essential oil has a detoxifying action. In massage oils, it can treat water retention and cellulite.

AIDS WEIGHT LOSS Inhaling lime essential oil has been shown to help to boost the metabolism and aid weight loss.

COMBATS OILY SKIN AND HAIR Used on the skin, diluted oil has a toning effect that can help clear oily and acne-prone skin. As part of a hair rinse, it can condition and remove excess oil from the scalp. For dandruff, try mixing lime juice in water and use it as a final rinse when you wash your hair.

ACTS AS AN ANTISEPTIC Lime oil is soothing and antiseptic. Apply the diluted oil to cold sores, insect bites, and cuts.

CLEARS THE MIND Lime essential oil has a refreshing and stimulating aroma, reputed to support creativity and clear thinking.

UPLIFTING CITRUS *continued*

▼ ORANGE *Citrus sinesnis*

REPAIRS AND PROTECTS SKIN Used in skin-care products, orange essential oil helps to promote collagen production and supports the skin's repair process. Its healing properties are attributed to the aromatic compound limonene, which is also a good antiseptic. Freshly squeezed orange juice is full of collagen-promoting vitamin C and antioxidants – drink it regularly to help skin from the inside.

TONES SKIN Seville, or bitter orange, yields petitgrain oil (see p77) from its leaves and twigs and neroli oil from its flowers. Both tone and condition the skin. Use orange floral water neat on the skin as a facial toner, or put it into a spray bottle and use as a facial spritz.

AIDS DETOX Used with a carrier oil during massage, orange essential oil can improve circulation and stimulate the lymphatic system, the bladder, and the kidneys, aiding the removal of toxins from the body.

ENHANCES SENSE OF WELL-BEING The oil has a sweet, uplifting scent that is both energizing and revitalizing. The scents of neroli and petitgrain oils can also enliven the senses.

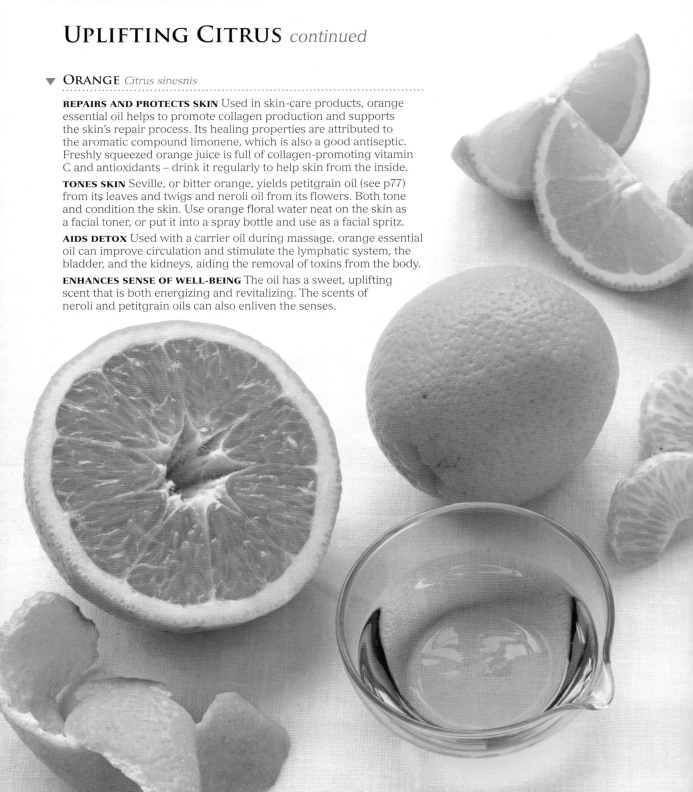

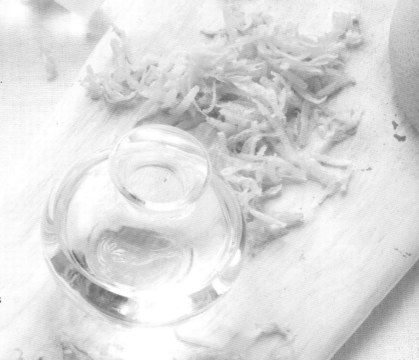

◀ **MANDARIN AND TANGERINE**
Citrus nobilis and Citrus tangerina

COMBATS OILY SKIN Mandarin and tangerine essential oils have astringent properties that are good for combatting oily skin and acne.

TONES SKIN Both oils can be used in body creams or massage oils to treat stretch marks and to help tone loose skin, for example, after weight loss.

AIDS DETOX Used with a carrier oil during massage, mandarin and tangerine oils can aid lymphatic drainage.

ENHANCES SENSE OF WELL-BEING Of all the citrus oils, mandarin has the sweetest aroma and is gentle and calming. Relaxing, warming, and soothing, the oil has a calming effect on the nerves and is especially good for fractious children and pregnant women. If you are feeling a bit nauseous, mandarin may also help to calm your stomach. Tangerine has a light, sweet citrus aroma, with similar therapeutic benefits.

BERGAMOT *Citrus aurantium bergamia* ▶

TONES SKIN Bergamot oil is particularly beneficial for combination or oily skin, where it exerts a balancing effect. Bergamot contains the compound bergaptene, which increases the risk of sunburn. Make sure you use oils that are bergaptene-free. Used in skin-care products, bergamot essential oil is suitable for all skin types.

ACTS AS AN ANTISEPTIC The oil has antiviral and antibacterial properties, making it ideal for you to dab, diluted in a base oil, onto cold sores and acne.

CONDITIONS AND SOOTHES SKIN Bergamot oil has a soothing effect on dry, itchy skin and can help to improve the appearance of scars.

ENHANCES SENSE OF WELL-BEING These oranges have a very sour fruit but a deeply scented rind. The fruit is what gives Earl Grey tea its unique scent. Used in aromatherapy, it is a balancing and calming oil with a fruity and uplifting scent.

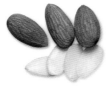

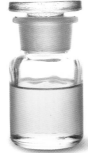

NUT OIL
Almonds are fruits rather than true nuts. The oil, pressed from the fruit seed, is suitable for all skin types.

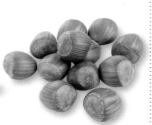

GROUND NUTS
This makes a gentle and vitamin E-rich exfoliant that removes dead skin cells and promotes natural skin regeneration.

ALMOND *Prunus amygdalus dulcis*

Vitamin-rich almonds produce an all-purpose oil that is gentle enough for babies and **soothing** for sensitive skin.

WHAT IS IT GOOD FOR?

CLEANSES AND CONDITIONS SKIN
A light oil for sensitive, irritated, or dry skin, that prevents moisture loss and relieves inflammation. It provides the skin with a thin barrier against the elements, nourishing and mantaining suppleness. Ground almond can cleanse and exfoliate.

NOURISHING MASSAGE Almond oil is absorbed slowly, making it a perfect lubricant for massage. It works well on its own as a base oil, but blends well with other prunus oils, such as apricot and peach kernel.

PROTECTS FROM THE SUN The oil has a low SPF against the sun's rays. Do not use this alone as a sunscreen.

NUT OIL
Full of vitamins and minerals, this oil has a slightly astringent action.

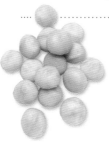

NUTS
Hazelnuts are rich in protein and healthy fats that nourish skin.

HAZELNUT *Corylus avellana*

Hazelnuts produce a mild, **nourishing** oil with a gentle **astringent** action that is especially good for oily skin or skin in need of repair.

WHAT IS IT GOOD FOR?

CONDITIONS AND SOOTHES SKIN
Hazelnut oil is suitable for sensitive skin, and even babies' skin. It makes skin soft and supple, and is astringent, so is great for those with oily skin who still want to moisturise. It can also help balance oily and combination skins.

REPAIRS AND PROTECTS SKIN
Deeply penetrating, hazelnut oil can be used in home-made products to treat rough or damaged skin. Blend it with rosehip seed oil to treat scars and stretch marks.

CONDITIONS HAIR Hazelnut oil can add balancing and conditioning properties to hair oils.

NUTS
The selenium, zinc, and essential fatty acids in macadamia nuts help the body burn fat more efficiently.

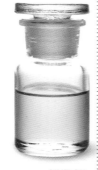

NUT OIL
Pressed from a native Australian nut, macadamia nut oil is similar to human sebum, which helps to balance the skin.

MACADAMIA *Macadamia ternifolia*

Nutrient-dense macadamia nuts produce an oil with **protecting** and healing properties. It is especially good for sun-damaged skin.

WHAT IS IT GOOD FOR?

REPAIRS AND PROTECTS SKIN
The macadamia nut has the highest amount of monounsaturated fats of any nut and contains around 22 per cent skin-repairing, omega-7 palmitoleic acid. A silky, emollient oil, its fatty acid and sterol (plant hormone) content helps to repair the skin's barrier function and stop water loss from the skin. It is especially suitable for sun-care formulations, and is also great for conditioning hair.

COMBATS SIGNS OF AGEING
Regenerating, moisturising, and hydrating, macadamia oil is rich in palmitoleic acid, which helps to delay skin- and cell-ageing.

NEEM *Melia azadirachta*

Neem seeds produce an oil that is **antiseptic** and **moisturising**. The oil can treat infections, skin eruptions, and inflammation.

SEED OIL
Pressed from the fruit and seeds of the tree, neem oil is highly antiseptic. A little goes a long way.

WHAT IS IT GOOD FOR?

CONDITIONS AND SOOTHES SKIN
Two anti-inflammatory compounds are found in neem oil – nimbidin and nimbin. They have been shown to ease eczema and psoriasis.

COMBATS SIGNS OF AGEING
Neem oil prevents and softens the appearance of wrinkles.

ACTS AS AN ANTISEPTIC Neem oil is useful for treating cold sores, as it prevents the virus from entering and infecting the cells.

ACTS AS AN INSECT REPELLENT A powerful insecticide, neem oil has become a staple of many natural head-lice treatments and mosquito repellents.

SEEDS
Neem seeds yield a medicinal oil for external use, but they must not be eaten raw as they can be toxic.

ARGAN *Argania spinosa*

A **nourishing** and exotic multi-purpose oil from Morocco. Argan oil can be used to **condition** and **protect** both hair and skin.

SEED OIL
Argan oil has a similar fat content to olive oil. It's a "dry" oil – which means it is light and absorbs quickly.

WHAT IS IT GOOD FOR?

REPAIRS AND PROTECTS SKIN Argan oil is rich in skin-loving fatty acids, sterols, and antioxidants, and is especially high in vitamin E. Great for scars, stretch marks, and sun-damaged skin. Before going to bed, apply a very small amount of argan oil to lips, to heal and repair at night.

CONDITIONS AND SOOTHES SKIN
Apply a little argan oil to skin and nails to replenish and revitalize. To spread the oil easily, apply it with damp hands. Regular application can significantly reduce greasiness and improve the appearance of oily skin.

CONDITIONS HAIR The oil is a great conditioner for dry or damaged hair.

SEEDS
The seeds of the argan fruit are pressed to produce a rich oil with a nutty aroma and taste.

JOJOBA *Simmondsia chinensis*

Protective jojoba produces an oil with renowned **revitalizing** and **moisturising** properties. It is recommended for all skin types.

SEED OIL
Jojoba is not a true oil, but is a liquid wax. It is extremely stable, and rich in proteins and minerals.

WHAT IS IT GOOD FOR?

CLEANSES AND CONDITIONS SKIN
Jojoba oil makes a great make-up remover for all skin types, helping to lift and dissolve dirt and oil that clog pores. The deeply penetrating oil also helps to soften hard, rough skin and skin conditions such as psoriasis and eczema.

REPAIRS AND PROTECTS SKIN
Jojoba oil is easily absorbed and has a structure similar to human sebum. It helps mature or weather-exposed skin to retain moisture.

CONDITIONS HAIR AND SCALP
Use jojoba oil on its own as a conditioning treatment for dry hair and scalp. It is also reputed to stimulate hair growth.

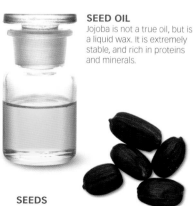

SEEDS
The seeds from jojoba shrubs were traditionally pounded to produce a healing salve.

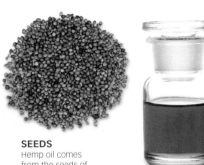

SEEDS
Hemp oil comes from the seeds of an "industrial" hemp variety, which retain the plant's nutrients.

SEED OIL
Hemp seeds produce the best oil, although the whole plant can be pressed for oil.

HEMP *Cannabis sativa*

Hemp contains **hydrating** essential omega-fatty acids, in a ratio similar to human skin. It produces a **balancing** oil for all skin types.

WHAT IS IT GOOD FOR?

REPAIRS AND PROTECTS SKIN
Hemp oil is good for most skin types. It is very good at helping the skin to retain moisture. Refined hemp oil is colourless and mostly odourless, making it suitable for a variety of cosmetic uses. It is added to many sun-care lotions and other products for use when the skin is exposed to extreme temperature changes.

CONDITIONS AND SOOTHES SKIN
An exceptionally rich oil high in essential fatty acids and proteins. Light and non-greasy, it is an excellent natural emollient and moisturiser for dry, inflamed, or weathered skin.

SEED OIL
The omega-3 alpha-linolenic acid (ALA) in flaxseed oil has a powerful anti-inflammatory action, whether taken internally or applied to the skin.

SEEDS
Flaxseeds are rich in plant hormones called lignans, which have a mild estrogenic action as well as antioxidant qualities.

FLAX *Linum usitatissimum*

These seeds are **nourishing** and **rejuvenating**, especially for dry skin. Choose organic oil that has been cold-pressed and unfiltered.

WHAT IS IT GOOD FOR?

COMBATS SIGNS OF AGEING The omega-3 protein found in flaxseed oil helps protect and rejuvenate skin cells, brighten dull-looking skin, and smoothen the appearance of wrinkles.

CONDITIONS AND SOOTHES SKIN
Flaxseed oil helps seal moisture into the skin, making it a great treatment for dry skin conditions. Its anti-inflammatory action is helpful for skin problems like eczema and psoriasis. The seeds contain skin-loving essential fats, so enjoy them as part of a healthy diet.

TREATS ACNE The oil is suitable for cleansing and conditioning oily or acne-prone skin and rosacea.

ESSENTIAL OIL
Castor oil is a thick, heavy oil best used in a blend. Add to carrier oils at a 10–15 per cent dilution.

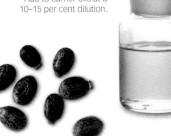

NUTS
The castor plant gets its name from its use as a replacement for castoreum, a perfume base made from the dried perineal glands of beavers.

CASTOR *Ricinus communis*

Castor seeds produce a heavy vegetable oil that **conditions** and provides a **protective** barrier on the skin that helps to aid **repair**.

WHAT IS IT GOOD FOR?

CONDITIONS AND SOOTHES SKIN The oil is used in cosmetic formulations to treat dry, chapped skin.

CONDITIONS HAIR AND SCALP
Many hair and skincare products use castor oil as it is a good conditioner for dry, brittle hair.

REPAIRS AND PROTECTS SKIN
Castor oil is often added to cosmetics because of its rich, emollient qualities. In particular, it provides a useful barrier against water loss for very dry skin.

APRICOT *Prunus armeniaca*

Apricot seeds produce a **skin-softening** oil for all skin types. It is a **soothing** oil that helps to maintain supple, moisturised skin.

WHAT IS IT GOOD FOR?

CONDITIONS AND SOOTHES SKIN
Apricot kernel oil brings relief to dry, inflamed, and prematurely ageing skin. It forms a light barrier against environmental damage.

CLEANSES AND TONES SKIN The oil helps lift and dissolve dirt and hard sebum, which can clog pores.

COMBATS SIGNS OF AGEING
Apricot kernel oil softens and helps improve skin elasticity and smooth out fine lines.

NOURISHING MASSAGE As apricot kernel oil absorbs more slowly into the skin than some oils, it is great for massage and skin serums.

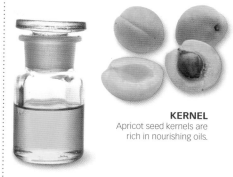

KERNEL
Apricot seed kernels are rich in nourishing oils.

KERNEL OIL
An emollient oil that helps soothe and condition the skin. If apricot oil is not available try peach kernel oil instead – they have the same qualities.

GRAPESEED *Vitis vinifera*

Grapeseeds yield a **soothing** oil for acne-prone or sensitive skin. The oil penetrates deeply, making it **conditioning** for dry skin.

WHAT IS IT GOOD FOR?

TONES SKIN Rich in linoleic acid (omega-6), this mildly astringent oil helps tighten, tone, and condition the skin.

SOOTHES SENSITIVE SKIN A wonderful, mild oil for those with skin sensitivities. It is non-allergenic and so is a good substitute for nut

oils, for those who may be allergic to nuts.

TREATS ACNE Acne-prone and oily skins benefit from grapeseed oil because of its astringent properties.

NOURISHING MASSAGE Grapeseed oil leaves the skin with a satin-like finish. It is used as a massage and emollient oil in premature infants.

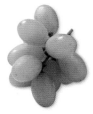

FRUIT
When pressed, grapeseeds yield a luxurious oil for culinary and cosmetic purposes.

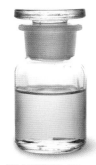

GRAPESEED OIL
A silky, non-greasy oil rich in antioxidants, vitamins, and minerals. Nourishing to all skin types.

WHEATGERM *Triticum vulgare*

Rich in antioxidants, wheatgerm yields an oil that can encourage natural cellular **repair**, restore skin's **vitality**, and prevent fine lines.

WHAT IS IT GOOD FOR?

COMBATS SIGNS OF AGEING
Wheatgerm oil revitalizes the skin, helping to prevent the development of lines around the eyes and mouth.

REPAIRS AND PROTECTS SKIN The oil is useful for preventing stretch marks during pregnancy and is a great

treatment for burns, sores, and other skin problems.

CONDITIONS AND SOOTHES SKIN
A nurturing oil rich in antioxidants, skin-protecting vitamin E, and beta-carotene. Ideal for use as a massage and skin-conditioning oil.

WHEATGERM
The germ is the kernel at the centre of a wheat seed from which a new wheat sprout develops. It is the most nutritious portion of wheat.

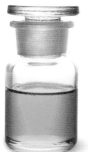

WHEATGERM OIL
Wheatgerm oil has the highest vitamin E content of any seed oil. It has a distinctive aroma and a thick, sticky consistency.

RICH WAXES AND BUTTERS

Waxes and butters add **moisturising** properties to cleansers and body and face creams. They have a much longer-lasting barrier effect on the skin than oils, making them particularly effective in **hydrating** formulations that protect dry, rough, or cracked skin. By acting as a **barrier** on the skin, they can prevent moisture loss and promote **natural healing**.

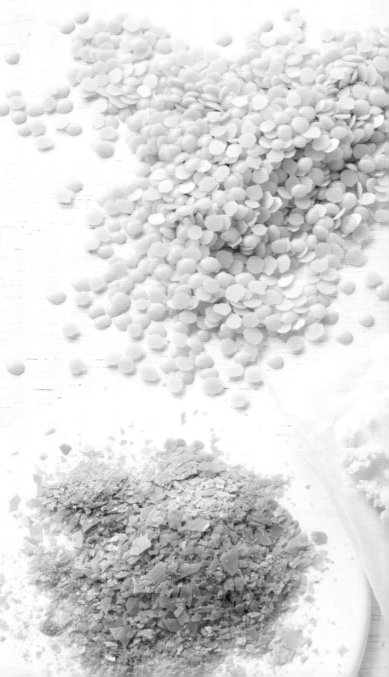

CANDELILLA *Euphorbia cerifera* ▶

SUITABLE FOR VEGANS Candelilla wax is made from a desert plant of the same name, making it vegetarian and vegan. It is often used to replace other non-vegan waxes, such as beeswax.

CONDITIONS AND SOOTHES SKIN Candelilla is used to make barrier products, such as lip balms, because it is an emollient wax that prevents moisture loss from the skin. It has an anti-inflammatory action that helps calm itchy skin conditions and may help reduce the appearance of blemishes.

REPAIRS AND PROTECTS SKIN Rich in nutrients and fatty acids, and not too heavy on the skin, candelilla wax is great for when the skin needs a little extra moisture and protection.

CARNAUBA *Copernicia cerifera* ▶

CONDITIONS AND SOOTHES SKIN A common ingredient in lipsticks and lip balms, carnauba wax creates a protective barrier that helps lips retain moisture and keeps them soft. An odourless hypoallergenic wax suitable for all skin types, it is especially good for sensitive skin.

ADDS TEXTURE AND SHINE TO COSMETICS Carnauba wax is a common thickening agent in cosmetics. As it is the hardest of all the natural waxes, and has a high melting point, small quantities added to products like lipsticks and lip balms help products remain solid yet flexible.

◀ **COCOA BUTTER** *Theobroma cacao*

REPAIRS AND PROTECTS SKIN Cocoa butter is a "dry" wax and a good emollient, which means it acts as a barrier to prevent water loss and helps keep skin soft. It supports collagen production, and thus can help prevent wrinkles and stretch marks and improve skin elasticity and tone.

SOOTHES SENSITIVE SKIN A mild wax that is suitable for most skin types. As it is an occlusive – capable of slowing down evaporation of water from the skin – it may not be suitable for facial use for those prone to acne and spots since it could clog pores.

CONDITIONS AND SOOTHES SKIN The butter is a natural emulsifier and softener for skin and hair. It has incredible moisturising and conditioning properties, which make it an ideal ingredient for skin and hair preparations.

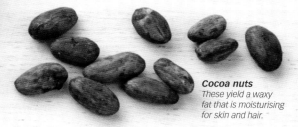

Cocoa nuts
These yield a waxy fat that is moisturising for skin and hair.

◀ **SHEA NUT BUTTER** *Butyrospermum parkii*

CONDITIONS AND SOOTHES SKIN Shea nut butter is a superb moisturising ingredient with excellent healing properties. It is rich in vitamin A, which helps improve skin conditions such as eczema, psoriasis, skin allergies, and blemishes. It is especially good for dry and damaged skin.

REPAIRS AND PROTECTS SKIN A gentle and effective moisturiser, shea nut butter contains oleic acid, a saturated fatty acid that is highly compatible with the sebum naturally produced by our skin. It is readily absorbed and is said to help in the absorption of other active ingredients. Adding shea butter to shaving cream formulations can help you to get a smoother shave.

COMBATS SIGNS OF AGEING An excellent addition to skin-care products, the butter contains 5–10 per cent phytosterols – plant hormones that help stimulate skin-cell growth. It also contains vitamin E, a natural antioxidant that helps protect the skin from free-radical damage.

MYRRH *Commiphora myrrha*

The **antiseptic** qualities of myrrh help to repair wounds that are slow to heal. It helps to **condition** dry and damaged skins and is an important **anti-ageing** treatment that delays the appearance of wrinkles and other signs of skin ageing. Used in aromatherapy, it has a **stimulating** and **strengthening** effect on the emotions.

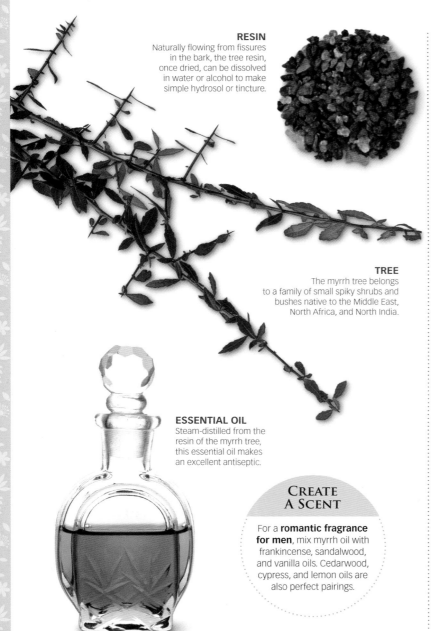

RESIN
Naturally flowing from fissures in the bark, the tree resin, once dried, can be dissolved in water or alcohol to make simple hydrosol or tincture.

TREE
The myrrh tree belongs to a family of small spiky shrubs and bushes native to the Middle East, North Africa, and North India.

ESSENTIAL OIL
Steam-distilled from the resin of the myrrh tree, this essential oil makes an excellent antiseptic.

CREATE A SCENT

For a **romantic fragrance for men**, mix myrrh oil with frankincense, sandalwood, and vanilla oils. Cedarwood, cypress, and lemon oils are also perfect pairings.

WHAT IS IT GOOD FOR?

CONDITIONS AND SOOTHES SKIN Myrrh oil is a great ingredient to speed up the healing process of chapped and cracked skin. Add to lip balms and salves to boost their effectiveness.

ACTS AS AN ANTISEPTIC Myrrh oil has long been used to treat many kinds of skin eruptions, including acne, athlete's foot, and weeping eczema. This non-irritating oil can also be dabbed directly on small areas where there are cuts, sores, burns, wounds, and skin infections such as cold sores.

COMBATS SIGNS OF AGEING Long regarded as a skin preserver, myrrh oil is often added to high-end cosmetics and toiletries to help prevent wrinkles and other signs of skin ageing.

TEETH AND GUM CARE Myrrh oil makes an excellent antiseptic mouthwash ingredient to treat infection or inflammation, including mouth ulcers, pyorrhoea, sore throat, bleeding gums, bad breath, and oral thrush.

ENHANCES FOCUS Use myrrh oil in aromatherapy to get in touch with your sense of purpose or strengthen your resolve to overcome difficulties.

EASES ACHES AND PAINS An aromatherapy massage with myrrh oil can help relieve painful periods. You could also place some resin in a muslin bag and allow it to dissolve in your bath water.

Myrrh is an anti-ageing treatment that delays the appearance of wrinkles.

BENZOIN *Styrax benzoin*

The **antiseptic**, **healing**, and **calming** properties of benzoin make it perfect for skin formulations. It is also a common ingredient in incense-making and perfumery as a fixative, which slows the evaporation of the scent, helping it to last longer.

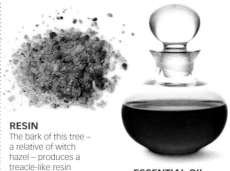

RESIN
The bark of this tree – a relative of witch hazel – produces a treacle-like resin prized in perfumery.

ESSENTIAL OIL
Extracted from the resin, the oil has a sweet, warm, vanilla-like aroma, and antiseptic properties.

WHAT IS IT GOOD FOR?

REPAIRS AND PROTECTS SKIN
Benzoin oil is a good remedy for dry, irritable, itchy, and chapped skin. It is often added to cosmetic preparations to relieve these conditions.

ACTS AS AN ANTISEPTIC Benzoin oil is a good addition to balms and ointments for healing cuts and wounds. Do not apply neat to the skin.

TREATS ACNE Added to skin salves, ointments, and lotions, the oil can help to heal acne and other skin eruptions.

COMBATS SIGNS OF AGEING The oil gives mature skin a general boost by increasing elasticity, which is why it is often found as an ingredient in natural anti-ageing products.

EASES ACHES AND PAINS Benzoin oil has a stimulating effect that helps to improve circulation. Added to a massage oil, it can help ease stiff muscles and the pain of arthritis and rheumatism.

ENHANCES SENSE OF WELL-BEING The oil has a calming effect on both the nervous and digestive systems, and can also help to ease symptoms of depression.

CREATE A SCENT

Make your own **spicy oriental fragrance** by combining benzoin oil with frankincense, sandalwood, ylang ylang, patchouli, rose, and bergamot oils.

CINNAMON *Cinnamomum zeylanicum*

This spice has a long history of uses – from the incense used in religious ceremonies to a **warming** foot massage. It brings **antiseptic** properties to cosmetics and has a **stimulating** aroma – but use sparingly. Do not apply neat and *avoid during pregnancy*.

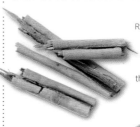

BARK
Rich in antioxidants and a first-class antiseptic and digestive aid, cinnamon keeps the stomach happy and skin healthy.

WHAT IS IT GOOD FOR?

ACTS AS AN ANTISEPTIC Cinnamon oil is effective against a broad range of bacteria, viruses, and parasites, especially lice and scabies.

EASES ACHES AND PAINS The oil has a warming action and treats chills and poor circulation to the extremities. It is a useful treatment for rheumatism, especially when the pain is aggravated in cold, damp weather.

RELIEVES STRESS Cinnamon oil helps to fight exhaustion and lift feelings of depression and weakness.

EAT YOURSELF BEAUTIFUL

Cinnamon Sprinkle the energy- and antioxidant-rich powder on oat porridge, roast vegetables, or toast. Use it to give a rich flavour to stews and preserves. You could use a cinnamon stick to stir hot chocolate or milky coffee.

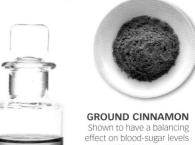

GROUND CINNAMON
Shown to have a balancing effect on blood-sugar levels – resulting in more energy and better skin.

ESSENTIAL OIL
Obtained by steam distillation of the bark and leaves, this strong, warming oil should be used with care.

FRANKINCENSE *Boswellia thurifera syn. B. carteri*

The **toning** and **rejuvenating** properties of frankincense make it one of the most important oils for **invigorating** the complexion, particularly for mature skin, and **repairing** skin damage. It has **antiseptic** and **anti-inflammatory** qualities, which make it useful for **healing** wounds. Its distinctive aroma has a **soothing** effect on the nervous system that can both **uplift** and **calm**.

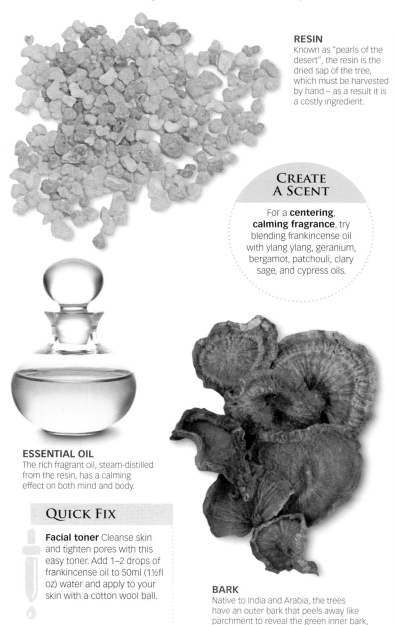

RESIN
Known as "pearls of the desert", the resin is the dried sap of the tree, which must be harvested by hand – as a result it is a costly ingredient.

CREATE A SCENT

For a **centering**, **calming fragrance**, try blending frankincense oil with ylang ylang, geranium, bergamot, patchouli, clary sage, and cypress oils.

ESSENTIAL OIL
The rich fragrant oil, steam-distilled from the resin, has a calming effect on both mind and body.

QUICK FIX

Facial toner Cleanse skin and tighten pores with this easy toner. Add 1–2 drops of frankincense oil to 50ml (1½fl oz) water and apply to your skin with a cotton wool ball.

BARK
Native to India and Arabia, the trees have an outer bark that peels away like parchment to reveal the green inner bark, which is the source of the aromatic sap.

WHAT IS IT GOOD FOR?

REPAIRS AND PROTECTS SKIN Boswellic acid gives frankincense oil an anti-inflammatory, skin-healing action, which is why it has become such a popular ingredient in skin-care products.

COMBATS SIGNS OF AGEING Frankincense oil has a rejuvenating effect, especially on mature skin. It minimizes wrinkles and fine lines, and reduces the appearance of scars and blemishes.

TONES SKIN The astringent quality of frankincense oil has an overall toning effect on the skin. A 5-minute steam facial (see opposite) can help cleanse pores, increase circulation, and tighten skin.

ACTS AS AN ANTISEPTIC Use frankincense oil topically to help heal wounds and skin ulcers. Remember to dilute it, as it should not be used neat on skin.

RELIEVES STRESS The essential oil is a popular choice in aromatherapy, as it can relieve anxiety, calm and lift the spirit, increase energy and focus, and aid meditation.

EASES ACHES AND PAINS The boswellic acid in frankincense is a powerful anti-inflammatory. Topical application as part of a massage oil blend or lotion can help reduce swelling and ease arthritis and rheumatic pain.

CANCER-FIGHTING PROPERTIES Preliminary studies have shown that the compounds found in frankincense may have a role to play in the fight against many types of cancer, including skin cancer.

ENHANCES SENSE OF WELL-BEING The oil has aromatherapeutic value, helping to increase contentment and positivity.

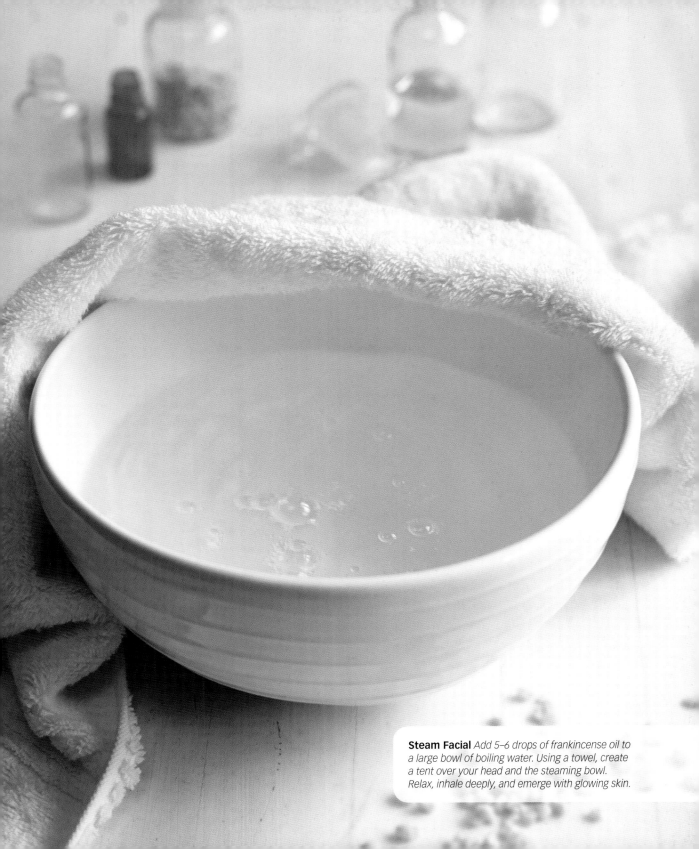

Steam Facial *Add 5–6 drops of frankincense oil to a large bowl of boiling water. Using a towel, create a tent over your head and the steaming bowl. Relax, inhale deeply, and emerge with glowing skin.*

EUCALYPTUS *Eucalyptus globulus*

This flowering tree provides a **warming** and **antiseptic** oil great for **relieving aches** and pains as well as **healing infections** such as mouth ulcers and insect bites and stings. It has a **toning** quality that makes it useful for treating problems such as spider veins. Although its aroma is slightly medicinal, it has been shown to help **increase concentration** and **dispel depression**.

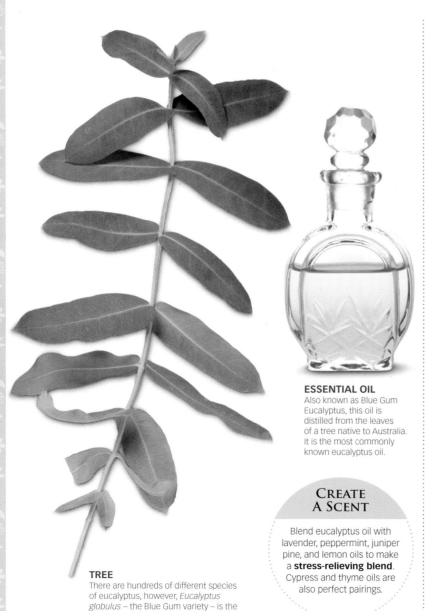

ESSENTIAL OIL
Also known as Blue Gum Eucalyptus, this oil is distilled from the leaves of a tree native to Australia. It is the most commonly known eucalyptus oil.

CREATE A SCENT

Blend eucalyptus oil with lavender, peppermint, juniper pine, and lemon oils to make a **stress-relieving blend**. Cypress and thyme oils are also perfect pairings.

TREE
There are hundreds of different species of eucalyptus, however, *Eucalyptus globulus* – the Blue Gum variety – is the most widely cultivated and produced.

WHAT IS IT GOOD FOR?

ACTS AS AN ANTISEPTIC Dab eucalyptus oil directly onto the skin to heal infections, wounds, herpes, and ulcers, and treat insect bites and stings. It is also helpful in removing lice and treating fungal infections such as athlete's foot. A related variety, *Eucalyptus citriodora*, has a lemony aroma, and is also highly antiseptic, but is more cooling in its action.

TONES SKIN Eucalyptus oil stimulates circulation, increasing the flow of blood to affected areas. It helps minimize the appearance of spider veins and varicose veins. For oily or acne-prone skin, try a cleansing and toning facial steam with a few drops of eucalyptus oil.

EASES ACHES AND PAINS Use eucalyptus oil to treat rheumatism and arthritis, especially when symptoms are worse due to cold and damp weather. The *Eucalpytus citriodora* variety is very useful for muscle and joint pains.

ENHANCES FOCUS AND MEMORY Eucalyptus oil has a refreshing effect and treats tiredness, poor concentration, headaches, and debility. *Eucalpytus radiata* is a milder form of eucalyptus, especially suitable for children and people with a low vitality, such as those recovering from illness.

Use eucalyptus oil to treat rheumatism and arthritis, especially in cold and damp weather.

TEA TREE *Melaleuca alternifolia*

A must-have oil for your first-aid kit, tea tree is a first-class **antiseptic** and a valuable addition to salves and ointments for **healing wounds and sores**. It has **stimulating** properties that strengthen the immune system and help the body **fight infection**. Generally non-irritant, use neat tea tree oil on small areas of the skin, such as on spots, but discontinue use if there is any sign of irritation.

WHAT IS IT GOOD FOR?

ACTS AS AN ANTIFUNGAL Tea tree oil is an excellent antifungal for the treatment of fungal diseases such as athlete's foot and ringworm.

ACTS AS AN ANTIBACTERIAL For cold sores, warts, and verrucae, dab on the oil daily. It inhibits the bacteria found in wounds and those which cause boils and abscesses.

REPAIRS AND PROTECTS SKIN An ingredient in the same family, Niaouli oil *(Melaleuca viridiflora)* is primarily used to treat skin complaints and respiratory illnesses. It is also helpful in steam inhalations for acute infections such as colds, flu, rhinitis, and sinusitis.

HEALS CUTS, SCRAPES, AND BRUISES Tea tree oil helps skin heal by stimulating the formation of scar tissue.

TREATS ACNE The oil has an antibacterial and toning action on acne-prone skin. Apply a small amount neat to spots or use in a facial steam.

COMBATS DANDRUFF A stimulating scalp massage with tea tree oil helps combat dandruff and bring balance to oily hair.

COMBATS BODY ODOUR Soaps, body powders, and deodorants containing tea tree oil are excellent at fighting body odour.

TEETH AND GUM CARE Use well-diluted tea tree oil as a mouthwash to treat bad breath, mouth ulcers, and gum infections.

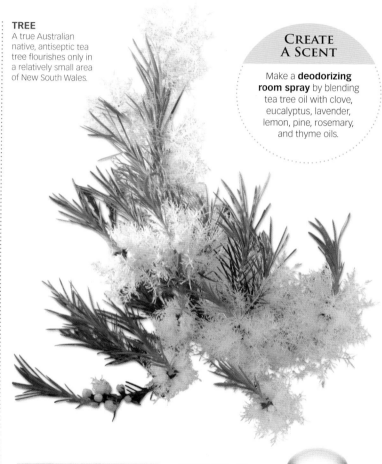

TREE
A true Australian native, antiseptic tea tree flourishes only in a relatively small area of New South Wales.

CREATE A SCENT

Make a **deodorizing room spray** by blending tea tree oil with clove, eucalyptus, lavender, lemon, pine, rosemary, and thyme oils.

QUICK FIX

Antiseptic wash Use a 10 per cent solution (mix 1 part tea tree oil to 10 parts water) for rinsing and cleansing infected wounds and sores on mucous membranes, as well as for treating lice.

ESSENTIAL OIL
Steam-distilled from the leaves of the tree, the essential oil is a clear liquid with a pleasant, though slightly medicinal, scent, reminiscent of eucalyptus.

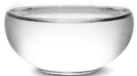

CEDARWOOD *Cedrus atlantica*

One of the oldest known essential oils, cedarwood is **toning** and **rejuvenating** for tired complexions. Its combination of **antiseptic** and **astringent** properties makes it good for **balancing** oily skin and hair, and helping to **heal** infections and skin eruptions. Its scent is **uplifting** and excellent in the aromatherapeutic treatment of nervous tension, anxiety, depression, and lethargy.

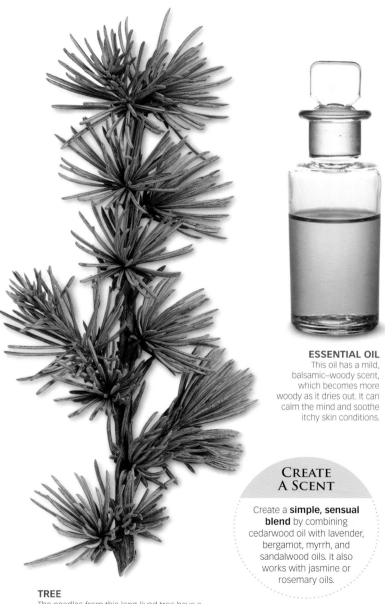

ESSENTIAL OIL
This oil has a mild, balsamic–woody scent, which becomes more woody as it dries out. It can calm the mind and soothe itchy skin conditions.

TREE
The needles from this long-lived tree have a scent that is earthy and grounding. The bark is the source of a thick essential oil.

CREATE A SCENT

Create a **simple, sensual blend** by combining cedarwood oil with lavender, bergamot, myrrh, and sandalwood oils. It also works with jasmine or rosemary oils.

WHAT IS IT GOOD FOR?

CONDITONS AND SOOTHES SKIN
Cedarwood oil is the richest source of aromatic compounds called sequiterpines, which are highly anti-inflammatory. This makes the oil useful for red, inflamed skin conditions. Use it diluted with a base oil to avoid skin irritation.

REPAIRS AND PROTECTS SKIN The oil can also be used to heal wounds and treat athlete's foot and skin ulcers.

COMBATS OILY SKIN AND HAIR The oil can balance oily or acne-prone skin. It is also a good treatment for oily hair. A few drops in water can make a quick astringent hair rinse, or add to a base oil such as olive oil and leave on for a conditioning pre-shampoo hair treatment. It helps treat dandruff and seborrheic dermatitis, too.

AIDS DETOX Cedarwood oil helps stimulate the flow of lymph fluid, reduces water retention, and aids the removal of toxins from the body.

SOOTHES ACHES AND PAINS Added to a massage oil, the warming properties of cedarwood oil help relieve pain from exertion and for conditions such as arthritis.

RELIEVES STRESS Cedarwood oil is soothing and uplifting in the treatment of nervous tension, chronic anxiety, depression, and tiredness. It clears the air and aids focus.

The oil is useful for balancing oily or acne-prone skin.

SANDALWOOD *Santalum album*

Sandalwood has been used since ancient times, mainly in rituals and religious ceremonies. Evidence shows that its **rejuvenating** and **protective** effect on skin is due to its **antiseptic** and **anti-inflammatory** properties. It is particularly good for dry or damaged skin, and as a mild **astringent** it has a **balancing** action on oily skin as well.

WHAT IS IT GOOD FOR?

CONDITIONS AND SOOTHES SKIN The anti-inflammatory properties in sandalwood oil make it extremely soothing for dry, dehydrated, itchy, or inflamed skin. Buy ready-blended, or dilute with a suitable base oil before applying to the skin.

COMBATS OILY SKIN Sandalwood oil has a mild astringent quality that is useful for balancing oily or acne-prone skin.

REPAIRS AND PROTECTS SKIN The oil can help reduce the appearance of scars and blemishes. Some evidence suggests it can help protect the skin against UV damage.

ACTS AS AN ANTISEPTIC Useful for conditions like acne and razor burn, the oil soothes, relieves the itch, and inhibits the bacteria which causes breakouts and rashes.

ACTS AS AN ANTIDEPRESSANT Sandalwood oil dispels depression and anxiety, aids sleep, and helps to restore vitality and energy.

ACTS AS AN APHRODISIAC Sandalwood's uplifting and energetic effects have earned it a reputation as an aphrodisiac.

PROTECTS FROM THE SUN In scientific tests, sandalwood oil has demonstrated the ability to prevent skin cancers caused by both UV radiation and toxic chemical exposure. Scientists are now considering this ingredient as a potential natural sun-screening agent.

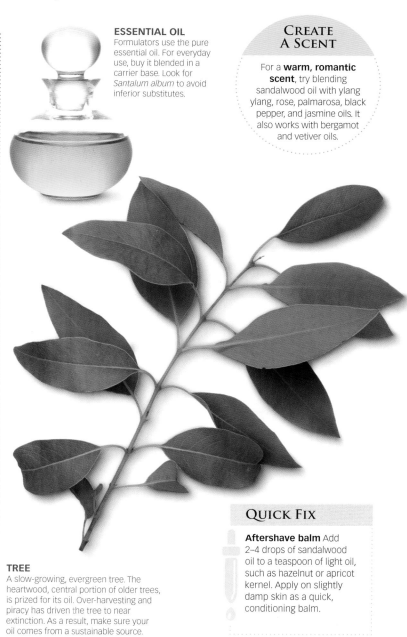

ESSENTIAL OIL
Formulators use the pure essential oil. For everyday use, buy it blended in a carrier base. Look for *Santalum album* to avoid inferior substitutes.

CREATE A SCENT

For a **warm, romantic scent**, try blending sandalwood oil with ylang ylang, rose, palmarosa, black pepper, and jasmine oils. It also works with bergamot and vetiver oils.

TREE
A slow-growing, evergreen tree. The heartwood, central portion of older trees, is prized for its oil. Over-harvesting and piracy has driven the tree to near extinction. As a result, make sure your oil comes from a sustainable source.

QUICK FIX

Aftershave balm Add 2–4 drops of sandalwood oil to a teaspoon of light oil, such as hazelnut or apricot kernel. Apply on slightly damp skin as a quick, conditioning balm.

CYPRESS *Cupressus sempervirens*

Generally known as a **warming** and **uplifting** oil, cypress can also be **soothing** and **relaxing**. It is great for **relieving muscular aches and pains**. It also has a **stimulating** effect on the circulatory system and a powerful **toning** action on skin and veins. Its fresh aroma is reminiscent of walking through a pine forest.

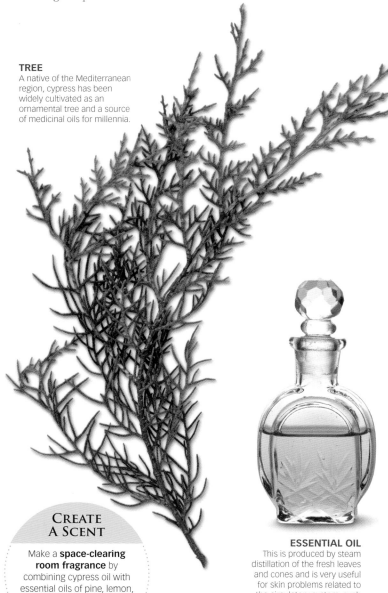

TREE
A native of the Mediterranean region, cypress has been widely cultivated as an ornamental tree and a source of medicinal oils for millennia.

WHAT IS IT GOOD FOR?

TONES SKIN Cypress oil has a toning action on the venous system that makes it useful for treating varicose veins, haemorrhoids, and broken capillaries. It is suitable for oily and over-hydrated skin and also for areas of loose skin, for example, after losing weight. Do not use undiluted on the skin; instead use it diluted in water (for instance, a bath or facial steam) or a carrier oil.

AIDS DETOX The very astringent oil is useful in massage blends, as it can treat water retention and help to reduce cellulite. It can stimulate circulation and help remove toxins.

COMBATS BODY ODOUR The astringent quality of cypress oil is also helpful for those suffering from excessive perspiration. It has a strong deodorizing effect, so is good for relieving foot odour.

EASES ACHES AND PAINS Added to a massage oil blend or lotion, cypress oil can help relieve muscle cramps and period pains.

RELIEVES STRESS Cypress oil refreshes and tones the nervous system and can be used to treat nervous strain and weariness brought about by stress.

Cypress oil can treat water retention and help to reduce cellulite.

CREATE A SCENT

Make a **space-clearing room fragrance** by combining cypress oil with essential oils of pine, lemon, lavender, ginger, juniper, and geranium.

ESSENTIAL OIL
This is produced by steam distillation of the fresh leaves and cones and is very useful for skin problems related to the circulatory system, such as varicose and spider veins.

PETITGRAIN *Citrus aurantium var. amara*

Along with neroli from the flowers and orange from the rind of the fruit, petitgrain is another beneficial oil obtained from the orange tree. One of its most valuable properties for the skin is its **balancing** effect on oily skin and hair. It has an **antiseptic** and **toning** quality useful for problem skin. Its **relaxing** aroma helps **calm** body and mind.

WHAT IS IT GOOD FOR?

CLEANSES AND TONES SKIN Apply petitgrain oil in a lotion or facial toner – it helps to balance greasy skin by reducing the overproduction of oil. It can also be added to rinses to control greasy hair and scalp.

STRENGTHENING MASSAGE Its toning action is more than skin deep. Used in a massage oil, for example, it can help strengthen and tone the digestive system.

REVITALIZES SKIN Like its relative neroli, petitgrain oil can help to lift a dull or tired complexion and is often added to skin formulas for this purpose. Buy the real thing – petitgrain can be adulterated with distillates from other citrus trees. Make sure you are buying *Citrus aurantium var. amara*, sometimes called "Neroli petitgrain".

ACTS AS AN ANTISEPTIC You can use petitgrain oil to help clear up acne, pimples, and other types of skin eruptions. It helps keep wounds clean and protected while they heal. Apply diluted oil to the problem areas.

COMBATS EXCESSIVE PERSPIRATION Petitgrain oil has an astringent action and can be used to control excessive perspiration. Its antibacterial properties also help control body odour. As a result, it makes a good ingredient for natural deodorant products or those you make at home.

RELIEVES STRESS Petitgrain oil has a sedative action that makes it useful for treating anxiety, nervous exhaustion, and stress-related conditions. It is particularly good for when you are feeling panicked or angry, as it helps to relax the body, ease breathing, and slow a rapid heartbeat.

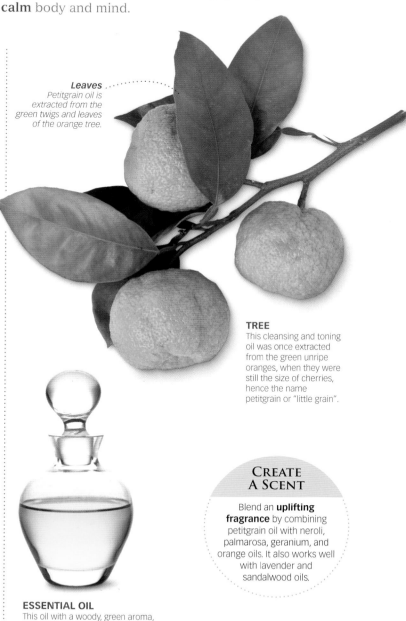

Leaves
Petitgrain oil is extracted from the green twigs and leaves of the orange tree.

TREE
This cleansing and toning oil was once extracted from the green unripe oranges, when they were still the size of cherries, hence the name petitgrain or "little grain".

ESSENTIAL OIL
This oil with a woody, green aroma, can revitalize a dull complexion. It is an essential ingredient in classic eau de Cologne.

CREATE A SCENT

Blend an **uplifting fragrance** by combining petitgrain oil with neroli, palmarosa, geranium, and orange oils. It also works well with lavender and sandalwood oils.

DAIRY

Used externally as cleansers and masks, fresh dairy products can help to **hydrate** and **refresh** the complexion. As part of a healthy diet, there is evidence that organic milk products, which contain calcium and vitamin D, help the body to burn calories more efficiently and maintain a steady weight. Their healthy fats can also help to **lower blood pressure**.

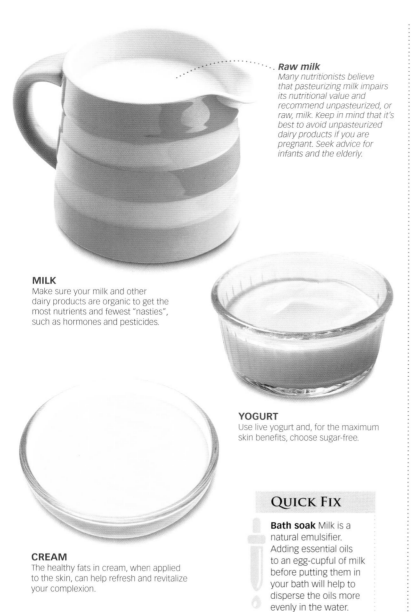

Raw milk
Many nutritionists believe that pasteurizing milk impairs its nutritional value and recommend unpasteurized, or raw, milk. Keep in mind that it's best to avoid unpasteurized dairy products if you are pregnant. Seek advice for infants and the elderly.

MILK
Make sure your milk and other dairy products are organic to get the most nutrients and fewest "nasties", such as hormones and pesticides.

YOGURT
Use live yogurt and, for the maximum skin benefits, choose sugar-free.

CREAM
The healthy fats in cream, when applied to the skin, can help refresh and revitalize your complexion.

QUICK FIX

Bath soak Milk is a natural emulsifier. Adding essential oils to an egg-cupful of milk before putting them in your bath will help to disperse the oils more evenly in the water.

WHAT IS IT GOOD FOR?

CONDITIONS AND SOOTHES SKIN Adding whole milk to your bath will help to soften skin and calm dry, itchy skin complaints.

TREATS ACNE More and more cosmetic companies are using the probiotics found in dairy as an ingredient in masks, creams, and cleansers. Research has shown that the good bacteria, such as *L. acidophilus*, in these products can prevent "bad" bacteria from colonizing skin and causing breakouts.

REPAIRS AND PROTECTS THE BODY Half the fat in milk is saturated fat, but the other half has healthy fat, such as oleic acid (found in olive oil), palmitoleic acid, and conjugated linoleic acid (CLA). Whole, organic, and grass-fed dairy is much higher in antioxidants and healthy omega-3 fatty acids, which can help improve skin, hair, and nail health. Non-organic dairy products, on the other hand, can contain genetically modified growth hormones and traces of antibiotics and pesticides.

METABOLIC BOOST Dairy products contain a novel form of vitamin B3 (niacin), which may help maintain a steady weight and improve energy expenditure. The calcium in dairy foods also increases the metabolism of fat.

DIGESTIVE HEALTH Live cultures in yogurt can improve the microflora of the gut, aiding digestion, immunity, and the metabolism of nutrients necessary to maintain glowing skin.

EAT YOURSELF BEAUTIFUL

Non-dairy options If you want to enjoy the benefits of "good bacteria" but you're allergic or intolerant to dairy, you can still get friendly bacteria in your diet with fermented foods such as miso, tofu, kimchi, sauerkraut, or goat's milk.

OATS *Avena sativa L.*

Oatmeal has both **anti-inflammatory** and **antioxidant** properties, and is an ideal ingredient to **protect** and **soothe** all skin types.

WHAT IS IT GOOD FOR?

CLEANSES AND CONDITIONS SKIN
Whether eating it or applying it, oatmeal is a skin-nourishing treat. It improves digestion and draws toxins from the skin. Ground or colloidal oatmeal can be used as a face scrub to remove dead skin cells and reveal a smoother complexion.

Tired skin can be hydrated and rejuvenated with oatmeal.

REPAIRS AND PROTECTS SKIN
You can use oats for treating skin problems like eczema, sunburn, and allergic reactions. If you are suffering from itchy skin, a handful of oatmeal in a muslin bag in your bath will moisturise skin and relieve the itch.

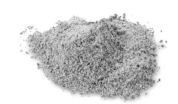

COLLOIDAL OATMEAL
Colloidal oats can be added to cosmetic formulations or dissolved in a bath to make a soothing soak.

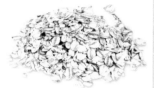

WHOLE OATS
Apart from their fibre content, oats are rich in healthy fats and antioxidant nutrients.

WHEAT BRAN *Triticum vulgare*

Used in exfoliating products, bran is considered to be an **antioxidant** as well as having **skin-conditioning** properties.

WHAT IS IT GOOD FOR?

COMBATS SIGNS OF AGEING Wheat bran helps hydrate mature skin and protect from free-radical damage. Research has shown that wheat bran is also a source of the free-radical fighting ferulic acid – a substance valued in anti-ageing face products.

CONDITIONS AND SOOTHES SKIN
Wheat bran gently cleanses and adds an emollient quality to products for sensitive skin, eczema, and psoriasis.

PROTECTS FROM THE SUN Wheat bran extracts have UV-absorbing properties that can help protect the skin during sun exposure. Always test on a small patch of skin first.

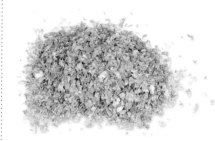

WHEAT BRAN
Wheat bran is what is left over after wheat grains are refined. It is rich in protein, B vitamins, and minerals. A good source of non-soluble fibre, it helps food move through the digestive tract efficiently.

SUGAR *Sucrose*

A natural humectant, sugar helps to **hydrate** by drawing moisture to the skin. It is also a gentle but effective **exfoliant**.

WHAT IS IT GOOD FOR?

CLEANSES AND CONDITIONS SKIN
Sugar contains both glycolic acid and alpha-hydroxy acids (AHAs), which help remove dead skin cells – even without scrubbing – and have a balancing effect on the skin.

EXFOLIATES SKIN Sugar granules have more rounded edges than salt

crystals and are therefore more suitable for sensitive skin. For your face, never use any harsh exfoliant – try icing sugar instead.

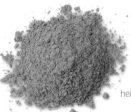

BROWN
Contains more of the natural antibacterial properties and glycolic acid than other sugars to help rejuvenate skin.

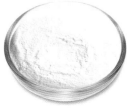

ICING
Retains the glycolic acid and alpha hydroxyl acids of granulated sugar, but is gentler on the skin.

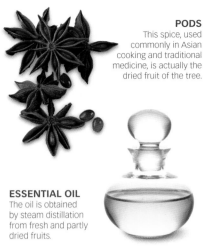

PODS
This spice, used commonly in Asian cooking and traditional medicine, is actually the dried fruit of the tree.

ESSENTIAL OIL
The oil is obtained by steam distillation from fresh and partly dried fruits.

STAR ANISE *Illicium verum*

With a strong scent of liquorice, star anise is a potent **antiseptic** and **deodorant** with a range of **skin-balancing** properties.

WHAT IS IT GOOD FOR?

ACTS AS AN ANTISEPTIC Star anise oil helps to fight bacteria or fungus on the skin. It can be used to treat head lice and mites.

COMBATS BODY ODOUR Star anise oil is often added to soaps to alleviate body odour. It makes for a natural breath freshener.

COMBATS OILY SKIN Star anise oil has a balancing effect that can be useful for treating oily skin.

RELIEVES STRESS Star anise oil has a sedative action that calms, slows the heart rate, and aids sleep. It blends well with citrus oils, cedarwood, citronella, lavender, petitgrain, or rosewood.

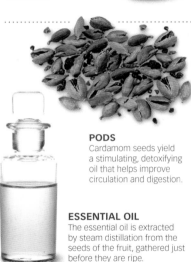

PODS
Cardamom seeds yield a stimulating, detoxifying oil that helps improve circulation and digestion.

ESSENTIAL OIL
The essential oil is extracted by steam distillation from the seeds of the fruit, gathered just before they are ripe.

CARDAMOM *Elettaria cardamomum*

An **antiseptic** oil used in natural **mouthwashes** and **deodorants**, cardamom also has a **stimulating** effect on circulation.

WHAT IS IT GOOD FOR?

COMBATS BODY ODOUR Cardamom oil is a great addition to body and foot deodorants. It kills the bacteria that causes odour.

TEETH AND GUM CARE As a mouthwash, cardamom oil helps to kill germs that cause gum disease and bad breath.

AIDS DETOX The oil in a massage can boost circulation, aid the removal of toxins, and has a mild diuretic action.

ENHANCES SENSE OF WELL-BEING Cardamom oil can help calm an upset stomach and has a refreshing effect when feeling fatigued.

ACTS AS AN APHRODISIAC The oil is also reputed to be an aphrodisiac.

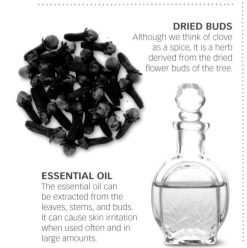

DRIED BUDS
Although we think of clove as a spice, it is a herb derived from the dried flower buds of the tree.

ESSENTIAL OIL
The essential oil can be extracted from the leaves, stems, and buds. It can cause skin irritation when used often and in large amounts.

CLOVE *Eugenia caryophyllata*

Clove oil is **antiseptic** with **analgesic** properties. Always dilute well – it should constitute no more than 1 per cent of the final mixture.

WHAT IS IT GOOD FOR?

TREATS ACNE Clove essential oil can help to kill the bacteria that causes acne. Its anti-inflammatory action can also help reduce painful inflammation and redness of pimples.

TEETH AND GUM CARE Clove oil is a useful antiseptic for maintaining healthy teeth and gums. It can help reduce pain from swollen gums and toothache.

ENHANCES FOCUS Clove oil enhances concentration.

ACTS AS AN APHRODISIAC Clove essential oil has aphrodisiac effects.

BLACK PEPPER *Piper nigrum*

Adds a **warming** and spicy note to cosmetics and aromatherapy blends. Used in small amounts topically, it is also **antiseptic** and **invigorating**. Black pepper has pain-relieving properties, making it an ideal addition to massage oils to ease sore muscles and joints.

CREATE A SCENT

Make a **spicy, stimulating scent** by combining black pepper oil with essential oils of patchouli, vanilla, rosewood, lavender, grapefruit, and bergamot.

WHAT IS IT GOOD FOR?

EASES ACHES AND PAINS Black pepper oil has anti-inflammatory properties. It is a great addition to products for tired, aching limbs and sore muscles.

HEALS CUTS, SCRAPES, AND BRUISES Black pepper oil's stimulating effect on circulation can help speed the healing of bruises. It also has an anti-bacterial action.

RELIEVES STRESS Black pepper oil aids focus and can help combat listlessness and mental fatigue.

EAT YOURSELF BEAUTIFUL

Black pepper This spice adds more than just flavour to your food. Research has shown that its main constituent, piperine, is antioxidant, anti-inflammatory, and an anti-microbial and can help protect the digestive tract from disease.

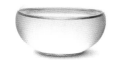

ESSENTIAL OIL
The essential oil is steam-distilled from the dried, crushed, unripe fruit. It can be irritating on the skin unless used well diluted.

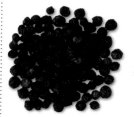

PEPPERCORNS
Peppercorns are the dried fruits of a climbing vine native to Indonesia.

SALT *Sel*

Salt adds a **cleansing**, **hydrating**, and **soothing** element to skincare products. Look for pure salts that do not have additives like anti-clumping agents or iodine. When used in cosmetics, salt acts as a thickener, emulsifier, and **preservative**.

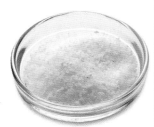

DEAD SEA SALT
Dead sea salt is rich in skin-loving minerals that can help heal skin conditions like eczema and psoriasis. Source it sustainably.

WHAT IS IT GOOD FOR?

CONDITIONS AND SOOTHES SKIN Salt helps the skin retain its natural moisture balance. It acts like a humectant, drawing moisture to the skin.

REPAIRS AND PROTECTS SKIN Mineral salts such as dead sea salt, which are rich in magnesium and calcium, improve hydration by strengthening the barrier function of the skin. They have a balancing action on oily or acne-prone skin.

AIDS DETOX A soak in salt water can help draw toxins from the skin, improving its appearance.

TEETH AND GUM CARE Warm water and salt make a great mouthwash to help relieve and heal sore or bleeding gums.

SEA SALT CRYSTALS
Obtained by evaporation from sea water, the crystals can condition and soothe skin.

Salt improves hydration by strengthening the skin's barrier function.

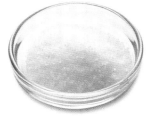

EPSOM
Particularly rich in magnesium sulphate, epsom salt is great for relieving muscle aches and pains.

ALCOHOL *Ethanol*

Alcohol is a good natural **preservative**. It also acts as a **fixative** for essential oils and is a natural **solvent**, useful for home-made tinctures (see p41). For home-made cosmetics, use a high-proof (90 or higher) food-grade alcohol such as vodka or brandy.

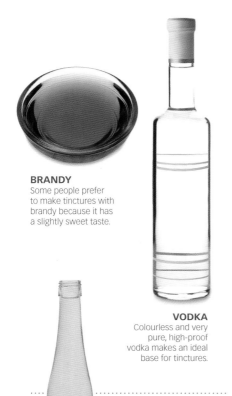

BRANDY
Some people prefer to make tinctures with brandy because it has a slightly sweet taste.

VODKA
Colourless and very pure, high-proof vodka makes an ideal base for tinctures.

WHAT IS IT GOOD FOR?

ACTS AS A SOLVENT Alcohol is mainly used to help dissolve and blend essential oils more effectively. It makes a great base for body sprays and natural perfumes. For tinctures, it dissolves the active constituents of a herb into liquid form.

ACTS AS AN ANTISEPTIC Alcohol makes a safe antiseptic for cleaning cuts and grazes. Added to home-made cosmetics it also acts as a useful preservative that prevents the build-up of harmful bacteria.

CONDITIONS HAIR AND SCALP Try putting 4 teaspoons of crushed rosemary, or one large sprig of the fresh herb, into 250ml (9fl oz) vodka. Leave it to infuse overnight, then strain through a sieve or coffee filter. Massage the liquid into your scalp and allow to dry. Shampoo as normal or simply rinse with cool water.

Alcohol is less harmful to skin than synthetic preservatives, such as parabens.

DISTILLED OR WHITE VINEGAR
A clear, refined, fermented mild vinegar made from distilled alcohol, which comprises around 5–8 per cent acetic acid in water. It is great for most beauty uses.

CIDER VINEGAR
Made from cider or apple musk, this is a living food often sold with the "mother" – a cloudy mass of friendly bacteria – in the bottle.

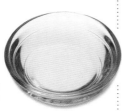

VINEGAR *Acetic acid*

An inexpensive and traditional home beauty product that is **astringent**, **deodorizing**, and **antiseptic**. Taken internally, it has a **balancing**, **alkalizing** effect on the body. It can also **condition** and soothe red or inflamed skin conditions.

WHAT IS IT GOOD FOR?

CONDITIONS AND SOOTHES SKIN Adding vinegar to your bath water can help soothe dry, itchy skin conditions like eczema and allergic reactions. Also good for sunburn, bites, and stings.

TREATS ACNE Vinegar has a balancing effect on oily or acne-prone skin. Applied neat it can help kill bacteria and dry up spots.

CONDITIONS HAIR AND SCALP Rinsing your hair in vinegar removes any product build-up and leaves hair soft and conditioned. It is also a good treatment for itchy scalp and dandruff.

EAT YOURSELF BEAUTIFUL

Apple cider vinegar Drink 1–2 tablespoons of apple cider vinegar in water each morning to help detox and alkalize the body, which helps to keep skin clear. It may also help to improve metabolism.

WATER *Aqua*

Beyond its **hydrating** properties, water is also a natural solvent and mild **cleanser** and **toner** that brings a light, **cooling** effect to products. Use mineral or filtered water in your home-made products.

WHAT IS IT GOOD FOR?

CLEANSES AND TONES SKIN Cool water has a tightening and toning effect on the skin and can help to improve circulation. In addition, water-based products, or water and oil emulsions, feel light on the skin and are easily absorbed.

CLEANSES SKIN The hot water in a steam facial can help to open pores and clear troublesome skin conditions. For additional skin benefits, add a few drops of an essential oil to your steam facial, such as frankincense or eucalyptus.

Studies have shown that while "soft" water may leave skin feeling less dry, drinking "hard" water, which is rich in calcium and magnesium, is better for your heart and bones.

EAT YOURSELF BEAUTIFUL

Water Make sure you drink at least 2 litres (3½ pints) water each day to help maintain efficient kidney function and remove toxins and waste that can make your skin look dull.

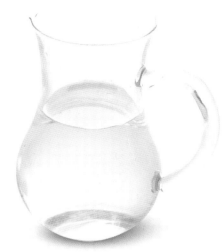

WATER
Water hydrates us on the inside and keeps us clean on the outside. These days tap water can contain a lot of industrial pollutants. Even a simple countertop filter can help remove these.

CLAY *Phyllosilicates*

A natural treatment that **tones** the skin, **stimulates** circulation, and **revives** the complexion as it removes dirt, oil, and dead skin cells. In products, mix clay first with floral or herbal waters, or aloe juice for best results. A little base oil can be added to the final mixture.

KAOLIN CLAY
Also called China clay, kaolin is rich in calcium, silica, zinc, and magnesium. Gently absorbent in masks and other cosmetics for sensitive skin.

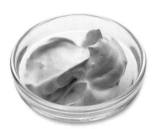

WHAT IS IT GOOD FOR?

AIDS DETOX Clay helps stimulate circulation and draw toxins and impurities from the skin.

CLEANSES AND TONES SKIN It has a deeply cleansing effect, especially on oily or acne-prone skin. It also has a tightening and toning effect that helps improve the appearance of sagging or puffy skin and large pores. When you do not want to – or cannot – use soap, try dissolving a little clay in bath water. This will both cleanse and soothe the skin.

CONDITIONS AND SOOTHES SKIN
Clay can be soothing in cases of eczema or sunburn or for insect bites and stings.

BENTONITE CLAY
Bentonite is a mineral-rich combination of montmorillonite and volcanic ash. It is very absorbent and great for oily skin and scalp.

Instead of soap, you could try dissolving a little clay in bath water.

GREEN CLAY
Made from sea clay, it is highly absorbent. Great for masks but also compresses or poultices to draw impurities from the skin.

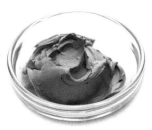

FACE

WHATEVER YOUR SKIN TYPE OR AGE, SHOW YOUR **BEAUTIFUL** FACE TO THE WORLD WITH **HEALTHY** SKIN-CARE HABITS AND A RANGE OF GREAT **NATURAL** PRODUCTS – WHETHER YOU BUY THEM OR MAKE THEM YOURSELF.

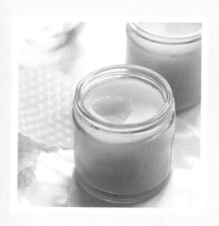 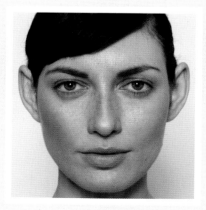 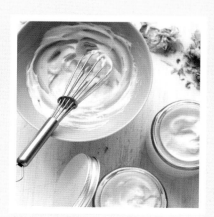

WHAT'S YOUR SKIN TYPE?

Identifying your skin type is a great starting point to use to plan a skincare regime and make adjustments to your lifestyle and diet. You probably have some idea of your skin type – maybe you've taken a quiz, looked at a comparison chart, or had a beauty consultation. However, it is a good idea to review it regularly, as your type is likely to change over time.

IDENTIFY YOUR TYPE

Your skin type is not set in stone and should be seen as more of a guideline than a rule. However, this simple flowchart helps to determine your basic type.

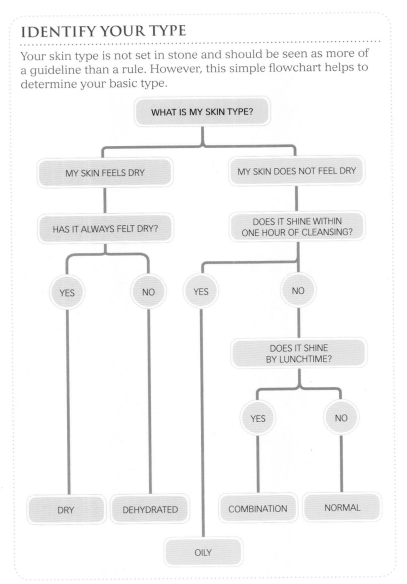

WHAT IS NORMAL?

Many of us try everything we can to change our skin type to "normal". From a beauty perspective, normal skin is shorthand for skin that is blemish-free, glowing, resilient when temporarily exposed to external challenges such as sun and wind, balanced between too oily and too dry, and toned in a way that defies age – at least for a little while.

Everything we do to improve our skin is geared towards getting our skin to that magical "normal" state, but the truth is that knowing your skin type is only a starting point. It's a basic guideline that can help you choose skin-care products as well as help you to make lifestyle decisions, such as how much sun exposure you should have.

Identifying your skin type is a helpful starting point when learning how to care for your skin.

INFLUENCES ON YOUR SKIN

Hereditary factors determine a great deal about our skin type, as well as its colour, tendencies, and susceptibility to certain skin problems. We can often use this knowledge of our family history in preventative care. For example, if you know your mother had fair skin and it was prone to sunburn, and you have a very similar skin type to her, you can take special precautions.

However, inheritance is not the whole story. Diet and skin-care routines are also important factors in the health of the skin. Skin types can change throughout your life too, most dramatically during periods of hormonal upheaval such as puberty, pregnancy, and menopause.

As a living organ, the skin is dynamic and responds to what's going on both inside and outside your body. If you think you have "sensitive skin", you may be reacting to a dietary allergen or, more commonly, an irritant in a cosmetic or toiletry. Remove the allergen and your skin type may become something else entirely.

NORMAL SKIN

Normal skin is soft, smooth, supple, and not prone to eruptions. It should also have a healthy glow. It requires a low-maintenance daily regime of regular cleansing and the use of a light moisturiser to keep the skin looking clear and healthy. As you grow older, normal skin can become prone to dryness and therefore requires a richer moisturiser.

Herbal healers Elderflower, marshmallow, marigold, and lavender
Essential oils Geranium, lavender, palmarosa, frankincense, and rose

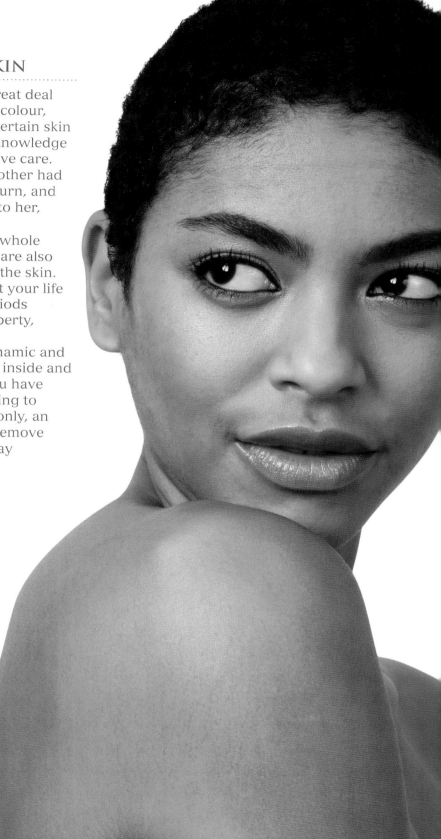

Skin Care: The Basics

Whatever skin type you have, it benefits from regular attention, care, and a daily regime. The skin on your face is thin and delicate compared to the rest of your body, so be careful with it. Find products and a regime that suit you, referring to the skin type information in this chapter. If you have normal skin, you could also follow the detailed regime for radiant skin on pages 92–93.

CLEANSE

Cleanse your skin thoroughly, morning and night. Do not use harsh cleansers or scrub vigorously. Use certified organic products to ensure that your cleanser is free from many of the harsh detergents and preservatives that may irritate your skin, and rinse well. If you use an oil-based cleanser, try a muslin or microfibre cloth to remove all traces of make-up and grime, as well as traces of cleanser. Gently pat the skin dry, rather than rubbing it.

TONE

Although many think that applying toner is optional, it is an important step, whether you use a simple herbal water or floral water, or something more complex. A good-quality organic toner – one rich in nourishing herbal extracts and antioxidants, and free from alcohol and harsh preservatives – helps to rebalance the skin after washing and prepares the skin for your moisturiser. If you exercise, refresh your face with toner afterwards. Sweat can clog your pores, making your skin look blotchy and aggravating existing skin conditions, such as acne.

MOISTURISE

All skin types need moisture, even skin prone to oiliness and/or acne. A good moisturiser helps to keep skin healthy, toned, and supple. Choose a moisturiser that suits your skin. Normal or combination skin only needs a light lotion, whereas skin prone to dryness benefits from a rich cream. Oily skin responds best to a gel-based product. Whatever your skin type, at night, you should use a nourishing serum to help restore skin as you sleep. Use certified organic products to ensure your skin gets everything that it needs, and none of the synthetic chemicals that it doesn't.

APPLY A MASK

A good facial mask once or twice a week is more than just a treat. It can deep cleanse, rejuvenate, rebalance, and intensely nourish the skin, leaving it feeling bright and radiant. Avoid harsh or synthetic masks with unnecessary colours and preservatives. Instead, make a simple mask yourself from mineral clays (see recipes, pp128–31), or choose products made from high-quality herbal extracts with antioxidant properties, as well as skin-loving ingredients like essential fatty acids that can help to reinforce the skin's natural defence and repair mechanisms.

EXFOLIATE

Gently exfoliate once or twice a week to lift dull, old skin cells and stimulate the production of new cells, mimicking the natural cycle of healthy skin (see pp14–15). Exfoliating reveals skin that is softer and more radiant, making your moisturiser and masks more effective. Use a good-quality scrub or polish that does not demand vigorous rubbing – this is counterproductive, especially for delicate facial skin. Avoid harsh chemical peels and opt for products that use natural ingredients, such as oats, crushed seeds, and clays.

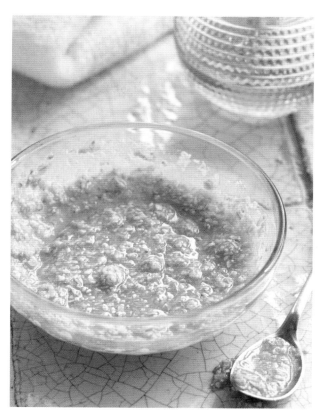

Make your own Honey and oat scrub (see pp122–23). It will exfoliate your face gently, leaving the skin soft, smooth, and hydrated.

PROTECT FROM THE SUN

Many face moisturisers contain sunscreen. If you spend most of your day indoors, this ingredient is not necessary – it simply adds to the chemicals on your skin. Most women apply their moisturiser only once in the morning. If you are outside all day, this renders the sunscreen useless as you must re-apply it regularly for it to be effective.

If you spend all day outdoors, a good-quality organic and mineral-based sunscreen is a must. This is the case even if it is cloudy or cold, as the sun's rays can reflect off water, sand, and snow. Far from a healthy glow, a tan is the skin's attempt to prevent sun damage. When a tan turns to a burn, that damage – which raises the risk of developing skin cancer – has been done.

THE TRUTH ABOUT SPF

Most of us are aware of the Sun Protection Factor (SPF), but very few of us understand how it works. You might think that SPF 30 gives you twice the protection of an SPF 15, but this is not the case, because the SPF scale is not linear. No sunscreen can block all the sun's rays, but if you have sensitive skin that is prone to burning, a few extra percentage points (see the scale, right) can make a difference. Never rely on sunscreen as your only method of protection; seek shade during the middle of the day, and wear protective clothing and a hat when you can.

THE SCALE

SPF 15
blocks 93% of UVB rays

SPF 30
blocks 97% of UVB rays

SPF 50
blocks 98% of UVB rays

DRY SKIN

Delicate and susceptible to flaking and fine lines, dry skin simply does not retain moisture well. It can produce uncomfortable symptoms, such as itchiness or tautness after washing. In rare cases, it leads to eczema, psoriasis, cracks, fissures, and infection. Dry skin is often a feature of genetics, but as we age, it is more common, as the skin produces less oil.

TRY...

Enjoy a gentle beauty regime. Use a sensitive cleanser that does not contain alcohol or fragrance, as these may contribute to dryness. When you wash your skin, rinse it with a generous quantity of tepid–warm water. Do not use hot water because it removes natural oils from your face that help to keep it hydrated. Gently exfoliate once a week to remove dead skin cells. Avoid salt and sugar scrubs and instead look for products that give a "soft" scrub, such as oatmeal – ideal as it will not stress the skin. Oatmeal also contains saponins (plant-based cleansers) that gently remove oil, dirt, and dead skin cells.

USE GENTLE and mild soaps or cleansers. Avoid deodorant soaps and products that contain alcohol, fragrance, retinoids, salicylic acid, or alpha-hydroxy acid (AHA) (see pp18–19).

GENTLY DRY your skin by patting with a towel. Do not scrub skin while bathing, or routinely use loofahs (sea sponges) or any other harsh exfoliating bath items.

MOISTURISE with a rich moisturiser immediately after bathing or washing your hands. Ointments or thick creams may work better than lotions, but they may take longer to soak in.

CHOOSE VEGETABLE OIL-based products instead of those based on mineral oils. Re-apply as needed throughout the day.

TRY A HUMIDIFIER and do not let indoor temperatures get too high.

WEAR GLOVES when you go outside in the cold or when you use household cleaning products.

TRY WEARING NATURAL FIBRES and use hypoallergenic laundry detergents as much as possible. Pay attention to everything that sits next to your skin.

VISIBLE LINES
Areas around the forehead and eyes are susceptible to fine lines and wrinkles.

RED OR DRY PATCHES
The cheeks and hairline are likely to be danger zones for patchy, dry, or inflamed skin.

DRY OR FLAKY SKIN
The nostrils may become particularly dry, especially during periods of cold weather.

QUICK FIX

Use virgin coconut oil to treat all dry skin conditions and improve skin health. Try applying it to the skin twice daily to calm inflammation and reduce water loss. Studies show that this affordable oil can help to treat atopic dermatitis – an allergic reaction that causes dry, inflamed skin.

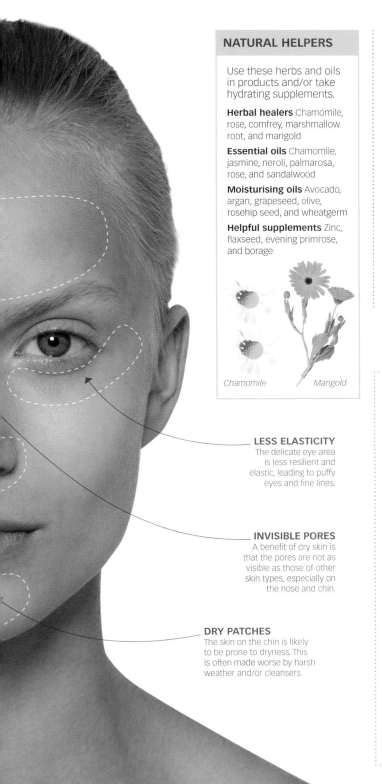

NATURAL HELPERS

Use these herbs and oils in products and/or take hydrating supplements.

Herbal healers Chamomile, rose, comfrey, marshmallow root, and marigold

Essential oils Chamomile, jasmine, neroli, palmarosa, rose, and sandalwood

Moisturising oils Avocado, argan, grapeseed, olive, rosehip seed, and wheatgerm

Helpful supplements Zinc, flaxseed, evening primrose, and borage

Chamomile   *Marigold*

LESS ELASTICITY
The delicate eye area is less resilient and elastic, leading to puffy eyes and fine lines.

INVISIBLE PORES
A benefit of dry skin is that the pores are not as visible as those of other skin types, especially on the nose and chin.

DRY PATCHES
The skin on the chin is likely to be prone to dryness. This is often made worse by harsh weather and/or cleansers.

AVOID...

If your skin is very dry, it often does not take much for it to become rough and scaly, especially on the backs of your hands, arms, and legs. However, there are key things to avoid that can help to alleviate the symptoms. When exposed to extreme heat or cold, dry skin can crack, peel, or become itchy, irritated, or inflamed. Although a necessary part of life for many of us, indoor heating and air-conditioning make it worse.

LIMIT BATHS and showers to 5–10 minutes. If your skin is very dry, bathe only once a day. Try to keep the temperature cool.

LIMIT EXPOSURE to extreme weather, such as wind, sun, or cold climates.

NEVER USE SUN BEDS as ultraviolet (UV) radiation from tanning beds and prolonged sun exposure can dry the skin.

EAT RIGHT FOR MY TYPE

Check any allergies to foods or chemicals. These may produce dry skin, or make it worse – so investigate this by making subtle changes to your diet.

Eat omega-3 fats (found in oily fish, olive oil, nuts, and seeds). These can help to boost skin hydration. There is scientific evidence that taking regular supplements of flaxseed or borage oil can significantly increase skin moisture and reduce rough patches.

Drink water – it is necessary for general skin health. It's not clear from the scientific evidence whether drinking extra water will help your skin retain more moisture, but it certainly helps make it more radiant. Make sure you drink at least 2 litres (3½ pints) of water per day.

A REGIME FOR... RADIANT SKIN

Our skin is a mirror to our overall health and well-being. Beautiful, healthy skin should not be a luxury to the few who can afford costly skin products – it is something all of us can have with good habits and careful choices. Regular use of natural skin-care products suitable for your skin type, and a good diet consisting of nourishing foods, can give you clear, dewy, and radiant skin.

EVERY DAY

1 CLEANSE

Use either a cream cleanser or a wash-off cleanser to remove make-up and grime. A good cleanser leaves the skin feeling clean but not dry or "tight".

HOW TO APPLY

Cleanse at the beginning and end of every day, following the instructions on your cleanser. Remove all traces of make-up.

2 TONE

Use a toner to refresh the skin, refine the pores, remove cleanser residue, and prepare the skin for moisturising. Toners should refresh the skin without causing dryness.

HOW TO APPLY

Twice a day, apply to cotton wool and sweep over the skin, especially over open pores.

3 APPLY SERUM

Serums, also known as concentrates, supply special nutrients to the skin, such as antioxidants or anti-ageing botanicals. They penetrate more deeply than a moisturiser. A good serum absorbs quickly without any tingling.

HOW TO APPLY

Apply before your moisturiser and/or make-up. Pat gently on the skin and allow it to sink in.

4 MOISTURISE

How rich your moisturiser should be depends on your skin type (see pp86–87).You could use a simple nut oil or a creamy lotion. Skin should feel soft and hydrated, not oily or tacky.

HOW TO APPLY

Use a light cream in the morning before you apply make-up, and a nourishing one after cleansing. Dab on dry areas. Avoid the eye area.

EVERY WEEK

APPLY A MASK

A mask deeply cleanses the skin, removing any grime. It also has a refining effect. Use a slightly astringent mask for oily skin and a moisturising mask for dry skin. It should leave your skin feeling clean and radiant and ready for a nourishing serum or moisturiser.

HOW TO APPLY

After toning, apply to the central panel of your face, then the cheeks. Leave on according to instructions – about 10 minutes – and rinse off.

SCRUB

Exfoliate your face to remove dead skin cells and refresh the skin, leaving it ready to absorb a serum or moisturiser. A good scrub or polish uses small granules to gently exfoliate the skin, without causing redness.

HOW TO APPLY

After toning, apply using your fingertips and small, circular movements around the face, avoiding the delicate eye area. Rinse off.

KEY BOTANICALS

This variety of natural plant extracts has stood the test of time and helps to promote radiant, healthy skin.

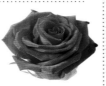

ROSE This helps the skin to retain moisture, has a soothing effect, and adds radiance, along with reducing any redness.

ALMOND OIL A light and easily absorbed oil, almond oil helps to balance the moisture in your skin, making it a wonderful natural moisturiser suitable for all skin types. It can help to improve your complexion and gives you that "youthful glow".

ARGAN OIL This contains high levels of vitamin E and fatty acids – perfect for healing many skin ailments as well as protecting against premature ageing caused by oxidation. Compounds, also known as plant sterols, improve skin metabolism, reduce inflammation, and promote excellent moisture retention.

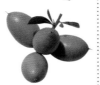

COCOA BUTTER This not only contributes to the taste of chocolate, but is also incredibly good for dry skin – both on your face and body – and adds a rich, creamy, and thick consistency to your lotions and creams. Rich in antioxidants, it softens, lubricates, adds flexibility, and reduces dryness.

SKIN SAVERS

• Create good daily habits – cleanse, tone, apply serum, and moisturise every day. This helps to keep skin youthful and prevents spots.

• A simple way to freshen up in the morning is by splashing your face with cold water before moisturising.

• Drink plenty of water throughout the day (at least 2 litres/3½ pints a day). This helps to keep the skin clear and hydrated from the inside.

• Physical exercise can help improve skin tone and maintain elasticity. It can also increase the blood flow to your skin, giving it a healthy glow.

Recipes to try:
Essential cleansing balm, p103;
Two-phase cleanser, p104;
Frankincense toner, p107;
Neroli facial spritzer, p107;
Cocoa butter moisturiser, p109;
Argan moisturiser, p110;
Green clay purifying mask, p131.

COMBINATION SKIN

When a complexion is oily in some places and normal–dry in others, it is known as combination skin. Those of us with combination skin may experience blemishes and breakouts at the same time as patches of dry, flaky skin. This skin type benefits from a "combination" approach to skin care, using one type of product and application technique on oily areas of the face, and another on drier areas. You may find that combination skin rebalances itself with simple adjustments to your routine.

TRY...

Many people with combination skin find that they can rebalance it. Are you using something that is too drying or oily, or which contains irritating preservatives, colours, or fragrances? Are you washing or scrubbing too much?

USE MILD CLEANSERS and gentle soaps. Avoid deodorant soaps and products that contain alcohol, fragrance, retinoids, salicylic acid, or alpha-hydroxy acid (AHA) (see pp18–19).

USE FLORAL WATER, such as rose or orange flower, as a natural toner.

MOISTURISE REGULARLY, but avoid heavy pore-clogging creams and opt instead for lighter lotions.

TRY WATER-BASED COSMETICS instead of oil-based ones. Most organic cosmetics use water in their formulas. Experiment with these to alleviate the oily areas on the face.

AVOID...

Oily or dry skin is sometimes caused by factors that are out of your control, such as your age, genetics, and hormonal changes. However, there are actions you can take to help.

RULE OUT HARSH PRODUCTS, such as non-gentle cleansers and exfoliants – these can make dry areas more dry and encourage oil production in oily areas.

DO NOT WEAR MAKE-UP TO BED – it can encourage spots and breakouts.

LIMIT EXPOSURE to the elements – use a mineral-based sunscreen when it's sunny and wrap up in the cold or wind.

NATURAL HELPERS

Make or buy products that include these herbs and oils. Taking a daily supplement may also help to balance your skin.

Herbal healers Rose, lavender, elderflower, dandelion, burdock, comfrey, yarrow, and calendula

Essential oils Geranium, ylang ylang, bergamot, lavender, palmarosa, frankincense, neroli, rose, and jasmine

Moisturising oils Hazelnut, jojoba, grapeseed, wheatgerm, and avocado

Helpful supplements Vitamin B-complex and zinc

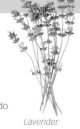

Lavender

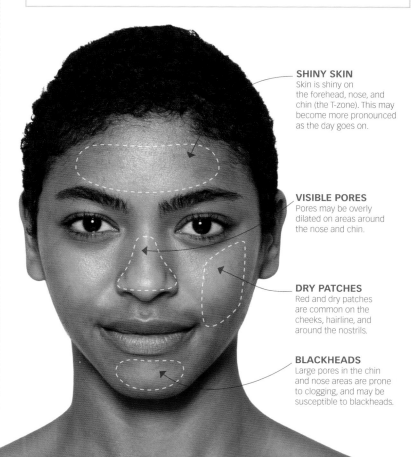

SHINY SKIN
Skin is shiny on the forehead, nose, and chin (the T-zone). This may become more pronounced as the day goes on.

VISIBLE PORES
Pores may be overly dilated on areas around the nose and chin.

DRY PATCHES
Red and dry patches are common on the cheeks, hairline, and around the nostrils.

BLACKHEADS
Large pores in the chin and nose areas are prone to clogging, and may be susceptible to blackheads.

SENSITIVE SKIN

Usually dry and prone to flaking, itching, and redness, sensitive skin is also susceptible to allergic reactions and broken capillaries. Anyone of any age or gender is capable of having sensitive skin, but genetics and cultural inheritance play a part. For instance, a number of skin conditions linked to sensitive skin – such as acne, eczema, psoriasis, and rosacea – tend to run in families, and those of Asian descent are especially sensitive to detergents.

TRY...

An allergy test with your doctor helps you to find out what your particular triggers are so you can avoid them. Even if the reasons turn out to be food allergies or intolerances, they can be made much worse by using harsh chemicals on your skin.

PATCH TEST unfamiliar products before you use them.

USE GENTLE natural, organic, and/or hypoallergenic products that are low-foaming and contain very few ingredients. Use them to wash and moisturise twice daily.

APPLY MOISTURISER while your skin is still moist and pat it dry.

AVOID...

The key approach to sensitive skin is "gently does it". Taking care of your skin means learning to avoid the things that can irritate it.

DO NOT TAKE HOT BATHS and showers. Showering or bathing once a day in warm water is frequent enough.

RULE OUT HIGHLY FRAGRANCED soaps, strong detergents, and harsh exfoliants and toners.

DO NOT WEAR MAKE-UP TO BED and if you can, avoid waterproof cosmetics, as these require harsh cleansers to remove.

LIMIT EXPOSURE to extreme temperatures – both indoors and out. Stay out of the sun when you can, and when you can't, use a good-quality mineral-based sunscreen.

NATURAL HELPERS

Make or buy products that include these herbs and oils. You may wish to take a daily supplement to help to calm the skin.

Herbal healers Calendula, oats, green tea, aloe, comfrey, marigold, chickweed, and marshmallow

Essential oils Chamomile, Roman chamomile, lavender, and rose

Moisturising oils Apricot kernel, avocado, almond, jojoba, wheatgerm, rosehip seed, and borage

Helpful supplements Probiotics, omega-3 fats, vitamins B5 and E

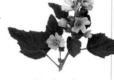

Marshmallow

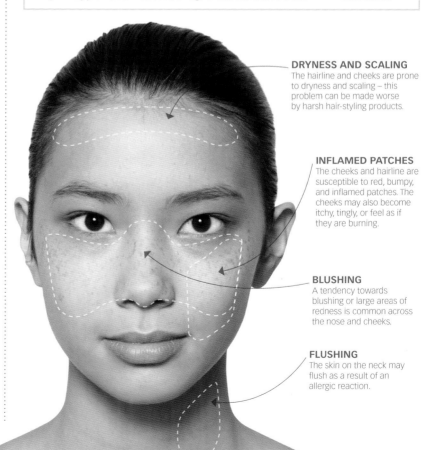

DRYNESS AND SCALING
The hairline and cheeks are prone to dryness and scaling – this problem can be made worse by harsh hair-styling products.

INFLAMED PATCHES
The cheeks and hairline are susceptible to red, bumpy, and inflamed patches. The cheeks may also become itchy, tingly, or feel as if they are burning.

BLUSHING
A tendency towards blushing or large areas of redness is common across the nose and cheeks.

FLUSHING
The skin on the neck may flush as a result of an allergic reaction.

OILY SKIN

Oily skin is often a matter of genetics or hormonal changes. The body produces hormones that lead to oily skin in adolescence, as well as during menstruation, pregnancy, and menopause. These changes trigger the body to produce more oil, which combines with dead skin cells to clog pores, but also moisturises and makes you less prone to wrinkles.

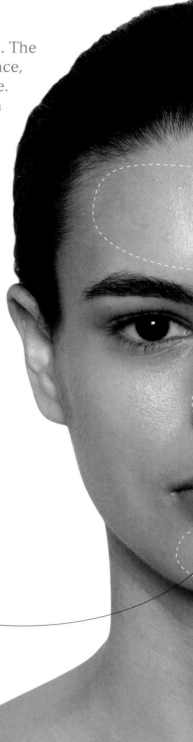

TRY...

Oily skin is likely to be a little lifeless, heavy, and prone to pimples and acne. You cannot do much about the hormonal changes that trigger oiliness, but there are lots of other changes you can make. Use a gently astringent beauty regime that helps to balance the skin and keep the pores clear.

CLEANSE TWICE DAILY, morning and night. Regular cleansing is a must in order to keep the pores clear and reduce a build-up of sebum. Do not scrub hard or make your skin "squeaky clean", and thoroughly rinse the product off the skin.

USE AN ASTRINGENT TONER, which helps to control oil and shine throughout the day. If you have been perspiring heavily, give your face a wipe with toner to ensure pores remain clear.

USE "NONCOMEDOGENIC" PRODUCTS – if they are labelled as such it means they do not contain any pore-clogging ingredients.

KEEP A SPRAY BOTTLE of gently astringent witch hazel herbal water or orange flower water on hand to spritz your face during the day.

TRY WATER-BASED COSMETICS instead of oil-based ones. Most organic cosmetics use water in their formulas. Experiment with these to alleviate the oily areas on the face.

MOISTURISE, as even oily skin needs hydrating. Choose light lotions over heavy creams or look for oil-free moisturisers.

ADJUST TO THE SEASONS as oiliness can change depending on the weather. Use a lighter cleanser in cold weather when skin is a bit dry, and use a deep-cleansing product in the warmer months.

WHAT'S CAUSING MY BREAKOUT?

In adulthood, acne and spots are linked to more than simply oily skin or normal hormonal changes. They can also be linked to poor diet or environmental toxins and may be a side effect of other conditions, such as sluggish liver function or polycystic ovaries. Although it may not seem an obvious trigger, stress could be the cause of your problem skin. Stress – whether physical or emotional – can cause oily skin and breakouts. In addition to your skin-care routine, make sure you find time to relax and de-stress.

BLACKHEADS, PIMPLES, AND OTHER BLEMISHES
The chin, nose, and forehead have large pores that are prone to clogging with dirt and oil. These areas may also be susceptible to blemishes.

NATURAL HELPERS

Use these herbs and oils in products. You can also try skin-balancing supplements.

Herbal healers Elderflower, witch hazel, yarrow, and lemongrass

Essential oils Cedarwood, cypress, vetiver, patchouli, orange, and lemon

Moisturising oils Hazelnut, jojoba, argan, and grapeseed

Helpful supplements Vitamins A, B3, and C, zinc, evening primrose, and probiotics

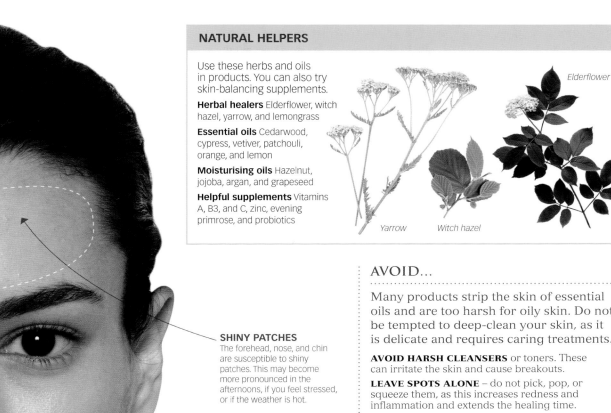

Elderflower

Yarrow   Witch hazel

SHINY PATCHES
The forehead, nose, and chin are susceptible to shiny patches. This may become more pronounced in the afternoons, if you feel stressed, or if the weather is hot.

ENLARGED PORES
The nose and chin may show enlarged pores. These contribute to excess oil production and hard-to-control areas of shine.

QUICK FIX

Clay masks temporarily draw oil and dirt from the pores, leaving oily skin looking fresher for several hours afterwards. As with any kind of skin treatment, you can overuse masks, so keep their use down to once or twice a month or before special occasions when you need your skin to look especially good.

AVOID...

Many products strip the skin of essential oils and are too harsh for oily skin. Do not be tempted to deep-clean your skin, as it is delicate and requires caring treatments.

AVOID HARSH CLEANSERS or toners. These can irritate the skin and cause breakouts.

LEAVE SPOTS ALONE – do not pick, pop, or squeeze them, as this increases redness and inflammation and extends the healing time.

DUMP THE GADGETS. Harsh electronic brushes or super scrubbers, marketed as quick ways to deep-clean skin, can strip the skin of oils and trigger higher oil production as the skin tries to rebalance itself.

EAT RIGHT FOR MY TYPE

Scientists struggle to determine whether certain foods can be conclusively linked to oily or problem skin. Many foods, such as chocolate, coffee, milk, or high-fat foods like French fries, have been linked to oily skin, but there is no consistent link between any food and problem skin.

Be healthy A diet that is high in fat, processed foods, sugar, salt, and additives may promote the kind of inflammation that leads to breakouts. Make sure you're getting all the nutrition you need to promote healthy skin (see pp126–27).

Consume probiotics Your skin reflects your gut health. Eating foods high in probiotics, such as yogurt, can balance oily skin.

Mature Skin

It is easy to fall into the trap of believing that the goal of mature skin care is to make you look younger. Exaggerated promises, such as "look 10 years younger overnight" or "quickly reduce all signs of ageing", sound too good to be true because they are. Looking healthy and the best you can for your age is a much more sensible and achievable goal.

TRY...

Your skin is the first organ in the body to show the signs of ageing. As a general rule, the more sensibly you care for your skin and your overall health throughout your life, the better you can withstand the ageing process. Alter your beauty regime to accommodate the changes in your skin.

MOISTURISE, DAY AND NIGHT. Buy products aimed at your particular skin type and needs.

A GOOD SUNCREAM can help to protect your skin. Opt for organic and mineral-based products without chemical contaminants.

LET YOUR SKIN BREATHE – go without make-up when you can, get plenty of fresh air to help oxygenate the cells of the skin, and exercise to encourage sweat and the release of toxins.

THE SKIN AROUND YOUR EYES is very delicate and becomes more so as you age. Use products specially designed for those areas – and pat them into the skin, without rubbing.

GET ENOUGH SLEEP – it costs nothing and studies show that lack of sleep can age your appearance by as much as 10 years.

FOR AN EXTRA BOOST when you really need to look your best, why not opt for a facial massage. You can book time with a professional therapist or learn how to do it yourself (see pp120–21).

QUICK FIX

To prevent or minimize the appearance of age spots, use a good-quality mineral-based sunscreen and choose organic products. Lemon and benzoin essential oils have skin-lightening properties. Look out for products containing liquorice (capable of lightening spots) and glycolic acid (a gentle exfoliant derived from citrus papaya).

THINNING
The skin around the eyes and cheeks becomes thinner as we age. This is linked to a loss of elasticity and a dryness that leads to lines and bags.

SAGGING, FINE LINES, AND WRINKLES
As collagen production drops, an associated loss of skin elasticity causes fine lines. Puffiness and bags are also common around the jawline, neck, eyes, and forehead.

FIGHT FREE RADICALS

Unstable molecules that attach to skin cells, free radicals are the main cause of premature skin ageing. The body produces them but pollution and synthetic chemicals increase exposure. Antioxidants help to neutralize free radicals, so choose products rich in vitamin E and make sure your diet contains plenty of fresh whole foods.

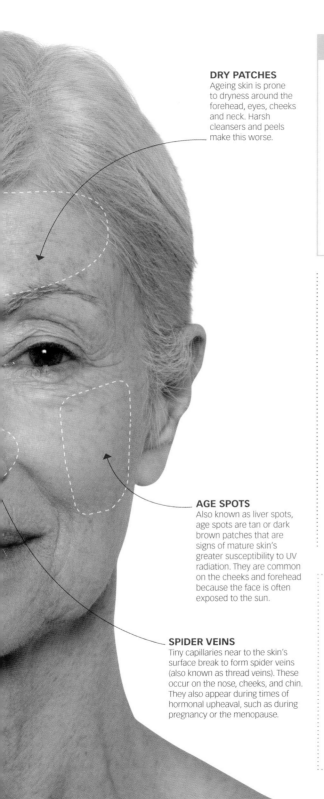

DRY PATCHES
Ageing skin is prone to dryness around the forehead, eyes, cheeks and neck. Harsh cleansers and peels make this worse.

AGE SPOTS
Also known as liver spots, age spots are tan or dark brown patches that are signs of mature skin's greater susceptibility to UV radiation. They are common on the cheeks and forehead because the face is often exposed to the sun.

SPIDER VEINS
Tiny capillaries near to the skin's surface break to form spider veins (also known as thread veins). These occur on the nose, cheeks, and chin. They also appear during times of hormonal upheaval, such as during pregnancy or the menopause.

NATURAL HELPERS

Use these herbs and oils in products or try taking daily supplements.

Herbal healers Rose, comfrey, marshmallow root, marigold, and white or green tea

Essential oils Frankincense, myrrh, rose, palmarosa, lavender, neroli, and patchouli

Moisturising oils Cocoa butter, apricot kernel, avocado, rosehip seed, and almond

Helpful supplements Vitamins A, C, D, and E, CoQ-10, evening primrose, selenium, and zinc

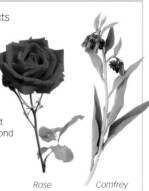

Rose   *Comfrey*

AVOID...

As we age, our skin undergoes changes – the collagen fibres that are the underlying support structure of the skin become twisted and matted, causing wrinkles and lines. There are some measures you can take to help slow down this inevitable process – the earlier you start, the better your skin will appear later in life.

DO NOT SCRUB THE SKIN as your cleanse. Use a gentle cleanser to remove dirt and make-up twice a day, rinse it thoroughly, and pat dry.

DO NOT SMOKE – it increases free-radical damage that causes premature skin ageing.

DO NOT DRINK TOO MUCH ALCOHOL because it can dry the skin and hasten the appearance of spider veins.

LIMIT SUN EXPOSURE, which hastens collagen damage. Use quality, mineral-based sunscreens and sun blocks.

DO NOT TAKE THE LABEL AS GOSPEL and choose products carefully. Some anti-ageing products, such as skin peels, can end up exaggerating the signs of skin ageing over time.

EAT RIGHT FOR MY TYPE

Drink water to stay hydrated and keep skin glowing.

Consume healthy fats, such as omega-3 fats (oily fish, nuts and nut oils, and egg yolks) and omega-6 fats (seed and seed oils, wholegrains, evening primrose, and borage oils).

Eat a rainbow. Bright-coloured organic fruit and vegetables, green tea, and dark chocolate are rich in antioxidants that help to fight free radicals.

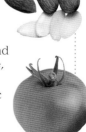

A REGIME FOR... ANTI-AGEING SKIN

A similar regime applies for both youthful and mature skin, but make a few refinements and pay closer attention to areas of wrinkles and delicate skin. Choose products with ingredients that have a high content of vitamins A and E, antioxidants, omega-fatty acids, collagen-boosting properties, and peptides, as these have all been proven to help reduce wrinkles and other signs of ageing.

EVERY DAY

1 CLEANSE

Choose a light, gentle cleanser to remove make-up and grime. A good cleanser will leave the skin feeling clean and soft.

HOW TO APPLY

Cleanse at the beginning and end of every day with a cotton wool pad, following the instructions on your cleanser. Remove all traces of make-up.

2 TONE

Refresh skin, refine pores, and remove residue with a toner that prepares the face for nourishing treatments. A slightly astringent toner has a non-drying, anti-wrinkle effect.

HOW TO APPLY

Twice a day, apply with cotton wool and sweep over the skin, especially over open pores.

3 APPLY SERUM

Serums supply collagen-boosting peptides and antioxidant botanicals. They penetrate more deeply than a moisturiser. Apply before your moisturiser or make-up. A serum should absorb quickly, without tingling.

HOW TO APPLY

Apply the serum to areas of skin that show signs of ageing. Allow to absorb.

4 MOISTURISE

Choose antioxidant and collagen-boosting cream with anti-ageing botanicals to protect and rejuvenate your skin. Use a light but nourishing cream, leaving your skin feeling soft, not oily or tacky.

HOW TO APPLY

Apply before make-up. Use gentle upward strokes, focusing on the edges of lips and eyes, and between the eyebrows.

5 USE NIGHT CREAM

Choose ingredients that nourish the skin and work overnight to boost collagen and reduce wrinkles. Antioxidants help to repair the skin from sun damage and ageing, and peptides will boost collagen. A suitable night cream should be nourishing and moisturising but should not feel too heavy.

HOW TO APPLY

Use before going to bed. Pat on and smooth into the skin, focusing on areas prone to wrinkling.

EVERY WEEK

APPLY A MASK

Nourish and cleanse the skin with a mask that removes grime. An anti-ageing mask should be rich in nutrients and supply antioxidants to the skin. A suitable mask leaves your skin feeling smooth, nourished, and clear.

HOW TO APPLY

After toning and before applying serum, smooth the mask over your skin and leave for 10–15 minutes before rinsing off gently with tepid water.

Recipes to try:
Frankincense toner, p107;
Argan moisturiser, p110;
Wild rose moisturiser, p111;
Frankincense day cream, p112.

KEY BOTANICALS

Some plants have antioxidant and anti-inflammatory effects that can provide anti-ageing properties.

FRANKINCENSE This essential oil has anti-inflammatory and anti-ageing properties. It will help to tone the skin, reducing fine lines and wrinkles. It also has a protective effect on healthy skin cells.

ROSEHIP SEED OIL Clinical studies have proven that regular use of this oil can reverse sun damage, and reduce wrinkles and age spots. It is naturally rich in vitamin A, retinol, and linoleic acid.

AVOCADO OIL Studies have found that this oil can mobilize and increase collagen in connective tissue, helping to keep skin soft, mobile, and more youthful-looking. It is rich in vitamins, lecithin, and essential fatty acids.

WHITE/GREEN TEA Excellent natural sources of antioxidants. Free radicals caused by sun damage, stress, and a poor diet, can damage the skin and cause it to age prematurely. By scavenging these free radicals, white and green tea protects the skin and helps to reverse some of the damage.

SKIN SAVERS

• Base both your diet and skin-care regime on antioxidant-rich plant extracts and anti-inflammatory omega-rich plant oils, and choose skin-care products that have proven benefits.

• Ensure that you get rest and relaxation. It is only while resting that your skin and body can repair itself.

• Protect your skin from excessive exposure to the sun – wear a hat, sunglasses, and use a sunscreen.

• Indulge in regular rejuvenating facials.

RECIPES FOR YOUR FACE

LOOK AFTER YOUR SKIN, LIPS, TEETH, AND EYES WITH THESE **CARING** RECIPES. EVERY RECIPE USES THE GOODNESS OF **NATURAL MATERIALS** WITH **BEAUTIFYING** INGREDIENTS THAT BENEFIT THE SKIN. BALMS, EMULSIONS, AND WATER-BASED MISTS FORM THE BASIS OF THIS HOME-MADE **SKIN-CARE** COLLECTION.

ESSENTIAL CLEANSING BALM

FOR ALL SKIN TYPES

Gently remove grime and dirt with this caring, **cleansing** balm. Sunflower oil and shea nut butter help to loosen oil and dirt, and lavender essential oil can cleanse and **heal** all skin types. The texture of the balm allows you to gently work it into the skin, **stimulating** circulation and removing make-up and everyday dirt from the skin. After use, remove with a muslin cloth or flannel.

INGREDIENTS

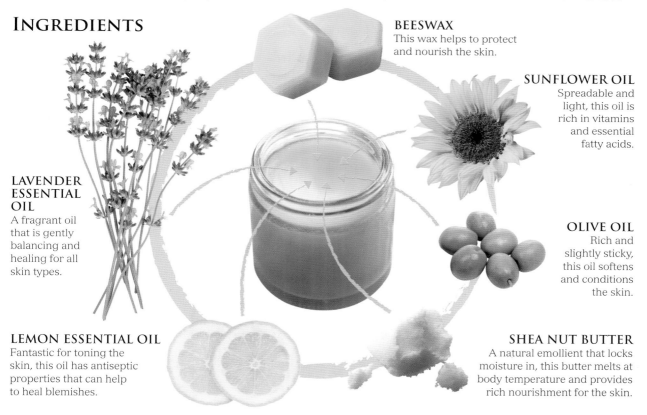

BEESWAX
This wax helps to protect and nourish the skin.

SUNFLOWER OIL
Spreadable and light, this oil is rich in vitamins and essential fatty acids.

LAVENDER ESSENTIAL OIL
A fragrant oil that is gently balancing and healing for all skin types.

OLIVE OIL
Rich and slightly sticky, this oil softens and conditions the skin.

LEMON ESSENTIAL OIL
Fantastic for toning the skin, this oil has antiseptic properties that can help to heal blemishes.

SHEA NUT BUTTER
A natural emollient that locks moisture in, this butter melts at body temperature and provides rich nourishment for the skin.

MAKES 140G (5OZ)

INGREDIENTS
90ml (3fl oz) sunflower oil
2 tsp olive oil
1 tbsp shea nut butter
1 tbsp beeswax
12 drops lavender essential oil
8 drops lemon essential oil

HOW TO MAKE

1 Heat all the ingredients, apart from the essential oils, in a bain-marie (see p133), until the wax has melted. Remove from the heat.

2 Add the essential oils as the mixture begins to cool.

3 Pour into a sterilized jar and leave to cool for 1–2 hours before using or placing the lid on. Store in a cool, dark place. Keeps for up to 3 months.

HOW TO APPLY

Massage a small, coin-size amount into the skin in small circular movements, paying particular attention to areas of congestion, for example around the nose. Work the product into the skin for 2 minutes and then remove with a clean muslin cloth or flannel and warm water.

Two-Phase Cleanser

FOR ALL SKIN TYPES

QUICK

The oil and water-based ingredients in this easy cleanser work in two stages – they **cleanse** the skin of oily dirt and make-up, and then **refresh** and **tone**. Ylang ylang and rose otto essential oils create an exotic scent with **balancing** and **hydrating** properties. Rose floral water **soothes**, is mildly **astringent**, and treats broken capillaries or areas of redness.

MAKES 100ML (3½FL OZ)

INGREDIENTS

75ml (2½fl oz) rose floral water
2 tsp glycerin
2 tsp almond oil
8 drops ylang ylang essential oil
4 drops rose otto essential oil

HOW TO MAKE

1 Combine the rose floral water and glycerin in a bowl.
2 Add the oil and the essential oils and mix well.
3 Pour the mixture into a sterilized bottle and place the lid on. Shake well before use. Store in a cool, dark place. Keeps for up to 6 weeks.

HOW TO APPLY

Using a cotton wool pad, sweep the cleanser across the brow, down the nose, and across the chin, before sweeping across the cheeks, avoiding the delicate eye area.

Exfoliating Cleansing Balm

FOR ALL SKIN TYPES

Purify, **soothe**, and **heal** your skin with this kaolin-rich balm. It has **exfoliating** properties that gently slough away dead skin cells. The combination of olive and coconut oils gently **cleanses** and **nourishes** the skin, leaving it smooth and fresh. Geranium not only lends a leafy-rosy aroma, but also balances the production of sebum – important for dry and acne-prone skin types.

MAKES 50G (1¾OZ)

INGREDIENTS

2 tbsp olive oil
1 tsp coconut oil
½ tsp beeswax
1 tbsp kaolin
6 drops geranium essential oil

HOW TO MAKE

1 Heat the oils and beeswax in a bain-marie (see p133) until the wax has melted. Remove from the heat.
2 Add the kaolin and stir well. As the mixture begins to cool, add the essential oil.
3 Pour into a sterilized jar. Leave to cool completely, for about 1 hour, before placing the lid on. Store in a cool, dark place. Keeps for up to 3 months.

HOW TO APPLY

Massage into the skin with small, circular movements. Remove with a muslin cloth or flannel and warm water. You could follow the balm with a toner, if required.

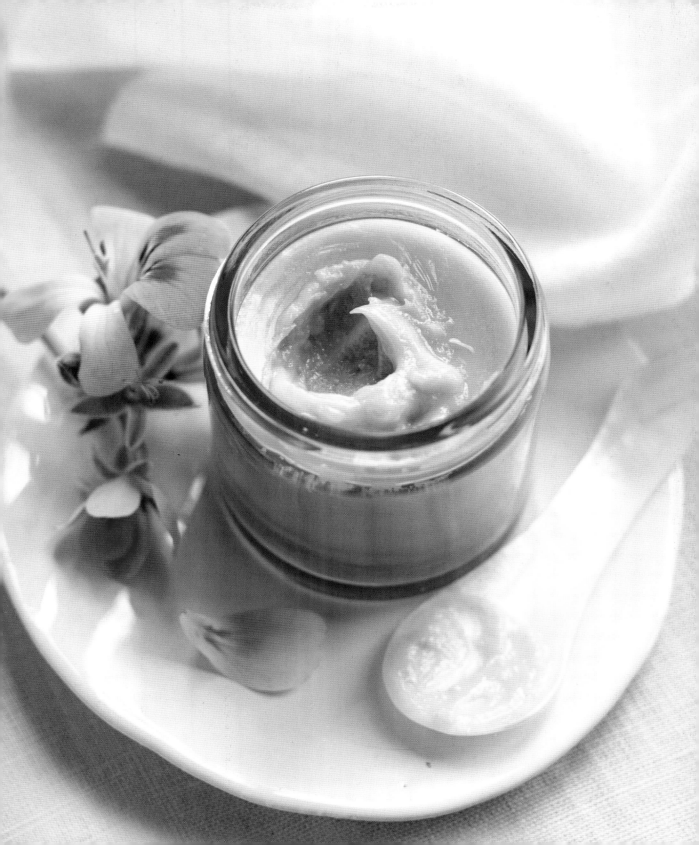

Rose And Aloe Vera Toner

FOR NORMAL AND DEHYDRATED SKIN

Hydrate and **refresh** the skin with a toner that has a simple rose petal infusion as its base. Rose is a natural **astringent** and helps to tighten pores, leaving skin feeling **smooth** and hydrated. It also has **calming** properties, which can help to soothe rosacea and eczema. Aloe vera is well known for **soothing** the skin and has a wonderful **cooling** affect. It can also **heal** and **moisturise**.

Ingredients

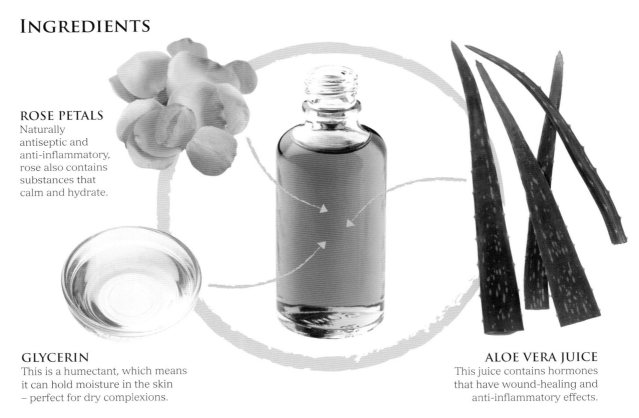

ROSE PETALS
Naturally antiseptic and anti-inflammatory, rose also contains substances that calm and hydrate.

GLYCERIN
This is a humectant, which means it can hold moisture in the skin – perfect for dry complexions.

ALOE VERA JUICE
This juice contains hormones that have wound-healing and anti-inflammatory effects.

MAKES 100ML (3¹/₂FL OZ)

INGREDIENTS
100ml (3½fl oz) mineral water
1 tbsp dried rose petals
1 tsp glycerin
1 tsp aloe vera juice

HOW TO MAKE

1 To make the rose petal infusion, boil the mineral water. Place the rose petals in a teapot or glass bowl and pour over the boiling water. Leave to steep for 10 minutes, then strain.

2 Add the glycerin and aloe vera juice to the infusion, and stir thoroughly. Pour into a sterilized bottle. Once cool, seal with a cap or atomizer. Store in the fridge. Keeps for up to 6 weeks.

HOW TO APPLY

Shake before use. After cleansing, apply to your face with cotton wool, avoiding the eyes. Alternatively, attach an atomizer for a facial spritz.

FRANKINCENSE TONER

FOR MATURE SKIN

The importance of frankincense in Egyptian skincare is well documented, and for good reason. The essential oil has wonderful properties, including being able to encourage cell turnover, promote the formation of scar tissue, and promote the **healing** of wounds – making it a great oil for mature skin. Myrrh essential oil can also heal the skin and has **anti-inflammatory** and **astringent** properties.

MAKES 100ML (3¹/₂FL OZ)

INGREDIENTS

75ml (2½fl oz) mineral water
1 tsp glycerin
3 drops frankincense essential oil
1 drop myrrh essential oil

HOW TO MAKE

1 Mix the mineral water and glycerin together in a bowl.
2 Add both the essential oils, and stir thoroughly. Pour into a sterilized bottle and place the lid on. Store in the fridge. Keeps for up to 6 weeks.

HOW TO APPLY

Use the toner after cleansing and whenever you need a refreshing, hydrating boost. Apply a few drops of toner to cotton wool and sweep across the forehead, down the nose, and across cheeks, to remove all traces of dirt and make-up. Use with an atomizer for a fresh facial mist.

NEROLI FACIAL SPRITZER

FOR ALL SKIN TYPES

When you've been exercising hard or enduring a long commute, a facial spritzer is the perfect choice to refresh your skin. Neroli oil and orange floral water are beautifully **fragrant** restorative remedies. They work on the nervous system to **alleviate stress and anxiety**, and **rejuvenate** dry skin. Bergamot has a **refreshing** citrus fragrance, an **antiseptic** action, and is great for use on oily skin.

MAKES 100ML (3½FL OZ)

INGREDIENTS

75ml (2½fl oz) mineral water
1 tbsp orange floral water
1 tsp glycerin
5 drops neroli essential oil
2 drops bergamot essential oil

HOW TO MAKE

1 Mix the mineral water and orange floral water together in a bowl.
2 Add the glycerin and essential oils, and stir thoroughly. Pour into a sterilized bottle, and attach the atomizer. Store in the fridge. Keeps for up to 6 weeks.

HOW TO APPLY

Spritz the face or body after cleansing and whenever your skin needs a refreshing, hydrating boost.

Palmarosa Facial Mist

FOR OILY AND COMBINATION SKIN

Balance and **refine** your skin with witch hazel and palmarosa essential oil. Witch hazel herbal water is astringent, and when combined with **soothing** and **healing** aloe vera juice, it can **rebalance** and **refresh** the skin. Palmarosa is **antiseptic** and **hydrating** and helps to balance levels of sebum, and lemon essential oil is **astringent** and **toning** – making a fragrant, effective toning mist for oily skin.

Ingredients

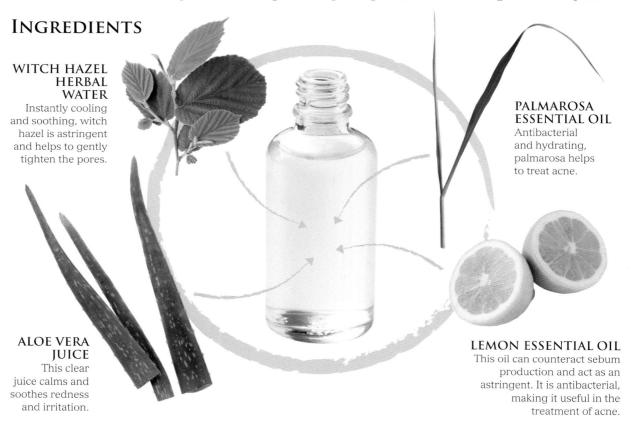

WITCH HAZEL HERBAL WATER
Instantly cooling and soothing, witch hazel is astringent and helps to gently tighten the pores.

PALMAROSA ESSENTIAL OIL
Antibacterial and hydrating, palmarosa helps to treat acne.

ALOE VERA JUICE
This clear juice calms and soothes redness and irritation.

LEMON ESSENTIAL OIL
This oil can counteract sebum production and act as an astringent. It is antibacterial, making it useful in the treatment of acne.

MAKES 60ML (2FL OZ)

INGREDIENTS
1 tbsp aloe vera juice
1 tbsp witch hazel herbal water
2 tbsp mineral water
2 drops palmarosa essential oil
1 drop lemon essential oil

HOW TO MAKE
1 Mix all the ingredients together in a bowl.
2 Pour into a sterilized bottle with an atomizer. Store in the fridge. Keeps for up to 6 weeks.

HOW TO APPLY
Shake before use. Use after cleansing or for a refreshing mist at any time. Either spritz directly onto the face, avoiding the eyes, or spritz onto cotton wool or a muslin cloth and gently wipe over the skin.

Cocoa Butter Moisturiser

FOR DRY SKIN

Blend deeply **nourishing** cocoa butter with almond and jojoba oils for a rich, **soothing** face cream. The essential fatty acids in almond and jojoba oils enrich and **nourish** the skin, improving its **suppleness**, while beeswax offers some additional **protection** and helps to prevent water loss. The result is an enriching moisturiser that locks moisture into the skin.

MAKES 100G (3½OZ)

INGREDIENTS

2 tsp cocoa butter
1 tsp almond oil
1 tsp jojoba oil
1 tsp beeswax
4 tbsp mineral water
1 tbsp emulsifying wax
1 tsp glycerin

HOW TO MAKE

1 Create an emulsion, as shown in the step-by-step technique below.
2 Once the mixture is smooth, pour into a sterilized jar and leave to cool for 1 hour. Once cool, either use the moisturiser or apply the lid. Store in the fridge. Keeps for up to 6 weeks.

HOW TO APPLY

Generously apply to the face and body, paying particular attention to dry patches. Massage into the face and neck with upward-sweeping movements, avoiding the delicate eye area.

Making An Emulsion

Cosmetic emulsions are basically a combination of oil and water-based ingredients, made physically stable by the addition of emulsifiers. Emulsions allow you to combine ingredients that are both oil-soluble and water-soluble, giving you the best of both worlds and enabling you to mix ingredients that would otherwise be very difficult to blend together. Emulsions form the basis of moisturisers and creams.

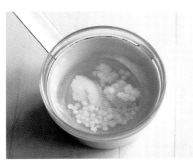

1 Place the cocoa butter, almond oil, jojoba oil, and beeswax in a glass bowl. Heat together in a bain-marie and remove from the heat once the wax has melted.

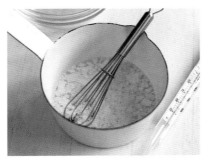

2 Using a thermometer, heat the mineral water in a saucepan to 80°C (175°F). Add the emulsifying wax and glycerin, and stir until the wax is fully dissolved. You may need to re-heat the water if it has not dissolved completely.

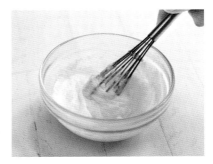

3 Add the hot oil mixture to the hot water mixture and, using a hand-held whisk or stick blender, whisk continuously until smooth. Continue to mix occasionally while the mixture cools.

Jasmine And Shea Nut Moisturiser

FOR DRY SKIN

Treat dry patches of skin with this aromatic cream. Shea nut butter **softens** and **nourishes**, and apricot oil **restores** and **soothes**. The cream especially suits hot, inflamed skin conditions, or burnt, wrinkled, or mature skin.

MAKES 100G (3½OZ)

INGREDIENTS

2 tsp shea nut butter
1 tsp avocado oil
1 tsp apricot oil
1 tsp beeswax
4 tbsp mineral water
1 tbsp emulsifying wax
1 tsp glycerin
6 drops jasmine absolute essential oil
2 drops geranium essential oil

HOW TO MAKE

1 Create an emulsion (see p109) by melting the butter, oils, and beeswax together in a bain-marie. Remove from the heat once the wax has melted.
2 Heat the mineral water in a saucepan to 80ºC (175ºF). Add the emulsifying wax and glycerin, and stir until the wax is fully dissolved.
3 Add the hot oil mixture to the hot water mixture. Using a hand-held whisk or a stick blender, whisk continuously until smooth.
4 Continue to stir occasionally as the mixture cools. Add the essential oils and mix well. Pour into a sterilized jar and leave to cool before placing the lid on. Store in the fridge. Keeps for up to 6 weeks.

HOW TO APPLY

Massage into the skin on your face and neck with upward-sweeping movements, avoiding the delicate eye area. Use day and night for soft, supple skin, paying particular attention to dry patches.

Argan Moisturiser

FOR DRY SKIN

Give skin a hydrating boost with this **nourishing** cream that locks moisture into the skin. Argan oil is known for its **moisturising** and nourishing properties. The shea butter also helps to nourish the skin, and vitamin-rich avocado oil can **soothe** dry, parched skin.

MAKES 100G (3½OZ)

INGREDIENTS

1 tsp shea nut butter
2 tsp argan oil
1 tsp avocado oil
1 tsp beeswax
4 tbsp mineral water
1 tbsp emulsifying wax
1 tsp glycerin
5 drops frankincense essential oil
2 drops neroli essential oil
1 drop bergamot essential oil

HOW TO MAKE

1 Create an emulsion (see p109) by melting the butter, oils, and beeswax together in a bain-marie. Remove from the heat once the wax has melted.
2 Heat the mineral water in a saucepan to 80ºC (175ºF). Add the emulsifying wax and glycerin, and stir until the wax is fully dissolved.
3 Add the hot oil mixture to the hot water mixture. Using a hand-held whisk or a stick blender, whisk continuously until smooth.
4 Continue to stir occasionally as the mixture cools. Add the essential oils and mix well. Pour into a sterilized jar and leave to cool before placing the lid on. Store in the fridge. Keeps for up to 6 weeks.

HOW TO APPLY

Apply to the face and neck with small, circular movements in an upward direction, avoiding the delicate eye area.

WILD ROSE MOISTURISER

FOR ALL SKIN TYPES

Restorative rosehip oil helps to **heal** and **revive** mature or scarred skin. It is rich in vitamins and antioxidants, with properties that can reduce scar tissue, hyperpigmentation, and wrinkles. The combination of essential oils helps to heal, **balance**, and **rejuvenate** the skin.

MAKES 100G (3½OZ)

INGREDIENTS
2 tsp shea nut butter
2 tsp rosehip seed oil
1 tsp beeswax
4 tbsp mineral water
1 tbsp emulsifying wax
1 tbsp rose water
1 tsp glycerin
2 drops geranium essential oil
2 drops rosemary essential oil
2 drops frankincense essential oil
2 drops patchouli essential oil
2 drops palmarosa essential oil

HOW TO MAKE

1 Create an emulsion (see p109) by melting the butter, oil, and beeswax together in a bain-marie. Remove from the heat once the wax has melted.
2 Heat the mineral water in a saucepan to 80°C (175°F). Add the emulsifying wax, rose water, and glycerin. Stir until the wax is fully dissolved.
3 Add the hot oil mixture to the hot water mixture. Using a hand-held whisk or a stick blender, whisk continuously until smooth.
4 Continue to stir occasionally as the mixture cools. Add the essential oils and mix well. Pour into a sterilized jar and leave to cool before placing the lid on. Store in the fridge. Keeps for up to 6 weeks.

HOW TO APPLY

Apply to the face and neck with small, circular movements in an upward direction, avoiding the delicate eye area.

AVOCADO AND HONEY MOISTURISER

FOR NORMAL AND DRY SKIN

Honey **softens**, **lubricates**, **nourishes**, **soothes**, and **protects** the skin. Enriching avocado oil is a vitamin-rich, **conditioning** oil. Also containing nourishing almond oil and fragranced with neroli and orange essential oils, this rich moisturiser is a treat for the delicate skin on your face.

MAKES 100G (3½OZ)

INGREDIENTS
2 tsp shea nut butter
1 tsp almond oil
1 tsp avocado oil
4 tbsp mineral water
1 tbsp emulsifying wax
1 tsp glycerin
1 tsp clear organic honey
5 drops orange essential oil
5 drops neroli essential oil

HOW TO MAKE

1 Create an emulsion (see p109) by melting the butter and oils together in a bain-marie. Remove from the heat once the butter has melted.
2 Heat the mineral water in a saucepan to 80°C (175°F). Add the emulsifying wax and glycerin, and stir until the wax is fully dissolved.
3 Add the hot oil mixture to the hot water mixture. Using a hand-held whisk or a stick blender, whisk continuously until smooth.
4 Add the essential oils and continue to stir as the mixture cools. Pour into a sterilized jar and leave to cool before placing the lid on. Store in the fridge. Keeps for up to 6 weeks.

HOW TO APPLY

Apply to the face and neck with small, circular movements, avoiding the delicate eye area. Start with a pea-sized amount and add more if required.

FRANKINCENSE DAY CREAM

FOR MATURE SKIN

Rejuvenate and **tone** the skin with this cream. It contains two essential oils known for their **anti-ageing** properties. Frankincense is rejuvenating and works synergistically with myrrh oil, which is regarded as a skin preserver. Together they can **delay wrinkles** and the signs of ageing.

MAKES 100G (3½OZ)

INGREDIENTS

1 tbsp cocoa butter
1 tsp argan oil
1 tsp beeswax
4 tbsp mineral water
1 tbsp emulsifying wax
5 drops frankincense essential oil
3 drops myrrh essential oil

HOW TO MAKE

1 Create an emulsion (see p109) by melting the butter, oil, and beeswax together in a bain-marie. Remove from the heat once the wax has melted.
2 Heat the mineral water in a saucepan to 80ºC (175ºF). Add the emulsifying wax and stir until the wax is fully dissolved.
3 Add the hot oil mixture to the hot water mixture. Using a hand-held whisk or a stick blender, whisk continuously until smooth.
4 Continue to stir occasionally as the mixture cools. Add the essential oils and mix well. Pour into a sterilized jar and leave to cool for 1 hour before placing the lid on. Store in the fridge. Keeps for up to 6 weeks.

HOW TO APPLY

Apply daily to clean, dry skin in an upward-circular motion, avoiding the delicate eye area.

SOOTHING FACE CREAM

FOR DRY AND SENSITIVE SKIN

Sensitive skin can react to stressful situations in your life, as well as certain products or ingredients. Reactions often lead to red patches, itchiness, or flaky skin. This cream is **anti-inflammatory**, **conditioning**, and **calming** due to **skin-repairing** calendula and a caring mix of essential oils.

MAKES 100G (3½OZ)

INGREDIENTS

1 tbsp cocoa butter
1 tsp calendula macerated oil
1 tsp beeswax
3 tbsp mineral water
1 tbsp emulsifying wax
1 tsp glycerin
1 tsp aloe vera juice
3 drops Roman chamomile essential oil
1 drop lavender essential oil
1 drop rose essential oil

HOW TO MAKE

1 Create an emulsion (see p109) by melting the butter, oil, and beeswax together in a bain-marie. Remove from the heat once the wax has melted.
2 Heat the mineral water in a saucepan to 80ºC (175ºF). Add the emulsifying wax and stir until dissolved. Add the glycerin and aloe vera juice.
3 Add the hot water mixture to the hot oil mixture. Using a hand-held whisk or a stick blender, whisk continuously until smooth.
4 Add the essential oils and continue to stir occasionally as the mixture cools. Pour into a sterilized jar and leave to cool before placing the lid on. Store in the fridge. Keeps for up to 6 weeks.

HOW TO APPLY

After cleansing, gently apply a pea-sized amount to the face and neck in small, circular movements, avoiding the delicate eye area.

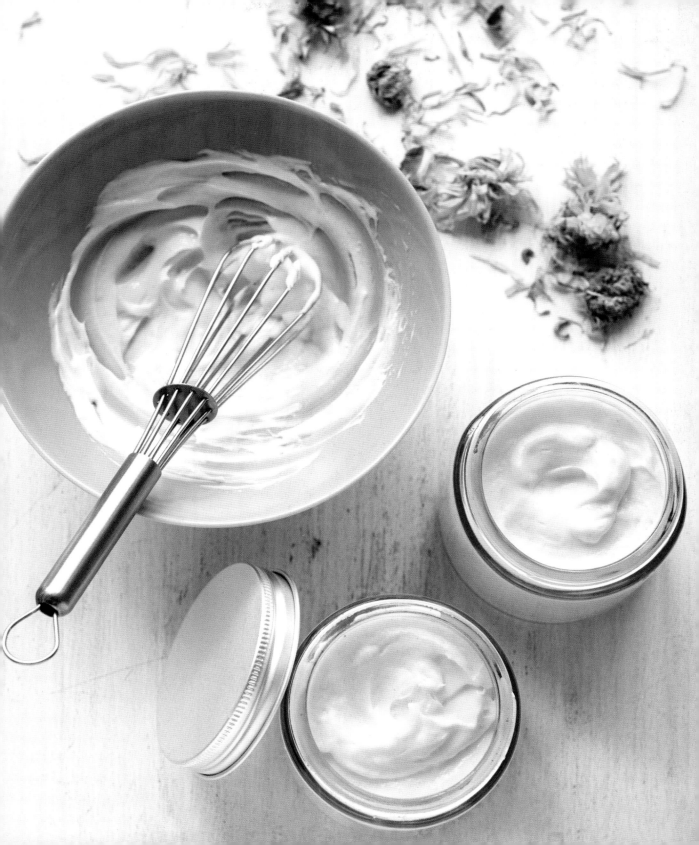

EVENING PRIMROSE MOISTURISER

FOR MATURE SKIN

Soothe, **cool**, and **rejuvenate** the skin with this cream. It features evening primrose oil, which is naturally rich in gamma-linolenic acid (GLA). GLA possesses natural **anti-inflammatory** and **skin-rejuvenating** properties, and can improve skin texture and smoothness.

MAKES 100G (3½OZ)

INGREDIENTS

200ml (7fl oz) mineral water
1 tbsp rose petals
2 tsp evening primrose oil
2 tsp jojoba oil
1 tsp beeswax
1 tbsp emulsifying wax
1 tsp glycerin
6 drops rose essential oil
4 drops patchouli essential oil
2 drops geranium essential oil

HOW TO MAKE

1 To make the infusion, boil the mineral water in a saucepan. Place the petals in a teapot and pour over the water. Steep for 10 minutes, then strain.
2 Create an emulsion (see p109) by melting the oils and beeswax together in a bain-marie. Remove from the heat once the wax has melted.
3 Reheat 4 tablespoons of the infusion in a separate pan to 80°C (175°F). Add the emulsifying wax and stir until the wax is fully dissolved. Add the glycerin and mix well. Add the infusion to the hot oil mixture. Using a hand-held whisk or a stick blender, whisk continuously until smooth.
4 Continue to stir occasionally as the mixture cools. Add the essential oils and mix well. Pour into a sterilized jar and leave to cool for 1 hour before placing the lid on. Store in the fridge. Keeps for 6 weeks.

HOW TO APPLY

Apply to dry skin in an upward-circular motion, avoiding the eye area.

NEROLI AND LEMON BALM NIGHT CREAM

FOR ALL SKIN TYPES

Support your skin as it naturally regenerates with this **hydrating** night cream. Jojoba oil forms a fine protective film on the skin, **softening** and **moisturising** it. With the added **nourishing** effects of shea butter and **uplifting** and **calming** neroli essential oil, this can replenish your skin as you sleep.

MAKES 100G (3½OZ)

INGREDIENTS

1 tsp shea nut butter
3 tsp jojoba oil
1 tbsp emulsifying wax
1 tsp beeswax
200ml (7fl oz) mineral water
1 tbsp chopped lemon balm
1 tsp glycerin
5 drops neroli essential oil
2 drops orange essential oil

HOW TO MAKE

1 Create an emulsion (see p109) by melting the butter, oil, wax, and beeswax together in a bain-marie. Remove from the heat once melted.
2 To make the infusion, boil the mineral water. Place the lemon balm in a teapot and pour over the water. Steep for 10 minutes, then strain.
3 Heat 4 tablespoons of the hot infusion in a separate pan to 80°C (175°F), then add the glycerin. Add the infusion to the hot oil mixture. Using a hand-held whisk or a stick blender, whisk continuously until smooth.
4 Continue to stir occasionally as the mixture cools. Add the essential oils and mix well. Pour into a sterilized jar and leave to cool before placing the lid on. Store in the fridge. Keeps for up to 6 weeks.

HOW TO APPLY

Massage into the face and neck with upward-sweeping movements, avoiding the eye area.

GERANIUM AND JOJOBA MOISTURISER

FOR OILY OR COMBINATION SKIN

This is a **balancing** cream for combination skin. Jojoba and geranium oils both encourage the regulation of the sebaceous glands, and palmarosa essential oil helps to balance sebum production. Palmarosa is also **antiseptic** and **hydrating**, making it useful in treating minor skin infections.

MAKES 100G (3½OZ)

INGREDIENTS

2 tbsp jojoba oil
3 tbsp mineral water
1 tbsp emulsifying wax
1 tsp glycerin
8 drops geranium essential oil
2 drops palmarosa essential oil

HOW TO MAKE

1 Create an emulsion (see p109) by heating the jojoba oil in a bain-marie. Remove from the heat once warm.
2 Heat the mineral water in a saucepan to 80°C (175°F). Add the emulsifying wax and glycerin, and mix well.
3 Add the hot oil to the hot water mixture. Using a hand-held whisk or a stick blender, whisk continuously until smooth.
4 Continue to stir occasionally while the mixture cools. Add the essential oils and mix. Pour into a sterilized jar and leave to cool before placing the lid on. Store in the fridge. Keeps for up to 6 weeks.

HOW TO APPLY

Massage into the face and neck with upward-sweeping movements, avoiding the eye area.

CHAMOMILE–CALENDULA MOISTURISER

FOR SENSITIVE SKIN

It is best to personalize moisturisers if you have sensitive skin. Minimize the number of ingredients you are putting on your skin with this gentle moisturiser. Calendula has traditionally been used for skin conditions. Like chamomile, it has **anti-inflammatory** and **wound-healing** properties.

MAKES 100G (3½OZ)

INGREDIENTS

1 tbsp cocoa butter
2 tsp calendula macerated oil
1 tsp beeswax
200ml (7fl oz) mineral water
1 tbsp dried chamomile flowers
1 tbsp dried calendula flowers
1 tbsp emulsifying wax
1 tsp glycerin

HOW TO MAKE

1 Create an emulsion (see p109) by melting the butter, oil, and beeswax together in a bain-marie. Remove from the heat once the wax has melted.
2 To make the infusion, boil the mineral water. Place the flowers in a teapot and pour the boiling water over. Steep for 10 minutes, then strain.
3 Heat 3 tablespoons of the infusion in a separate pan to 80°C (175°F), then add the emulsifying wax and glycerin. Stir until the wax is completely dissolved.
4 Add the hot emulsion mixture to the hot infusion mixture. Using a hand-held whisk or a stick blender, whisk continuously until smooth. Pour into a sterilized jar and leave to cool before placing the lid on. Store in the fridge. Keeps for up to 6 weeks.

HOW TO APPLY

Massage into the face and neck with upward-sweeping movements, avoiding the eye area.

BEAUTY BALM

FOR ALL SKIN TYPES

Use this indulgent facial balm to **revive** and **nourish** dull or tired-looking skin. Rich oils and shea nut butter help to prevent excessive water loss from the skin, keeping it supple and soft. The balm can **cleanse**, **exfoliate**, decongest, and enrich. It contains argan oil, a Moroccan treatment for skin and hair, and vitamin- and antioxidant-rich rosehip oil, which **regenerates** the skin and **improves** its tone.

INGREDIENTS

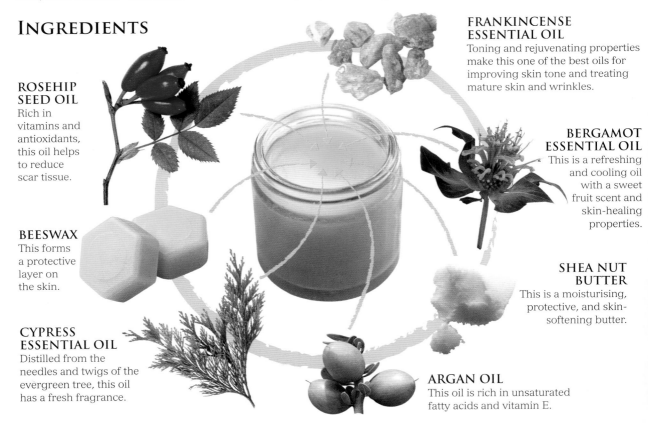

FRANKINCENSE ESSENTIAL OIL
Toning and rejuvenating properties make this one of the best oils for improving skin tone and treating mature skin and wrinkles.

ROSEHIP SEED OIL
Rich in vitamins and antioxidants, this oil helps to reduce scar tissue.

BERGAMOT ESSENTIAL OIL
This is a refreshing and cooling oil with a sweet fruit scent and skin-healing properties.

BEESWAX
This forms a protective layer on the skin.

SHEA NUT BUTTER
This is a moisturising, protective, and skin-softening butter.

CYPRESS ESSENTIAL OIL
Distilled from the needles and twigs of the evergreen tree, this oil has a fresh fragrance.

ARGAN OIL
This oil is rich in unsaturated fatty acids and vitamin E.

MAKES 100G (3½OZ)

INGREDIENTS

2 tbsp argan oil
2 tbsp rosehip seed oil
2 tbsp shea nut butter
1 tbsp beeswax
5 drops cypress essential oil
5 drops frankincense essential oil
5 drops bergamot essential oil

HOW TO MAKE

1 Heat the oils, butter, and beeswax, together in a bain-marie (see p133), until the wax has melted. Remove from the heat.
2 Add the essential oils and pour into a sterilized jar. Allow to cool for 1–2 hours, before using or applying the lid. Store in a cool, dark place. Keeps for up to 3 months.

HOW TO APPLY

Massage into the skin with circular movements. Leave on for an ultra-rich protective moisturiser, or use as a cleanser and remove with a damp muslin cloth or flannel, to polish away dead skin cells.

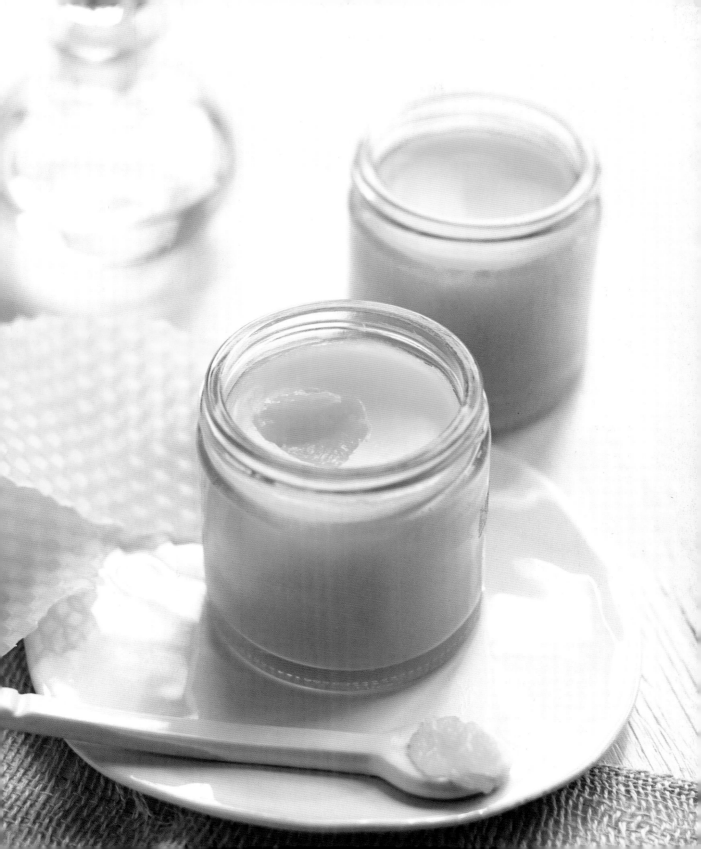

Palmarosa Facial Oil

FOR OILY OR COMBINATION SKIN

This blend of light grapeseed, **balancing** jojoba, and hemp oils helps to **revive** and restore the balance to oily or combination skin. Palmarosa essential oil has a sweet, rosy–floral odour and **antiseptic** properties. It is **hydrating** and helps to **normalize** sebum production. Zesty lemon essential oil is an **astringent**, tightening the pores and counteracting overproduction of sebum.

MAKES 90ML (3FL OZ)

INGREDIENTS

60ml (2fl oz) grapeseed oil
1 tbsp jojoba oil
1 tbsp hemp seed oil
5 drops palmarosa essential oil
2 drops bergamot essential oil
2 drops lemon essential oil
1 drop lavender essential oil

HOW TO MAKE

1 Pour the oils into a bowl. Add the essential oils and mix well.
2 Pour into a sterilized bottle and place a tight-fitting lid or dropper on. Shake well before use. Store in the fridge. Keeps for up to 3 months.

HOW TO APPLY

Apply a few drops to the fingertips and massage into the face and neck, using upward-sweeping motions, avoiding the delicate eye area. Use at night or under your everyday moisturiser if your skin is in need of additional hydration.

Brightening Facial Oil

QUICK

FOR ALL SKIN TYPES

Revive dull and tired skin with this **antioxidant-rich** facial oil. Rosehip oil has been found to be beneficial in tissue **regeneration** for conditions such as burns, facial wrinkles, and treatment of scars. Sea buckthorn oil is rich in essential fatty acids and carotenoids, making it a fantastic oil for **brightening** the skin. It may leave a slight yellowish tinge on the face, but it is easily washed off.

MAKES 60ML (2FL OZ)

INGREDIENTS

2 tbsp rosehip oil
1 tbsp wheatgerm oil
1–2 drops sea buckthorn oil
2 drops cypress essential oil
2 drops clary sage essential oil
2 drops rosemary essential oil
2 drops frankincense essential oil

HOW TO MAKE

1 Pour the oils into a bowl. Add the essential oils and mix well.
2 Pour into a sterilized bottle and place a tight-fitting lid or dropper on. Shake well before use. Store in the fridge. Keeps for up to 3 months.

HOW TO APPLY

Apply a few drops to the fingertips and massage into the face and neck, using upward-sweeping motions, avoiding the delicate eye area. Use at night or under your everyday moisturiser if your skin is in need of additional hydration.

Night-Time Facial Oil

FOR ALL SKIN TYPES

QUICK

Soothe your skin as you sleep with this luxurious, fragrant facial oil. Rich in essential fatty acids, this combination of vegetable oils **nourishes** and **smoothes** the skin as you sleep. The blend of essential oils in this recipe has beneficial actions on the skin: **skin-regenerating** patchouli oil, **balancing** ylang ylang oil, and **soothing** orange essential oil.

MAKES 100ML (3½FL OZ)

INGREDIENTS

1 tbsp pomegranate oil
2 tbsp macadamia seed oil
2 tsp castor oil
3 tbsp jojoba oil
2 drops benzoin tincture
1 drop cypress essential oil
1 drop clary sage essential oil
1 drop patchouli essential oil
1 drop ylang ylang essential oil
1 drop orange essential oil

HOW TO MAKE

1 Pour the oils into a bowl. Add the tincture and essential oils, and mix well.
2 Pour into a sterilized bottle and place a tight-fitting lid or dropper on. Store in the fridge. Keeps for up to 3 months.

HOW TO APPLY

Apply a few drops to the fingertips and massage into the face and neck, using upward-sweeping motions, avoiding the delicate eye area. Use at night to help nourish your skin while you sleep, especially if your skin is in need of additional hydration. You could use this oil as part of a 10-minute facial massage, as shown on pp120–21.

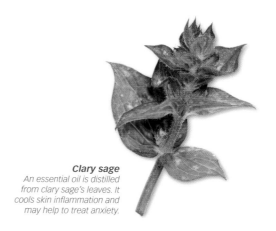

Clary sage
An essential oil is distilled from clary sage's leaves. It cools skin inflammation and may help to treat anxiety.

10-MINUTE FACIAL MASSAGE

A weekly facial massage can help to increase circulation, create an even skin tone, lift slack skin, and reduce puffiness. Before you begin, wash and dry your hands. Sit down on a chair comfortably and relax with your feet flat on the floor and your back supported. Throughout the process, always massage in an upwards direction.

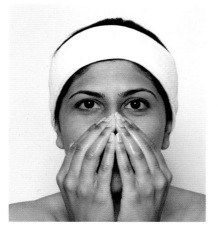

1 Choose a facial oil that is suitable for your skin type. Rub 3 drops of the oil between your fingertips. Hold your hands in front of your nose and inhale into your hands, then exhale deeply. Repeat 3 times.

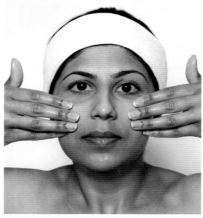

2 Spread the oil over the face, starting under the jaw and moving upwards towards the forehead with gentle but firm sweeping movements, avoiding the delicate eye area. Repeat 3 times.

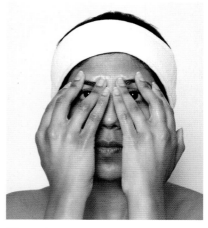

3 Evenly space out the fingertips of the index, middle, and ring fingers along the eyebrows. Gently press and release the fingertips. Move 1cm (¹⁄₃in) towards the hairline and repeat.

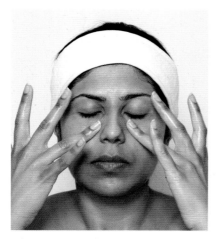

4 Draw spectacles around the eyes using ring fingers, starting from between the eyes. Repeat 3 times.

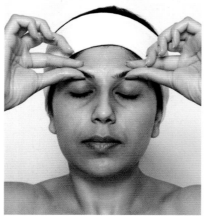

5 Pinch both of the eyebrows. Start from above the nose and move outwards towards the ears. Repeat 3 times.

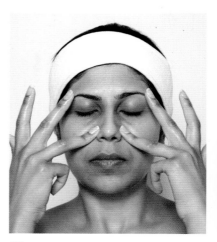

6 Using the ring fingers, apply small circular movements to the bridge of the nose, moving down towards the nostrils.

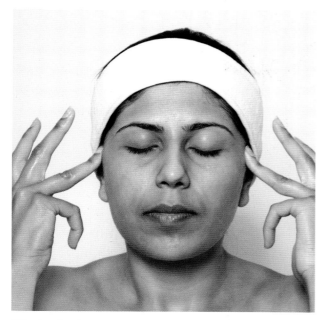

7 Using the ring fingers, apply very gentle pressure underneath the centre of the eyes, moving along the cheekbone towards the ears. Sweep fingers down your neck towards the shoulders.

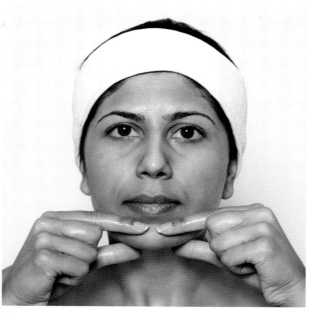

8 Pinch the chin using the thumb and forefinger of both hands, then sweep along the jaw towards the ears. This helps to invigorate the jaw.

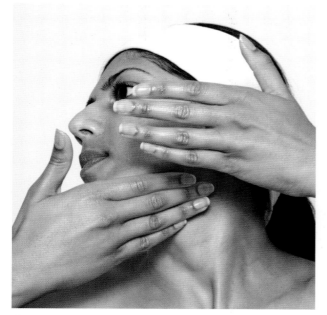

9 Gently tug the ear lobes, then, using both hands, invigorate the face using quick flicking movements with your fingers to get the blood pumping, moving across the jaw and up the cheeks.

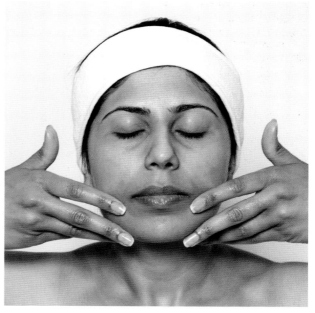

10 Finish with deep stroking movements using the full hand and fingers, starting under the jaw and sweeping up the cheeks, around the eyes, and up to the forehead. Repeat 3 times.

HONEY AND OAT SCRUB

FOR ALL SKIN TYPES

Boost the circulation and slough off any dead skin cells using this gentle scrub that leaves the complexion bright and radiant. Oats have skin **soothing**, **softening**, and **cleansing** properties and their mild action makes them perfect for treating dry or irritated skin. Honey has been used since ancient times as a **moisturiser** that also softens, lubricates, soothes, and **protects** the skin.

INGREDIENTS

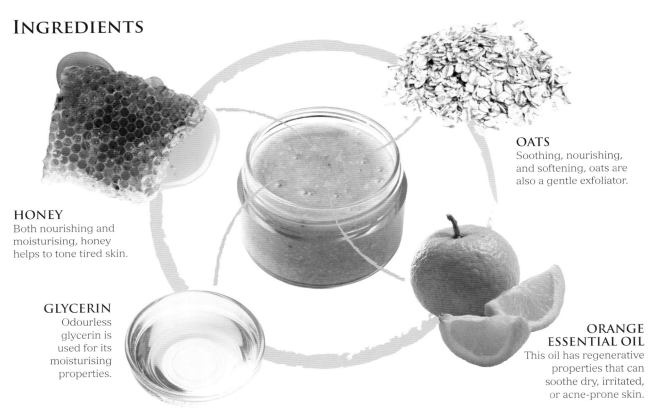

OATS
Soothing, nourishing, and softening, oats are also a gentle exfoliator.

HONEY
Both nourishing and moisturising, honey helps to tone tired skin.

GLYCERIN
Odourless glycerin is used for its moisturising properties.

ORANGE ESSENTIAL OIL
This oil has regenerative properties that can soothe dry, irritated, or acne-prone skin.

MAKES 50G (1¾OZ)

INGREDIENTS
1 tbsp jumbo oats
2 tbsp glycerin
1 tsp honey
4 drops orange essential oil

HOW TO MAKE

1 Using a mortar and pestle or a stick blender, grind the oats into a fine powder.

2 Transfer the oats to a bowl and add the remaining ingredients. Store in a sterilized jar with a tight-fitting lid in the fridge. Keeps for up to 6 weeks.

HOW TO APPLY

Gently massage the scrub into clean skin, avoiding the eye area, and rinse off with warm water. Pat skin dry with a clean towel.

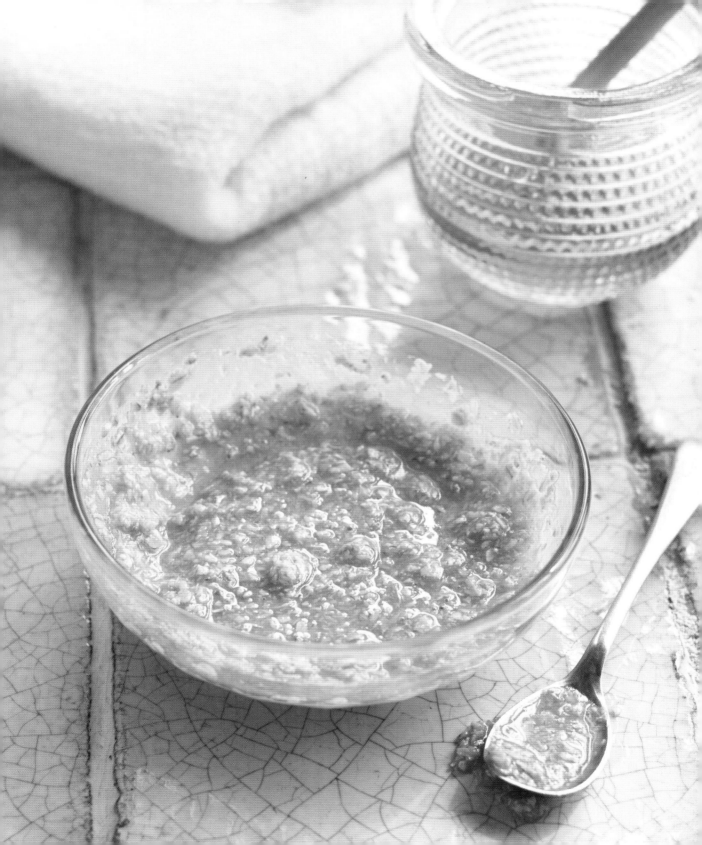

AVOCADO AND HONEY SCRUB

FOR ALL SKIN TYPES

The perfect recipe to use up store-cupboard basics, this scrub can **revitalize** a dull or tired complexion, while gently **exfoliating** and **nourishing** the skin. Honey has natural **cleansing** and **soothing** properties, and avocados are a good source of vitamins A and E, both of which help to maintain healthy skin. They are also rich in the essential fatty acid linoleic acid.

INGREDIENTS

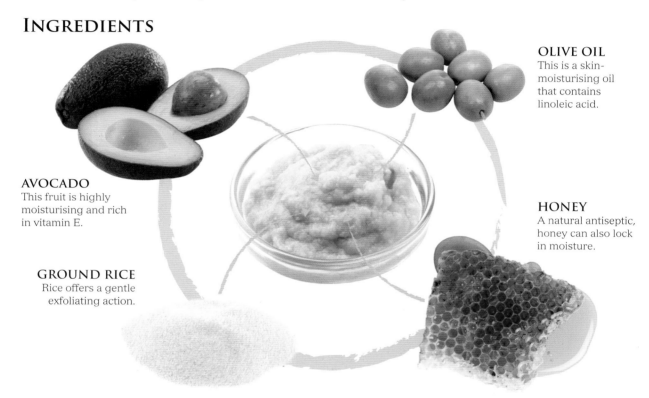

OLIVE OIL
This is a skin-moisturising oil that contains linoleic acid.

AVOCADO
This fruit is highly moisturising and rich in vitamin E.

HONEY
A natural antiseptic, honey can also lock in moisture.

GROUND RICE
Rice offers a gentle exfoliating action.

MAKES ENOUGH FOR ONE SCRUB

INGREDIENTS
½ ripe avocado
1 tsp honey
1 tbsp olive oil
1 tbsp ground rice

HOW TO MAKE

1 Mash the avocado in a bowl using a fork.

2 Heat the honey in a bain-marie (see p133). Add the oil and warm honey to the avocado, and mix together.

3 Add the ground rice and mix until you have a paste. Use immediately as it contains fresh ingredients and cannot be stored.

HOW TO APPLY

Gently massage the scrub into the skin, paying particular attention to areas of congestion. Leave on for 1–2 minutes then rinse off with warm water. Pat skin dry with a clean towel.

STRAWBERRIES AND CREAM SCRUB

FOR ALL SKIN TYPES

Use up the last few strawberries in the fridge to make this **exfoliating** mask. Antioxidant and vitamin-rich strawberries can have an instant **revitalizing** and **brightening** effect on the skin, helping to boost **radiance**. Jumbo oats are gently exfoliating. When they are mixed with mashed strawberries and **moisturising** single cream, the resulting scrub looks, feels, smells, and even tastes great.

MAKES ENOUGH FOR ONE SCRUB

INGREDIENTS
2 tbsp jumbo oats
2–4 ripe strawberries
2 tsp single cream

HOW TO MAKE

1 Using a mortar and pestle or a stick blender, grind the oats into a powder.

2 Mash the strawberries in a bowl using a fork. Add the oats and mix together.

3 Pour in enough cream to make a paste. Use immediately, as it contains fresh ingredients and cannot be stored.

HOW TO APPLY

Gently massage the scrub into the skin, avoiding the delicate eye area. If using as a mask, leave on the skin for 10 minutes. Gently remove with warm water. Pat skin dry with a clean towel.

ROSE FACIAL SCRUB

FOR ALL SKIN TYPES

Slough off dead skin cells and reveal bright new skin beneath with this facial scrub. Ground rice and oats create a gentle abrasive action suitable for **exfoliating** all skin types. The beautifully fragrant rose floral water **refreshes** and **cleanses** the skin and glycerin gives it a **moisturising** boost. The scrub will set quickly, so be generous with the coverage of the paste and have a thorough exfoliation.

MAKES ENOUGH FOR ONE SCRUB

INGREDIENTS
1 tbsp glycerin
1 tsp organic cornflour
2 tsp–1 tbsp rose floral water
1 tsp oats
1 tsp ground rice

HOW TO MAKE

1 Mix the glycerin and cornflour together in a bowl to make a paste.

2 Add the rose floral water, stirring continuously with a balloon whisk.

3 Using a mortar and pestle or a stick blender, grind the oats into a powder.

4 Add the ground oats and rice to the bowl, and stir until it becomes a paste. Add more rose water if the paste is too dry. Use immediately as it contains fresh ingredients and cannot be stored.

HOW TO APPLY

Gently massage the scrub into the skin, avoiding the delicate eye area, and remove with warm water. Pat skin dry with a clean towel.

EAT WELL FOR... CLEAR SKIN

Our skin is a visible indicator of our health and well-being. A poor diet, lack of nutrients or fluids, stress allergies, or inflammation can show up on the skin as spots, eczema, dullness, or premature ageing. If you want to transform the health of your skin, adapt your diet and you will see the effects in 1–2 weeks. Here are some dietary dos and don'ts and the key superfoods that can contribute to beautiful, healthy skin.

BOOST YOUR BASICS

GET YOUR 7-A-DAY Eat at least 7–10 portions of organic fruit and vegetables a day. This ensures you get enough vitamin C, which has an anti-inflammatory effect and can also boost collagen production. In addition, phytonutrients in fresh fruit and vegetables contain antioxidants that boost skin health and help to prevent skin ageing.

CHOOSE WHOLEGRAIN Whole wheat, oats, and brown rice contain the antioxidant vitamin E, which has a protective effect on skin cells.

DRINK WATER Drinking plenty of water is cleansing for your skin, and helps to rid your body of toxins. It can also help the skin to stay plump and hydrated.

TRY OMEGA-RICH OILS Keep your skin supple and healthy by including "good" oils in your diet, such as those found in fish, nuts, and seeds. Olive, hazelnut, hemp, and flaxseed oils are superb choices. Omega-rich oils also have an anti-inflammatory effect, which is important for clear skin.

EAT ORGANIC Containing fewer toxic pesticide residues, organic food is healthier because it is higher in certain important nutrients, such as zinc – an essential mineral for clear and healthy skin.

SUPERFOODS

Supplement a balanced diet with these superfoods – bursting with the vitamins, minerals, and antioxidants that your skin needs to repair itself, they can dramatically improve your complexion.

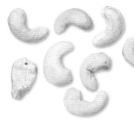

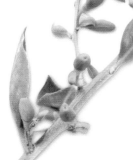

CASHEWS
These nuts contain a high level of protein to repair the skin and are a useful source of minerals, such as iron and zinc, that help to heal the skin.

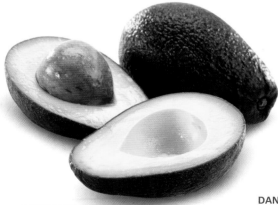

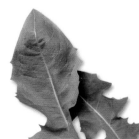

AVOCADOS
This fruit is high in omega-fatty acids, which help to maintain moisture in the epidermal layer of the skin, keeping it soft. They are also a source of oleic acid – involved in regenerating damaged skin cells and reducing inflammation, facial redness, and irritation.

DANDELION LEAVES
Eat fresh greens in a salad or make tea from the dried leaves. Dandelion leaves encourage healthy elimination, thus reducing outbreaks. They are also a source of carotenoids, flavonoids, vitamins A and C, and calcium, iron, and potassium.

GOJI BERRIES

This berry, once known as the "key to eternal youth" due to its regenerative properties, is a powerhouse of antioxidants, and contains vitamins A and E. Eating them can nourish the skin from the inside and help to protect against inflammation.

SAY NO TO...

PROCESSED FOODS These are full of pro-ageing unhealthy fats, salt, and sugars. A diet based on these foods is high in calories but low on the real nutrients your skin needs to stay clear and healthy.

SUGAR AND REFINED CARBOHYDRATES These can quickly make your blood-sugar level soar, triggering your body to produce the hormone insulin to help your cells absorb the sugar. Studies show that insulin plays a role in acne. Embracing a diet with a low-glycemic load can help to clear the skin – to do this, avoid sugar and refined carbohydrates, and completely cut out the worst culprits – fizzy drinks.

TOO MUCH DAIRY There is nothing wrong with a small amount of milk and dairy in a balanced diet, but if you suffer from acne or spots, it can be worth eliminating these from your diet for a while, as some people find that milk is pro-inflammatory. Studies show that going on a dairy-free diet can help eliminate acne.

SMOKING This is not a dietary recommendation but abstaining makes a massive difference to the health of your skin, because smoking wrecks the skin, causing dullness, congestion, and premature ageing.

FLAXSEEDS

These seeds contain the anti-inflammatory fatty acids that are necessary for maintaining healthy, clear skin. Flaxseed oil is particularly good at helping to reduce skin problems involving inflammation, such as eczema or acne. Sprinkle the cracked seeds or drizzle the oil over salads, soups, and stews.

BRAZIL NUTS

Good sources of zinc, brazil nuts also contain selenium, which supports immunity and helps wounds and skin to heal.

ALMONDS

These are high in vitamin E, an antioxidant nutrient that helps to improve the condition and appearance of your skin. Eat a few almonds every day or try almond milk as an alternative to cow's milk.

APPLES

Fresh apples contain vitamins A and C – both helpful for healing the skin and boosting healthy collagen. The compound pectin helps to balance blood sugar and encourage elimination so that skin remains clear.

Reviving Tomato Mask

QUICK

FOR ALL SKIN TYPES

Give your skin a **reviving** boost with this vitamin-rich mask. Tomatoes are great for the skin as they have **cooling** and **astringent** properties and are rich in skin-brightening vitamin C. Olive oil is commonly used in skin-care preparations because it is skin **softening** and **nourishing**. It is also rich in oleic acid and is great for **moisturising** dry skin.

MAKES ENOUGH FOR ONE APPLICATION

INGREDIENTS

1 medium-sized tomato
2 tsp cornflour
1 tsp olive oil

HOW TO MAKE

1 Hold the tomato steady and use a sharp knife to score an "X" through the skin at the base. Immerse completely in boiling water for about 20 seconds, or until the skin splits.

2 Using a slotted spoon, carefully remove the tomato from the water and immediately plunge it into a bowl of iced water to cool it.

3 When the tomato is cool enough to handle, use a paring knife to peel off the skin, starting at the base where the "X" was made.

4 Mash the tomato with a fork in a bowl and strain the seeds using a sieve.

5 Add the cornflour to make a paste. Pour the oil into the paste, and mix well. The paste should be thick enough for you to spread or brush evenly. Use immediately.

HOW TO APPLY

Apply the mask to freshly cleansed skin with the fingertips. Leave it on for 5 minutes and remove with warm water. Pat skin dry with a clean towel.

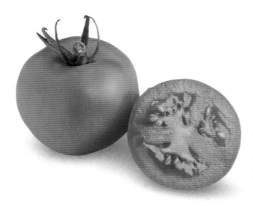

Tomato
Rich in beta-carotene and vitamin C, tomatoes are an incredible source of lycopene – a substance found to reduce the risk of cancer, protect the eyes and skin, and boost immunity.

AVOCADO AND BANANA MASK

FOR ALL SKIN TYPES

Fresh banana has a richly **moisturising** and **smoothing** effect on the skin. This recipe combines it with vitamin and mineral-rich fresh avocado, which has great **skin-conditioning** properties. Mix it with moisturising honey to give the skin a deeply **nourishing** treatment that can stay on the skin for 10 minutes. Close your eyes, relax, and allow the mask to work its magic.

MAKES ENOUGH FOR ONE APPLICATION

INGREDIENTS

½ ripe avocado
½ ripe banana
1 tsp honey
1 tsp rose floral water

HOW TO MAKE

1 Place the avocado and banana in a bowl and mash them with a fork to make a paste.

2 Add the honey and rose water to the paste, and mix well. The paste should be thick enough for you to spread or brush evenly. Use immediately.

HOW TO APPLY

Apply the mask to freshly cleansed skin with the fingertips, avoiding the delicate eye area. Leave it on for 10 minutes and remove with warm water. Pat skin dry with a clean towel.

ALOE VERA COOLING MASK

FOR ALL SKIN TYPES

Give your skin a moisture boost with this **cooling** combination of aloe vera, lavender essential oil, and kaolin clay. Aloe vera is commonly used as a **healing** and **moisturising** gel and is great for use on damaged skin. Kaolin clay helps to **purify** the skin by drawing out impurities, and glycerin provides the skin with moisture.

MAKES 30G (1OZ)

INGREDIENTS

1–2 tbsp aloe vera juice
1 tbsp glycerin
1–2 tbsp kaolin
2 drops lavender essential oil

HOW TO MAKE

1 Place the aloe vera juice, glycerin, and kaolin in a bowl. Using a hand-held whisk or a stick blender, whisk together to make a paste.

2 Add the essential oil to the paste and mix well. The paste should be thick enough for you to spread or brush evenly.

3 Add more aloe vera juice if the mixture is too thick, and more kaolin if the mixture is too runny. Use immediately or it may dry out.

HOW TO APPLY

Apply the mask to freshly cleansed skin with the fingertips or with a clean foundation brush, avoiding the delicate eye area. Leave on for 5 minutes, but do not allow to dry. Remove with warm water and pat skin dry with a clean towel.

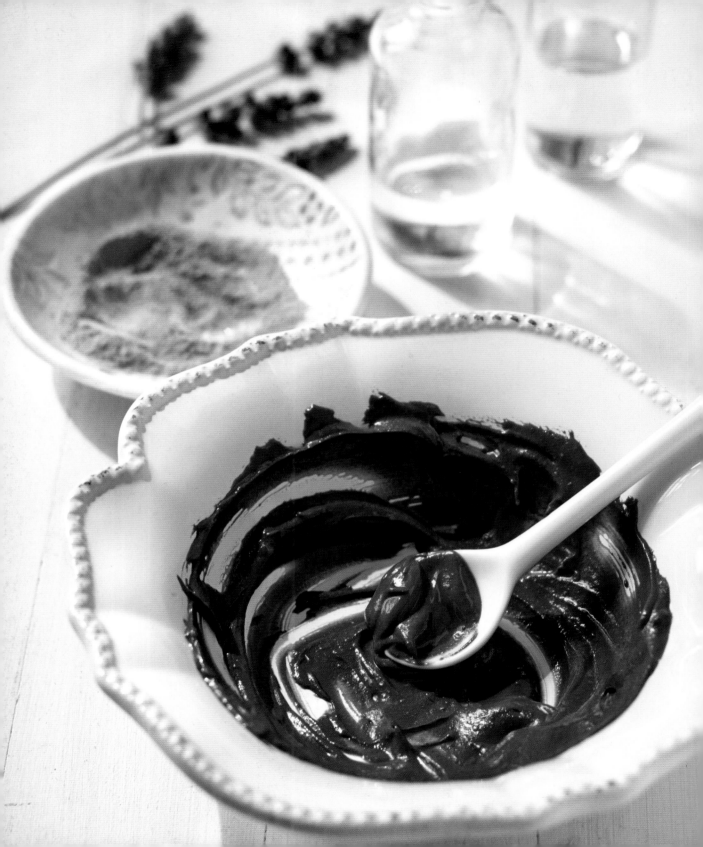

GREEN CLAY PURIFYING MASK

FOR ALL SKIN TYPES

Green clay has a natural ability to absorb, which makes it a useful ingredient for **cleansing** and absorbing excess oil. Used as the basis for a face mask, it helps to draw impurities from the skin. In combination with **nourishing** glycerin and **calming** lavender, this mask cleanses and balances the skin. It also has **toning** properties, which help to **refine** pores and **revitalize** the complexion.

MAKES ENOUGH FOR ONE APPLICATION

INGREDIENTS

1 tbsp powdered green clay
1 tbsp glycerin
1 tsp lavender floral water

HOW TO MAKE

1 Place the powdered clay, glycerin, and floral water in a bowl.
2 Using a fork, mix into a paste. The paste should be thick enough for you to spread or brush evenly. If the mixture is too runny add more clay. Use immediately or it may dry out.

HOW TO APPLY

Apply the mask to freshly cleansed skin with the fingertips or with a clean foundation brush, avoiding the delicate eye area. Leave on for 10 minutes, but do not allow to dry. Remove with warm water and pat skin dry with a clean towel.

Refine Your Pores

Underneath the surface of the skin are glands called sebaceous glands. These produce an oily substance known as sebum, which is excreted through the pores or the hair follicles. Maintaining clean, healthy skin pores is important for healthy skin. Clogged pores below the surface of the skin cause whiteheads and clogged pores on the surface of the skin cause blackheads. External factors, such as make-up, pollution, and oil-producing hormonal changes, can cause blocked pores. Use this purifying facial mask to deep cleanse and refine the pores, bringing the skin back into balance.

WITCH HAZEL AND ALOE VERA AFTERSHAVE SPLASH

FOR ALL SKIN TYPES

Calm, **cool**, and **refresh** freshly shaved skin with **healing** witch hazel herbal water and **soothing** aloe vera juice. Witch hazel herbal water is a traditional remedy made from a macerate of the freshly cut leaves and twigs of the *Hamamelis virginiana* tree, which are distilled before alcohol is added. It can calm inflamed skin conditions.

MAKES 100ML (3½FL OZ)

INGREDIENTS

3 tbsp witch hazel herbal water
3 tbsp aloe vera gel
2 tsp glycerin
5 drops tea tree essential oil
3 drops grapefruit essential oil
2 drops bergamot essential oil
1 drop lavender essential oil

HOW TO MAKE

1 Mix all the ingredients together in a bowl.
2 Pour into a sterilized bottle and place a tight-fitting cap or atomizer on. Store in the fridge. Keeps for up to 6 weeks.

HOW TO APPLY

Shake well before each use. Apply the aftershave splash after shaving, either with fingertips, or spritz all over the skin using an atomizer.

OLIVE SHAVING OIL

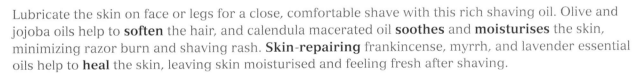

FOR ALL SKIN TYPES

Lubricate the skin on face or legs for a close, comfortable shave with this rich shaving oil. Olive and jojoba oils help to **soften** the hair, and calendula macerated oil **soothes** and **moisturises** the skin, minimizing razor burn and shaving rash. **Skin-repairing** frankincense, myrrh, and lavender essential oils help to **heal** the skin, leaving skin moisturised and feeling fresh after shaving.

MAKES 30ML (1FL OZ)

INGREDIENTS

2 tsp olive oil
2 tsp jojoba oil
2 tsp calendula macerated oil
5 drops frankincense essential oil
2 drops myrrh essential oil
1 drop lavender essential oil

HOW TO MAKE

1 Mix all the ingredients together in a bowl.
2 Pour into a sterilized bottle and place a tight-fitting lid or dropper on. Store in a cool, dark place. Keeps for up to 3 months.

HOW TO APPLY

Wet the area to be shaved with hot water. Rub 8–10 drops of the oil into the skin. If using on the face, shave in the direction of hair growth, rinsing the razor regularly. Rinse the shaved skin with cold water and pat dry with a clean towel.

COCONUT SHAVING BALM

FOR ALL SKIN TYPES

This ultra-rich shaving balm contains a combination of **nourishing** and **skin-smoothing** oils that **lubricate** the skin for a close and comfortable shave. Coconut oil **softens** the hair making it easier for the razor to glide along the skin. Sandalwood essential oil has **soothing** and **cooling** properties and is blended with **refreshing** neroli oil, which helps **reduce redness** and irritation.

MAKES 60G (2OZ)

INGREDIENTS

2 tbsp coconut oil
1 tsp sweet almond oil
1 tbsp sunflower oil
1 tsp shea nut butter
1 tsp carnauba wax
4 drops sandalwood essential oil
4 drops neroli essential oil
1 drop German chamomile essential oil

HOW TO MAKE

1 Make a balm, as shown in the step-by-step technique below.
2 Once the balm has cooled, it is ready for use. Place the lid on, and store in a cool, dark place. Keeps for up to 3 months.

HOW TO APPLY

Apply to clean, exfoliated skin. Wet the area to be shaved with hot water and apply a pea-sized amount of balm. Apply more balm if required. If using on the face, shave in the direction of the hair growth, rinsing the razor regularly. Rinse the shaved skin with cold water and pat dry with a clean towel.

MAKING A BALM

Balms are a simple combination of oils, butters, and waxes that nourish the skin and help to protect it from excess water loss. Make them using a bain-marie to gently melt the ingredients together. Balms set hard, making them practical and transportable. They don't contain water, so are safe from microbial attack.

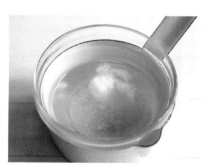

1 Place the oils, butter, and wax into a glass bowl. Fill a saucepan halfway with boiling water. Place the glass bowl on top, to form a bain-marie. Allow the ingredients to melt.

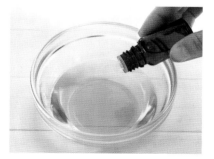

2 Remove the bowl from the heat, taking care as the glass will be hot. As the balm cools, add the essential oils and mix well.

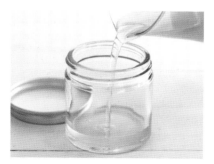

3 Pour into a sterilized jar and leave to cool for about 1 hour. The balm will change in colour, becoming more opaque as it cools.

COCONUT AND LIME LIP BALM

FOR ALL SKIN TYPES

This heavenly combination of coconut oil, shea nut butter, and almond oil **conditions** and **nourishes** the lips. Beeswax forms a protective layer on the delicate skin, helping the lips to retain water and remain **hydrated** and **smooth**. Refreshingly fruity lime and lemon essential oils smell delicious and have a mild **anti-microbial** effect.

MAKES 40G (1¼OZ)

INGREDIENTS

1 tbsp coconut oil
1 tsp shea nut butter
1 tsp almond oil
1 tsp beeswax
4 drops lime essential oil
1 drop lemon essential oil

HOW TO MAKE

1 Heat all the ingredients, apart from the essential oils, in a bain-marie (see p133) until the wax has melted. Remove from the heat.

2 Add the essential oils as the balm cools and mix well.

3 Pour into a sterilized jar and leave to cool for about 1 hour before placing the lid on. Store in a cool, dark place. Keeps for up to 3 months.

HOW TO APPLY

Apply to lips when they are dry and in need of moisture. Apply before bed to help lips to retain moisture as you sleep.

KISS-ME-SLOWLY LIP BALM

FOR ALL SKIN TYPES

This mixture of oils and waxes helps to keep lips silky smooth and **hydrated**. Shea butter lends its **moisturising** and **skin-protecting** properties to the recipe, and castor oil is **healing** and helps create a protective layer over the delicate skin on the lips. The mint adds a refreshing taste and scent, and a mildly **antiseptic** action.

MAKES 30G (1OZ)

INGREDIENTS

1 tbsp shea nut butter
1 tsp castor oil
1 tsp sunflower oil
1 tsp beeswax
4 drops peppermint essential oil

HOW TO MAKE

1 Heat all the ingredients, apart from the essential oil, in a bain-marie (see p133) until the wax has melted. Remove from the heat.

2 Add the essential oil as the balm cools and mix well.

3 Pour into a sterilized jar and leave to cool for about 1 hour before placing the lid on. Store in a cool, dark place. Keeps for up to 3 months.

HOW TO APPLY

Apply to lips when they are dry and in need of moisture. Apply before bed to help lips to retain moisture as you sleep.

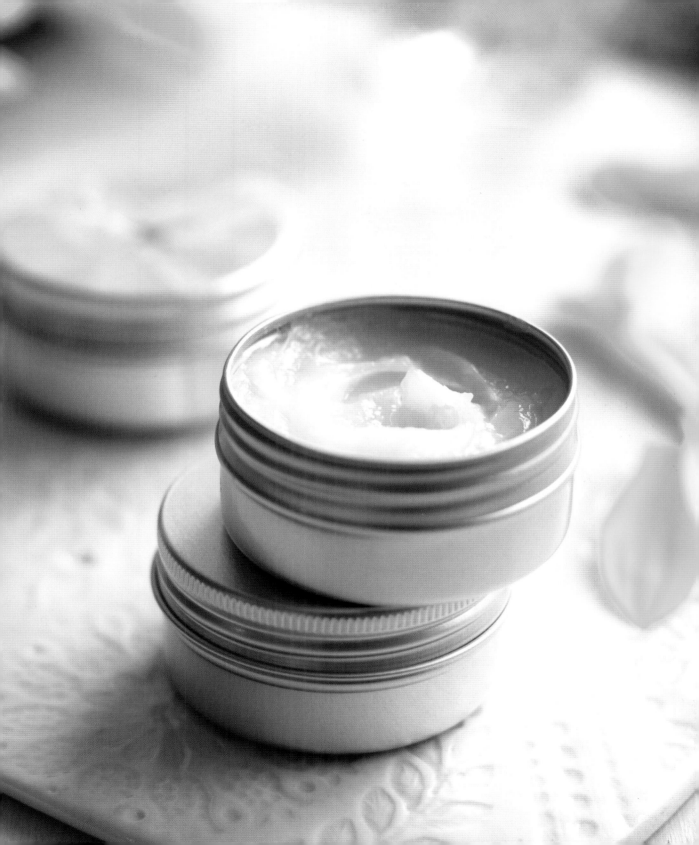

KIDS' CITRUS TOOTHPASTE

QUICK

FOR KIDS

Kids will love this citrus-flavoured toothpaste. It has gentle **antiseptic** and **cleansing** properties and is perfect for early dental care. Get the kids to help make it, bringing some fun into their daily routine. Bicarbonate of soda is gently **abrasive** and cleansing, and the blend of mandarin and bergamot oils has a sweet citrussy odour that is familiarly fruity.

MAKES 10G (¼OZ)

INGREDIENTS

2 drops glycerin
1 tsp bicarbonate of soda
6 drops mandarin essential oil
1 drop bergamot essential oil

HOW TO MAKE

1 Place all the ingredients in a small bowl. Add 1 teaspoon water and mix well to make a paste.
2 Makes enough for two applications. Store in the fridge and use in one day.

HOW TO APPLY

Scoop the paste onto your toothbrush and brush as usual. Do not swallow. Use twice a day.

HERBAL TOOTHPASTE

QUICK

FOR ALL

Most conventional toothpastes contain harsh cleansers like sodium lauryl sulphate (SLS), which can cause skin eruptions and allergies. This natural version has the same **cleansing** and **antiseptic** action without the risk of irritation. It contains a naturally **antiseptic** blend of essential oils that works to **protect** against bacteria and **maintain gum health**.

MAKES 15G (½OZ)

INGREDIENTS

2 drops glycerin
1 tsp bicarbonate of soda
1 tsp table salt
2 drops thyme essential oil
2 drops rosemary essential oil
2 drops sweet fennel essential oil

HOW TO MAKE

1 Place all the ingredients in a small bowl. Add 1 teaspoon water and mix well to make a paste.
2 Makes enough for two applications. Store in the fridge and use in one day.

HOW TO APPLY

Scoop the paste onto your toothbrush and brush as usual. Do not swallow. Use twice a day.

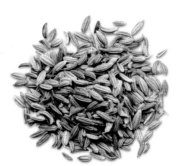

Fennel seeds
With its aniseed-like flavour and ability to treat gum disorders and sore throats, fennel is a perfect ingredient for toothpastes.

MINTY FRESH MOUTHWASH

FOR ALL

This minty mouthwash is alcohol and sugar-free, and is **healing** and **antiseptic** when used regularly. The combination of peppermint infusion and peppermint essential oil provides the sharp menthol fragrance, and tea tree is highly antiseptic. Myrrh's antiseptic qualities can help to treat sore gums, bad breath, and mouth ulcers.

MAKES 100ML (3½FL OZ)

INGREDIENTS

100ml (3½fl oz) mineral water
1 tbsp dried peppermint
1 drop peppermint essential oil
1 drop tea tree essential oil
1 drop myrrh essential oil
1 tsp table salt
1 tsp aloe vera juice
1 tsp glycerin

HOW TO MAKE

1 To make the infusion, boil the mineral water in a saucepan. Place the dried peppermint in a teapot or glass bowl and pour over the boiling water. Leave to steep for 10 minutes, then strain.

2 In a separate bowl, add the essential oils to the salt. Pour over the warm infusion and allow the salt to dissolve. Add the aloe vera juice and glycerin.

3 Pour into a sterilized bottle and leave to cool before placing a lid or atomizer on.

4 Shake well before each use. Store in the fridge. Keeps for up to a week.

HOW TO APPLY

Use twice a day to rinse your mouth after brushing teeth. Do not swallow.

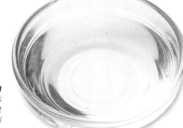

Glycerin
*Sweet in taste, glycerin acts as
a preservative. Unlike sugar, it
does not promote bacterial
growth and plaque formation.*

COOLING EYE MASK

QUICK

FOR ALL SKIN TYPES

Cooling, **soothing**, and **refreshing**, this eye mask helps to **tone** the delicate skin around the eye area and reduce puffiness or inflammation. Witch hazel herbal water is **astringent** and refreshing. The soothing properties of calendula tincture work in combination with aloe vera and witch hazel to **smooth puffy lines** and leave eyes feeling refreshed.

MAKES 20ML (4 TSP)

INGREDIENTS

2 tsp witch hazel herbal water
1 tsp aloe vera juice
1 tsp glycerin
1 tsp calendula tincture

HOW TO MAKE

1 Mix all the ingredients together in a sterilized mixing bowl.

2 Pour into a sterilized bottle and place the lid on. Store in the fridge. Keeps for up to a week.

HOW TO APPLY

Apply the eye mask to the bones around the eyes (the brow bone and cheekbone). Never apply on the lids or directly under the eyes as the skin there is very delicate. Leave it on the skin for 5 minutes, before removing gently with cotton wool pads, a damp flannel, or muslin cloth.

Rejuvenate Your Eyes

This simple sequence can refresh tired eyes. Repeat each of the following steps three times.

- Sitting comfortably, close your eyes and lightly cover them with clean hands, blocking out the light. Take three slow, deep breaths.
- Remove your hands and close your eyes tightly for 4 seconds, then open them for 4 seconds.
- Soak a muslin cloth in hot water, wring it out, and lightly press to your face. Lightly massage the eyebrows outwards from the nose.
- Soak the cloth in cold water, wring it out, and hold it over your face. Lightly massage the cheekbone and brow bone.
- Roll the eyes clockwise, then anticlockwise, blinking in between.
- Focus on a distant object for 10 seconds, then focus on a nearby object for 10 seconds without moving your head.
- Look up and down, then left to right.
- Gently hold the palms over closed eyes and take a deep breath.

REVITALIZING EYE MASK

FOR ALL SKIN TYPES

Our eyes are under constant strain, with overexposure to computer and television screens. **Revitalize** tired eyes with a combination of eyebright, witch hazel, and chamomile. Eyebright and witch hazel have **astringent** properties, which can help to **soothe** eyes at the end of the day and **tone** the delicate eye area. Chamomile works as an **anti-inflammatory**, which can **revitalize** overworked eyes.

MAKES 10ML (2 TSP)

INGREDIENTS

100ml (3½fl oz) mineral water
1 tbsp dried eyebright
1 tbsp dried chamomile flowers
1 tsp witch hazel herbal water
1 tsp glycerin

HOW TO MAKE

1 To make the infusion, boil the mineral water in a saucepan. Place the dried eyebright and chamomile flowers in a teapot or glass bowl and pour over the boiling water. Leave to steep for 10 minutes, then strain.

2 Add the witch hazel herbal water and glycerin to the infusion. Allow to cool. Pour into a sterilized bottle and place the lid on. Store in the fridge. Keeps for up to a week.

HOW TO APPLY

Apply the eye mask to the bones around the eyes (the brow bone and cheekbone). Never apply on the lids or directly under the eyes as the skin there is very delicate. Leave it on the skin for 5 minutes, before removing gently with cotton wool pads, a damp flannel, or muslin cloth.

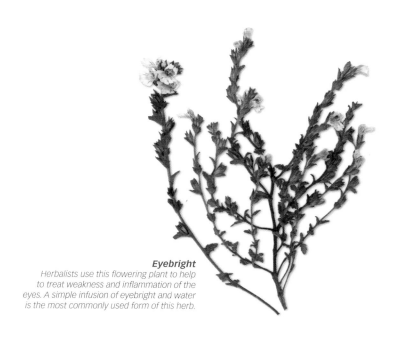

Eyebright
Herbalists use this flowering plant to help to treat weakness and inflammation of the eyes. A simple infusion of eyebright and water is the most commonly used form of this herb.

FACE Get The Look

DON'T BE AFRAID TO EXPERIMENT WITH MAKE-UP.
WITH THE RIGHT COMBINATION OF EASY-TO-LEARN
TECHNIQUES AND GOOD-QUALITY **NATURAL**
COSMETICS, ANYONE CAN **TRANSFORM** THEIR LOOK
OR SIMPLY **ENHANCE** WHAT IS ALREADY THERE.

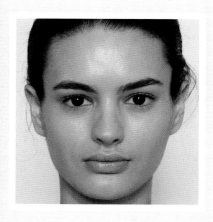 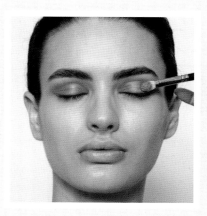 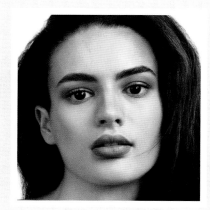

THE MAGIC OF MAKE-UP

Make-up is the ultimate quick fix and a fantastic way to temporarily transform your look. Many of us feel beautiful and confident when we wear make-up. It is possible to define cheekbones, accentuate or open up the eyes, even out the skin tone, and make lips look full or lashes look long. However, learning to love your face without make-up is the first step towards using make-up positively, as a means to bring out the best in your unique self.

POSITIVE MAKE-UP

Studies show that we still live in a world where most of us perceive women who wear make-up to have qualities that are lacking in those who don't wear it, such as greater competency in the workplace, trustworthiness, and likability. These perceptions can push us into tortuous, high-maintenance fixes – fake tan, false lashes, sculpted brows, and big hair – in order to look good. But there are easy, natural ways to look good and wear make-up that do not require hours of application and regular top-ups.

GO ORGANIC

Conventional make-up products are full of synthetic colours and fragrances, and harsh preservatives that can cause skin problems. It's worth investing in organic and natural cosmetics, which avoid these in favour of mineral colours and natural preservatives, such as vitamin E.

KNOW WHEN YOU DON'T NEED IT

Make-up has become such a part of our lives that many of us do not "choose" to wear it, in any real sense of the word. We wear it because we are expected to, or because we think it makes us look better, or because all the other women we know wear it. Make wearing make-up a positive choice. Ask yourself every once in a while: do I really need to wear make-up today?

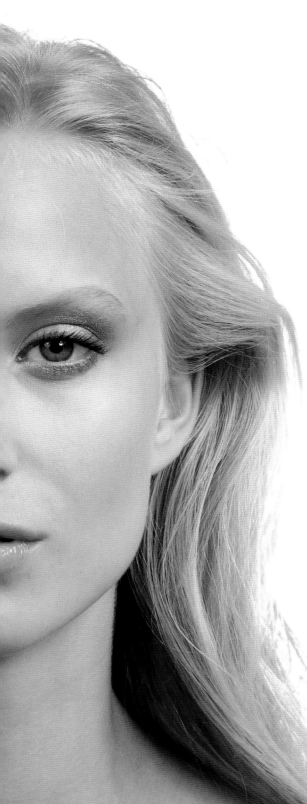

KEEP IT CLEAN

Clean your make-up brushes and other tools regularly to keep them free from harmful bacteria. Replace products regularly (even make-up has a sell-by date) and do not share them with others as this can pass viruses and bacteria from one person to another.

REMOVE MAKE-UP AT NIGHT

It may be tedious, especially if you are tired, but removing make-up is the best thing you can do for your skin, since night-time is when the skin repairs and renews itself. Incorporate a little light massage into your facial cleansing routine to help promote good circulation and enhance the tone and texture of your skin.

AVOID TANNING PRODUCTS

Although you might think that a fake tan is a better option than sunbathing, many products contain dihydroxyacetone (DHA), a chemical that, according to research, accelerates skin-cell death and has the potential to cause genetic alterations and DNA damage.

ACCEPT CHANGES

As you age, your skin tone changes and the colours you wore when you were younger don't look the same. Don't be afraid to refresh your look and palette from time to time to suit these changes. Be aware that too much make-up can make you look older – not younger.

USE MAKE-UP SENSITIVELY

If you have skin problems, the ingredients in your make-up could be the cause. If your skin is irritated and red, spending a few days without make-up can help it to recover faster. Re-introduce products one at a time to determine which products you are reacting to. Do not wear eye make-up if you have an eye infection and once this has cleared up buy new make-up to avoid re-infecting the area.

GET THE LOOK WATER

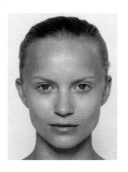

This fantastic daytime look represents water with healthy, dewy skin, and a focus on soft sheens and shimmering textures. Beautifully hydrated skin is essential, so take time to prepare it. For fresh, energized, and truly healthy-looking skin, thoroughly cleanse the skin, then apply a face mask for 10 minutes, followed by a hydrating serum, a moisturiser, and finally a facial oil. Before you begin, apply a flawless foundation base that creates a natural sheen (see pp152–53).

TOOLS

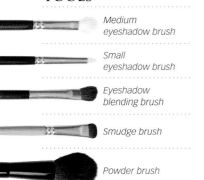

Medium eyeshadow brush

Small eyeshadow brush

Eyeshadow blending brush

Smudge brush

Powder brush

Lip brush

EXPERT TIPS

If you have close-set eyes, the highlight in the inner corner of the eye helps to widen them.

If you've applied too much bronzer, take a dry cotton wool pad and gently buff, removing the excess. Your bronzer should look healthy, not muddy.

If you have mature skin, use products with a very subtle shimmer as high shimmer textures can highlight fine lines.

EYES

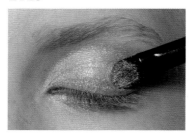

1 HIGHLIGHT Using a medium eyeshadow brush, apply a golden-coloured eyeshadow or cream eyeshadow all over the lid. You may wish to hold a tissue under the eye to stop any shadow from falling onto your cheeks.

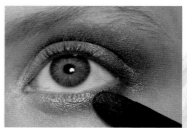

2 CONTOUR Take a small brush and dab a little shadow on the inner corner of the eye and along the lower lash line. Using the first brush, blend a deep gold shadow into the socket, the outer corner of the eye, and the lower lash line.

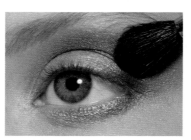

3 BLEND Make sure the two eyeshadow colours blend seamlessly. Take a clean blending brush and using soft, circular movements, blend the hues outwards towards the temple.

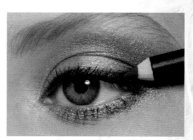

4 DEFINE Take a dark brown or bronze shimmer eyeliner and apply along the upper lash line. Blend using a smudge brush to define the eye. Curl the lashes and apply brown or black mascara.

CHEEKS

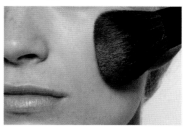

BRONZE The skin should look glowing and sun-kissed. Swirl a powder brush into the product. Tap off any excess. With large circular movements, apply to the skin, starting on the cheeks, then blending into the temples.

LIPS

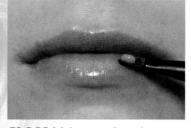

GLOSS Make sure there is no dry skin on your lips by brushing them with a soft toothbrush and applying lip balm. Choose a lip-gloss that is the same colour as your natural lip or just one shade lighter. Apply with a lip brush.

ADAPTING TO YOUR SKIN TONE

Eyeshadow Pale gold and rose gold suit pale skin tones; a more antique gold suits olive skin tones; and rich burnished gold suits darker skin tones.

Bronzer Tawny peach bronzers suit pale skin tones; caramel tones suit olive skin tones; and chestnut bronzers suit dark skin tones.

GET THE LOOK EARTH

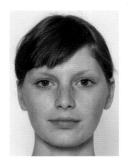

This look draws inspiration from Mother Earth and her "grounded" tones of umber, warm browns, toasted sand, and rich russets. Focus on the contour of the eye and blend well to create soft fluid lines. This look suits everyone, moves seamlessly from day to evening, and is easily adapted. It shouldn't be rushed, so set aside 30 minutes and enjoy some time out. Before you begin, apply a flawless foundation base (see pp152–53).

TOOLS

Blusher brush

Lip brush

Medium eyeshadow brush

Small eyeshadow brush

EXPERT TIPS

If you have deep-set eyes, look straight ahead when you apply the eyeshadow to the socket line. This helps you see where to place the product to "create" your socket. Apply the colour above where your eyelid finishes.

Don't apply too much dark eyeshadow. Load your brush and tap any excess onto the back of your hand. This technique allows you to have greater control over the amount of product you apply.

For a more dramatic look, apply eyeliner to the lower water line (this is the area just inside the eye).

ADAPTING TO YOUR SKIN TONE

Blusher If you are fair, choose a warm peach tone. Amber tones suit brunettes. Choose a rich terracotta for dark skin tones.

Lips The darker your hair and skin tone, the deeper the lip colour can go. A rose or peach colour suits pale skins, and dark skin tones can choose between warm nutty browns, cinnamon, and russet earthy tones.

CHEEKS

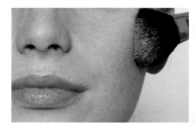

BLUSH Using a blusher brush, apply a warm peach colour to the centre of the cheekbones and blend outwards towards the temple, using soft, round movements.

LIPS

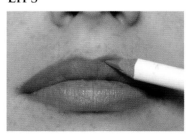

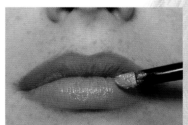

1 LINE Use a nude lip liner to line the lips. Starting at the cupid's bow, trace your natural lip line from the centre outwards. Blend the lip liner with a cotton bud to soften the edges.

2 COLOUR Using a lip brush, apply a peach-coloured lipstick. Blot with a tissue and then re-apply. A clear gloss over the top makes this look more glamorous.

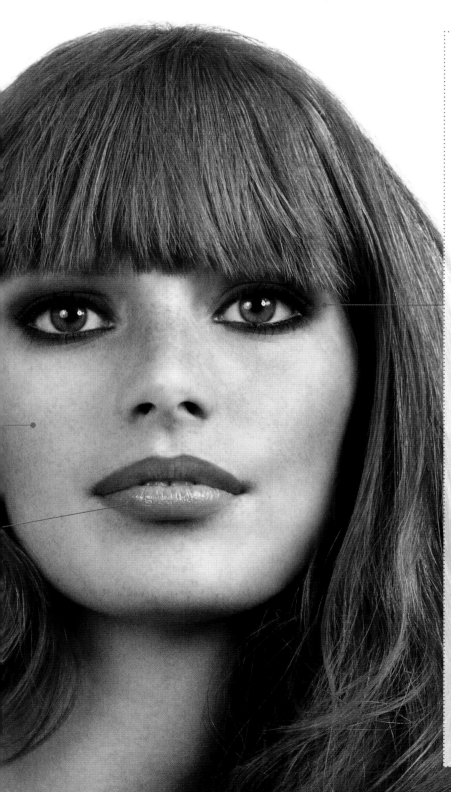

Eyes

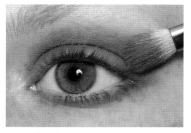

1 BASE Apply a tawny brown shadow over the entire eyelid and up into the socket line using a medium eyeshadow brush. Apply to the lower lash line with a small eyeshadow brush.

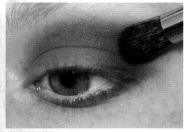

2 CONTOUR Using a medium brush, apply a dark hazelnut shade to the outer corner of the lid and blend into the crease of the socket line. Blend the colours using soft back and forth strokes. Apply dark brown mascara.

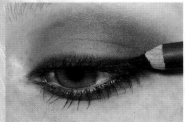

3 LINE Press a dark chocolate eyeliner into the eyelash roots, moving along the upper lash line. Go over this with a precise line, staying close to the lashes. Draw eyeliner along the lower lash line from the outer to the inner corner.

GET THE LOOK AIR

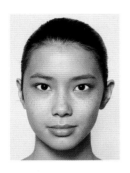

This fresh look requires light make-up. Air make-up is about suggestion and weightlessness, so use very little product and set aside around 10 minutes for crisp and pure results. The look works best with groomed brows, so brush them through with a clean mascara wand or brow brush. Before you begin, apply a foundation base (see pp152–53).

TOOLS

Medium eyeshadow brush

Small eyeshadow brush

Blusher brush

Lip brush

EYES

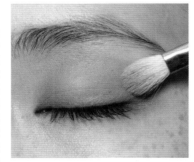

BASE Take a medium eyeshadow brush and apply rose mineral blusher over the eyelids. Blend above the eyelid and into the socket line. Using a smaller brush, apply the colour along the lower lash line.

EXPERT TIPS

To get the brow shape right, place a thin pencil or make-up brush along the side of the nostril, facing upwards, towards the brow. Do not bring the brow further in than this line. Then swing the pencil out from the side of the nostril to the outer corner of your eye. Do not bring the brow further out than where this line hits the brow.

Play with your cosmetics. Mineral blusher isn't the only versatile product. You could pat on a little lipstick on your cheeks as blusher, or use eyeshadow instead of brow powder.

ADAPTING FOR YOUR SKIN TONE

Mineral blusher Soft pink and peach colours work on pale skin tones; rose and tawny browns work well on medium skin tones; and russets, burnt sienna shades, and chestnut suit dark skin tones.

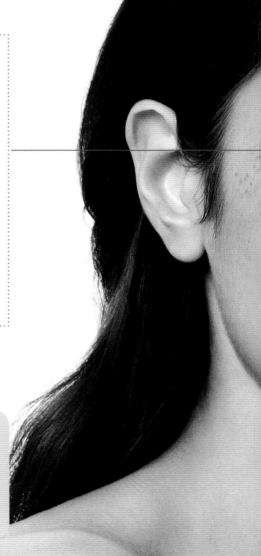

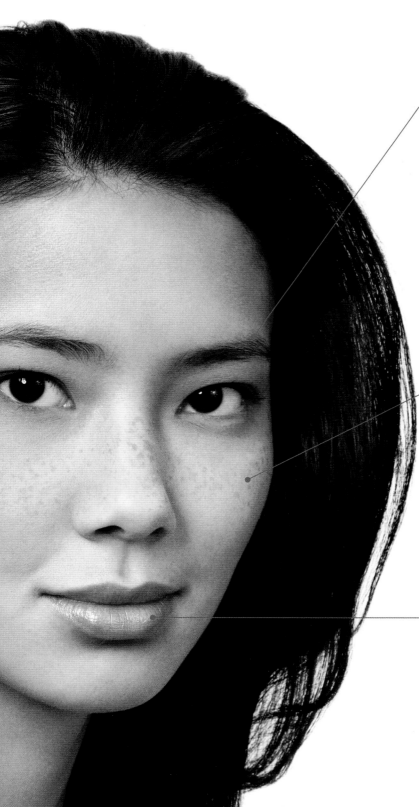

Brows
Where there are gaps in your eyebrows, apply a brow pencil or powder in a shade slightly lighter than your hair colour. A brow pencil gives a precise line. A small angled brush dipped in a brow powder gives a softer look.

CHEEKS

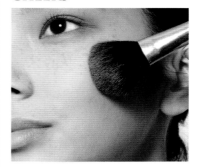

BLUSH Lightly swirl a blusher brush in the same mineral blusher used on the eyes. Tap off the excess. Start off light and build up to a lovely fresh glow. Use soft, circular movements starting in the centre of your cheek and blending back. Avoid getting any product in your hairline.

LIPS

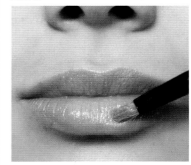

ENHANCE Add a touch of lip balm to help your lips look soft and hydrated. Using a lip brush, apply a pale rose–pink shade of gloss to subtly enhance them, making them look full and moisturised.

GET THE LOOK FIRE

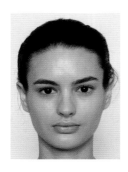

This dynamic and sensuous look focuses on the flaming lips. Rather than the classic brick red, this look explores natural berry tones. The finishing touch is delicately flushed cheeks. Smooth a brightening serum underneath your moisturiser to give the skin extra radiance. For evening wear, simply intensify the tones. Before you begin, apply a foundation base (see pp152–53).

TOOLS

Brow brush

Small angled brush

Medium eyeshadow brush

Small eyeshadow brush

Foundation brush

Lip brush

BROWS

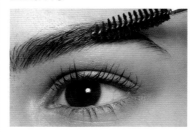

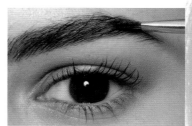

1 GROOM Comb through the brows using a brow brush or soft toothbrush. Hold in place with either brow gel or spritz hairspray onto the brow brush before combing through.

2 FILL IN Fill any gaps in the eyebrow with a small angled brush dipped in eyeshadow that is just a little lighter than your hair colour. Curl lashes and apply black or dark-brown mascara.

EXPERT TIP
If you use a cream blusher, it is best to apply it on top of liquid foundation or tinted moisturiser. Powder afterwards if necessary. A good way to remember this is "cream on cream, powder on powder".

ADAPTING TO YOUR SKIN TONE
Lip stain Medium and dark skin tones work well with rich plum or mulberry lip colours, whereas pale skin suits lighter berry tones.

EYES

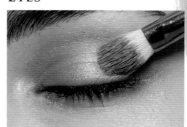

BASE Using a medium eyeshadow brush, apply a cream eyeshadow in taupe to the entire eyelid, blending to the outer corners. Using a small brush, apply along the lower lashes.

CHEEKS

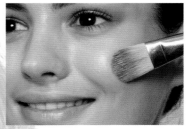

BLUSH Smile in order to find the "apple" of your cheek. Dab a small amount of raspberry cream blusher onto the centre of the "apple" and blend outwards using a foundation brush or your fingers.

LIPS

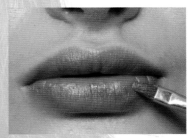

COLOUR Using a lip brush or your fingers, apply a deep berry colour onto the lips to create a "stain". Blot with a tissue.

10-MINUTE FLAWLESS FOUNDATION

The key to an even, flawless foundation is good skin. If you don't take care of your skin, make-up is hard to apply and won't last the day. If you follow a cleanse, tone, and moisturise routine, exfoliate twice a week, and use a mask when you can; you won't need to apply too much foundation and your skin will appear luminous and healthy.

LIQUID

Use an organic foundation to limit the toxins that make contact with your skin. Begin with foundation, blending thoroughly, before you apply concealer, powder, contouring powder, and highlights, if desired (see box, opposite).

THE RIGHT SHADE

Liquid foundation Apply a stripe of foundation along the side of your face and jawline. After a few seconds, if the colour is right for you, it will disappear and blend seamlessly into the skin. Don't be tempted to choose a shade darker than your neck. If you feel you are too pale, use bronzer on the neck and face.
Concealer Choose a concealer that has illuminating ingredients to lift any areas of darkness.
Contouring powder Use a matte powder in cool colours – taupe for pale skin tones, grey–brown for medium tones, and cool chocolate-brown for dark tones.

TOOLS

You need just a few tools to achieve a perfect base using liquid or powder products.

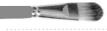
Foundation brush

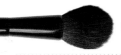
Powder brush

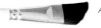
Angled brush

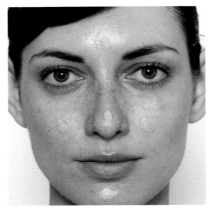

1 Dot a small amount of foundation onto your forehead, nose, chin, and cheeks and begin to blend with a foundation brush. You could also use your fingers or a sponge.

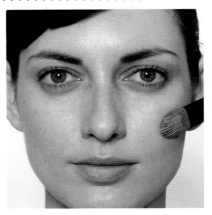

2 Continue to blend. If you find you have applied too much foundation, blot with a clean tissue. By the time you have blended out to the hairline there should be hardly any product left.

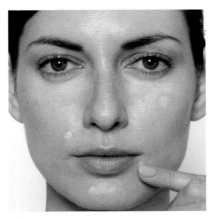

4 To conceal blemishes, use another concealer with a slightly thicker consistency. Apply with your finger, a cotton bud, or a small brush. Blend by patting gently with your ring finger.

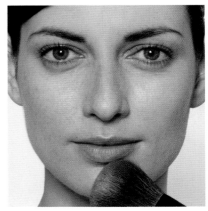

5 Dust lightly with powder where you need it. Most people need it on their T-zone (forehead, nose, and chin). Too much powder shows up fine lines and wrinkles, so use it sparingly.

HIGHLIGHTING

Emphasize the cheekbones, the inner corner of the eyes, the browbone, and the cupid's bow of the lips using a little highlighting powder that has a satin sheen. Beware that highlighting may accentuate fine lines and wrinkles.

MINERAL POWDER

Free from harmful ingredients, mineral powders adhere to the natural oils in the skin, allowing it to breathe. They are perfect for sensitive skin and won't irritate acne-prone skin. Before you apply the powder, moisturise your face, then wait a few minutes for the lotion to sink in. Follow this sequence with contours and highlights, if desired.

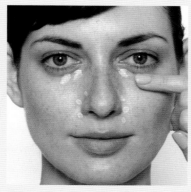

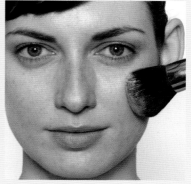

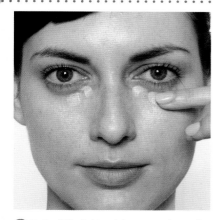

3 Dot a little lightweight concealer under the eye from the inner corner to three-quarters of the way across. Pat with the ring finger until the product blends seamlessly. Apply more if needed, but not too much or eyes can look puffy and dry.

1 Conceal blemishes and circles under the eyes, as shown in steps 3 and 4 opposite. To use mineral powder concealer, tap a little in the lid. Swirl a brush in the product, tap off excess, and gently sweep over the areas.

2 Mineral foundation goes a long way, so start by pouring only a little powder into the product lid. Swirl a large, dense powder brush in the powder. Tap off excess and sweep the brush on the cheekbone.

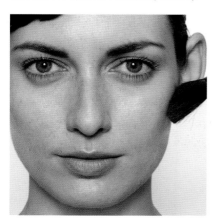

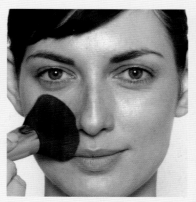

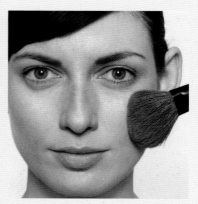

6 Use an angled brush to sweep contouring powder under the cheekbones. Stop directly below the outer corner of your eyes, otherwise it may look "muddy". Blend well. Finish by brushing on highlights, if desired (see box, above).

3 Using large, round swirling movements, buff the brush over your cheek all the way up to your forehead. Buff the other cheek, then down the nose and chin. The more you buff the greater the coverage.

4 Mineral foundation has a radiant sheen. If you have oily skin or think it looks reflective, use a setting powder for a matte finish. Dip a powder brush into a pressed or loose powder, tap off excess, and apply where necessary.

GET THE LOOK METAL

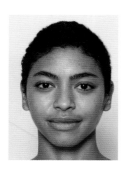

Metal's mutability and reflective properties create intense make-up looks. This is an easy, adaptable, and contemporary look. The skin is natural and fresh, and the eyes are bold. Hydrate your skin but don't allow it to get too dewy otherwise there will be too much shine. Metallic eyeshadow may drop onto the skin, and it is tricky to remove without disturbing your make-up, so apply it before your foundation (see pp152–53).

TOOLS

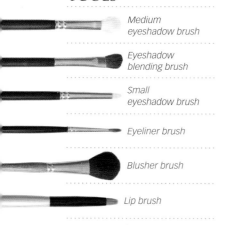

Medium
eyeshadow brush

Eyeshadow
blending brush

Small
eyeshadow brush

Eyeliner brush

Blusher brush

Lip brush

EXPERT TIPS

While applying eyeliner and mascara, look down into a mirror to make application easier. Use a cotton bud dipped in eye make-up remover to wipe off any mistakes.

If you have close-set eyes, don't add any black eyeliner. Instead use a cream kohl eyeliner to open up the eye.

EYES

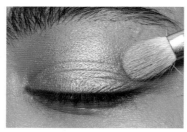

1 COLOUR Using a medium eyeshadow brush, apply a metallic copper shade over the lids, up to the socket line. Apply a deeper copper onto the outer corners of the eye. Blend using an eyeshadow blending brush.

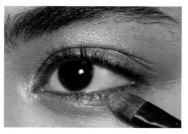

2 LASH LINE Apply the copper colour along the lower lash line and into the inner corner of the eye using a small eyeshadow brush. If you do not have a small brush, use a cotton bud.

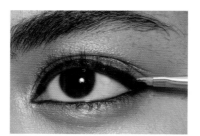

3 DEFINE Apply a kohl black pencil along the lower inner waterline. Dip an eyeliner brush into a black gel liner. Wipe the brush against your hand to remove excess. Trace along the roots of the upper lash line.

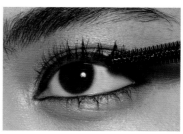

4 LASHES For curly lashes, use eyelash curlers. Apply black mascara. Wiggle the wand across the lashes from root to tip. Blink onto your finger to remove excess, then apply a second coat.

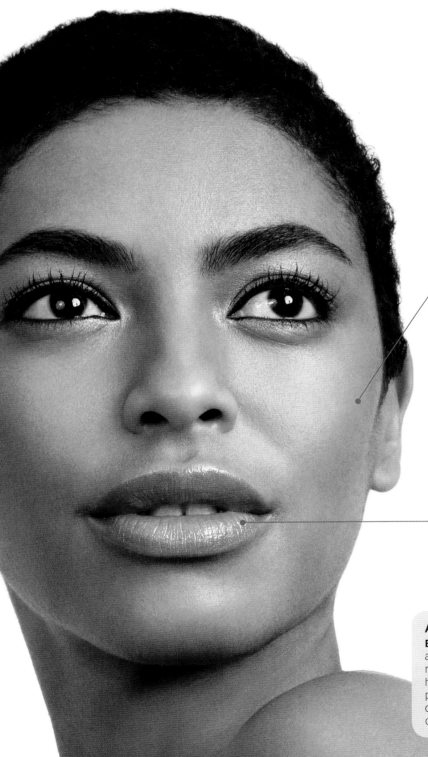

CHEEKS

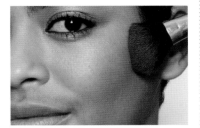

BLUSH Dip a blusher brush into a warm golden bronze shade and tap off any excess. Start lightly and gradually build up. Buff the blusher into the apples of your cheeks, blending out towards the temples.

LIPS

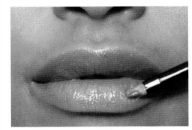

GLOSS Using a lip brush, glide a rose gold, copper, or bronze gloss along the lips. You can also use a lipstick mixed with a lip balm, which will create a similar effect.

ADAPTING TO YOUR SKIN TONE

Eyeshadow Mature skins work better with a slight sheen texture rather than highly reflective metallics, as the latter tend to highlight wrinkles and fine lines. Rose and pale gold look great on pale skin tones, while darker tones work beautifully with rich golds, coppers, and pewters.

GET THE LOOK WOOD

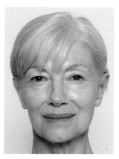

This is a sophisticated look, inspired by walking in the woods. Nature showcases an abundance of colours, yet at the same time the palette is subtle. This look uses neutral, muted tones which softly define and contour the eyes. Before you begin, apply liquid or mineral foundation, conceal under-eye dark circles and blemishes, and lightly powder (see pp152–53).

TOOLS

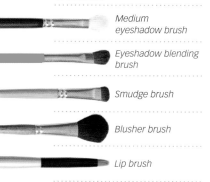

Medium eyeshadow brush

Eyeshadow blending brush

Smudge brush

Blusher brush

Lip brush

EXPERT TIPS

If you wish to create more definition, contour under the cheek bones using an angled brush and contouring powder. Mature women could contour along the jawline to disguise any slackening of the skin.

If you overdo the blusher, gently remove it with a cotton wool pad or apply a thin layer of foundation over the top.

If there is a harsh line of lip liner beneath your lipstick, buff and blend in the lip liner with a dry, clean lip brush.

EYES

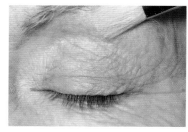

1 HIGHLIGHT Using a medium eyeshadow brush, apply a pale highlighter to the brow bone and dot it into the inner corners of the eye. This opens up and lifts the eye.

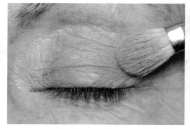

2 BASE Using a medium eyeshadow brush, apply medium beige-coloured eyeshadow all over the eyelid. Hold a tissue under the eye to catch any fallen shadow.

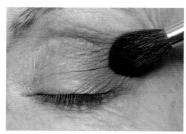

3 CONTOUR Take a charcoal grey or brown eyeshadow and work it into your socket line and into the outer corners of the eye. Blend using an eyeshadow blending brush.

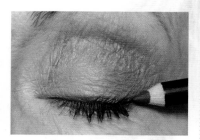

4 DEFINE Using a grey–brown pencil, draw along the upper lash line. Dot the liner on the lower lashes, from the outer corner to three-quarters of the way in. Blend the liner with a smudge brush. Curl lashes and apply mascara.

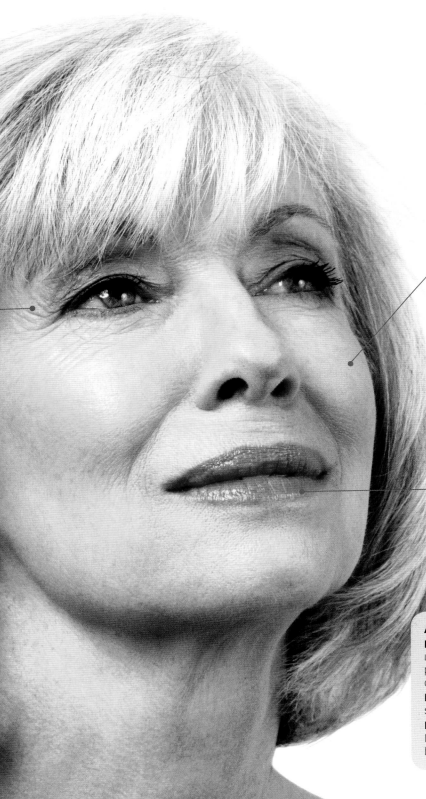

CHEEKS

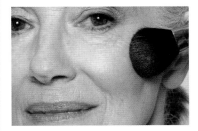

BLUSH Dip a blusher brush into a soft pink or coral blush and tap off any excess. Start lightly and gradually build up. Buff the blusher into the apples of your cheeks, blending out towards the temples.

LIPS

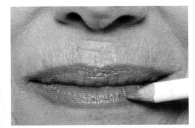

COLOUR Line the lips using a tawny brown or peach lip liner – starting at the cupid's bow, trace your lip line from the centre outwards. Using a lip brush, apply lipstick of the same colour over the top.

ADAPTING TO YOUR SKIN TONE

Eyeshadow To contour your eye make-up, use charcoal grey or brown eyeshadow for pale and medium skin tones, and deep-coffee colours for dark skin tones.

Blusher Choose a soft pink or coral for pale skin, or a warm bronze for dark skin tones.

Lip colour Use a tawny brown or peach lip liner for a pale skin tone, and rich chestnut-brown colours for medium-to-dark skin tones.

BODY

YOU DON'T NEED TO GO TO AN EXPENSIVE SPA TO ENJOY REVIVING AND **REVITALIZING** TREATMENTS. **PAMPER** YOURSELF WITH SIMPLE TECHNIQUES AND CREAMS, OILS, AND **NATURAL** EXTRACTS THAT LIFT THE SPIRIT, **NOURISH** YOUR SKIN, AND MAKE YOU FEEL GOOD ALL OVER.

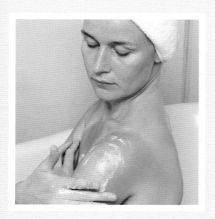
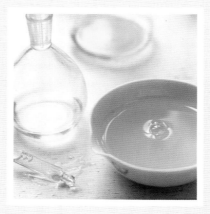
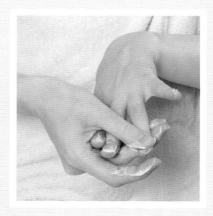

YOUR PAMPERING PACKAGE

We all need an indulgent night in every once in a while. Taking time out for regular pampering treatments helps you to feel great and improves the look and feel of your skin and hair. Create some quiet time where you can have the bathroom to yourself, and treat your body to an hour of pampering bliss and your mind to some valuable relaxation time. Tailor this pampering package according to your mood. You can start with a head massage and/or spa facial, or go straight to pages 164–65 for a full-body pampering session in the bath.

WHAT DO YOU NEED?

For an evening of blissed-out treatments, keep these items within easy reach.

EQUIPMENT

- Muslin cloth or flannel
- Cotton wool pads
- Hair band (optional)
- Tissues
- Foundation brush (optional)

PRODUCTS

- Conditioning hair oil, such as argan or coconut oil
- Facial oil, such as frankincense or orange flower
- Cleanser
- Toner
- Exfoliating facial polish
- Mask
- Eye cream or gel
- Body moisturiser
- Hand cream

HEAD MASSAGE

An ancient proverb states: "a healthy mind is medicine; no better prescription exists." The head, neck, and shoulders are an important energy centre within your body. If you are stressed or angry, tension can accumulate. Regular head massage can work to relieve the build-up of tension. It is a wonderfully relaxing treatment and can enhance the health of the scalp and promote hair growth.

Change into a dressing gown or wrap a towel around you, remove jewellery, and sit comfortably with your feet flat on the floor, shoulders back, and eyes closed. Breathe deeply in and out through the nose 3 times.

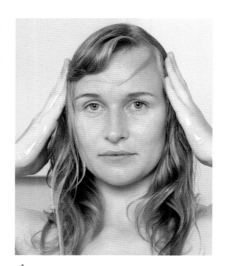

1 Pour oil into the palms and rub your hands together to warm the oil. Smooth the oil into the hair, starting at the top and working down the sides, then moving towards the front and the back.

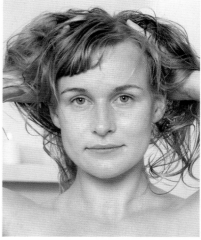

2 Once you have covered the whole head with oil, distributing it evenly, gently massage the whole of the head with thumbs and fingers in a simple shampooing motion.

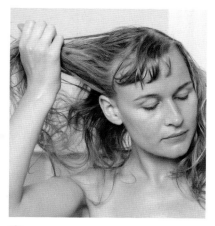

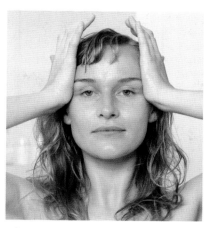

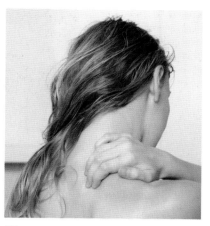

3 Grasp fistfuls of hair at the roots and gently tug from side to side, keeping the knuckles close to the scalp. This invigorates the hair roots.

4 Squeeze your temples with the heel of the hands or the fingertips and make slow, circular movements. Close your eyes and breathe deeply.

5 Massage the back of the neck by squeezing and rolling the muscles. Start at the top of the neck and work your way down. Repeat this movement 3 times.

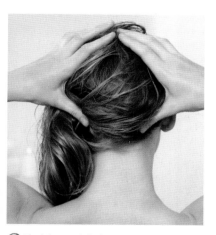

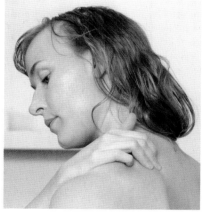

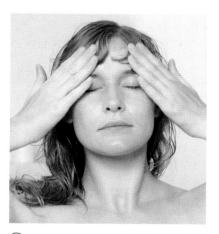

6 Find the occipital area at the back of the head. Place the left thumb under the left occipital area (see box below) and the right thumb under the right occipital area. Rub to release the muscles.

7 Place your right hand on your left shoulder, near the base of the neck, and squeeze. Work your way outwards along the shoulder and down the arm to the elbow. Repeat on the other side.

8 Rub your fingertips lightly all over the head and face. Relax for 5 minutes, before drinking a glass of water to hydrate.

WHAT IS THE OCCIPITAL AREA?

The occipital bone forms most of the back portion of the skull. It has a large opening where the spinal cord links with the brain. The occipital area is often the site of pain and "tension headaches". Mobility of the muscles in this area with gentle massage can help to ease headaches and relieve pain.

NEXT...

Either wash out the oil using your usual shampoo or, to extend your pampering session, wrap your hair in a warm towel and indulge in a spa facial (over the page) and/or a full-body pamper in the bath (see pp164–65). The oil will continue to give your hair an intense, nourishing treatment.

SPA FACIAL

Turn on some soothing music, pour yourself a glass of cold water, and settle into a relaxing facial that will rejuvenate your skin. Use your favourite natural skin-care products, referring to the instructions carefully. Before you start, gather all the products and equipment. If your hair isn't already wrapped in a warm towel, pull your hair away from your face with a hair band.

1 PREPARE

Wash your hands. Place a towel over your lap so you can use it to wipe off any excess product. Sitting comfortably with your feet flat on the floor in front of a mirror, pour 3 drops of facial oil into the palm of your hand, rub palms together, and hold over the nose. Close your eyes and take 3 deep breaths to relax.

2 CLEANSE

Apply a cleanser to your fingertips and massage into the skin with small, circular movements, paying attention to the chin, forehead, and around the nose. Start under the jaw and work up towards the eye area. Remove the cleanser with warm water and a muslin cloth or flannel. Start at the forehead and finish under the jaw.

3 TONE

Apply a cooling toner to 2 cotton wool pads. With a cotton pad in each hand, sweep the toner up over the jaw, across the chin, up your cheeks, and across the forehead. Leave the toner on your skin for a few minutes to evaporate or soak in.

4 EXFOLIATE

5 APPLY A MASK

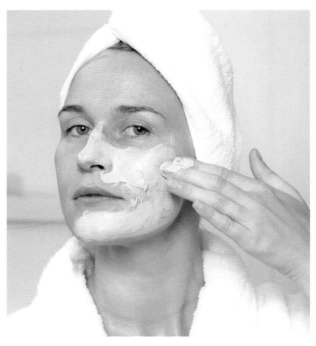

Apply an exfoliating face polish to your fingertips and gently massage it into the skin using small, circular movements. Start with the jaw and finish with the forehead, paying attention to the chin, forehead, and the area around your nose. Avoid the delicate eye area. Remove the exfoliator with warm water and a muslin cloth or flannel. Repeating step 3, remove traces of your exfoliating face polish with toner on 2 cotton pads, sweeping up over the jaw to the forehead.

Apply a mask to your face with the fingertips or a clean foundation brush, starting with the jaw and moving up to the forehead, leaving the eyes free from product. Leave on according to the manufacturer's directions (about 10 minutes). In the meantime, apply your eye product (see step 6).

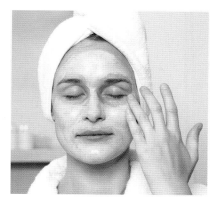

6 APPLY EYE CREAM OR GEL

Gently pat an eye cream or gel around the eyes using your ring finger, without getting too close to the eyes. Afterwards, soak 2 cotton wool pads in cold water and place over the eyes. Relax for 5 minutes. Remove the eye pads and replace the cold water with fresh warm water. Relax for another 2 minutes.

7 RINSE

Gently remove all traces of the mask with clean warm water. Swipe a muslin cloth or flannel across the face, avoiding the delicate eye area. Dab gently with a clean towel to dry the skin – it is important that the skin is completely dry before you apply the massage oil. Make sure you thoroughly rinse the mask from the muslin cloth or flannel before you use it again.

8 MASSAGE

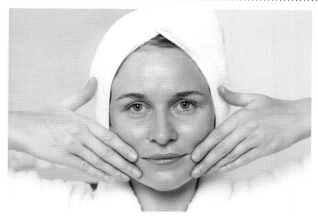

1. Apply a facial oil to your fingertips. Warm it between the hands and sweep up the face from the jaw, around the eyes, and up over the forehead. Repeat 3 times.

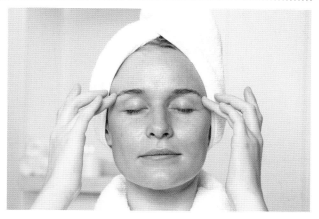

2. Using your ring fingers, gently draw spectacles around the eyes, starting from between the eyes and working out towards the ears. Repeat 3 times.

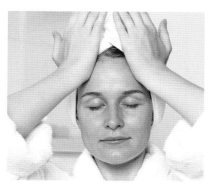

3. Gently pinch the eyebrows, starting from between the eyes. Using flat palms and a firm pressure, iron the forehead from brow to hairline.

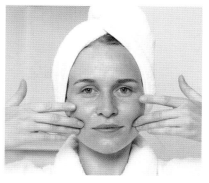

4. Sweep your fingertips up the face from the jaw, around the eyes, and over the forehead. Repeat 3 times. Blot excess oil with a tissue.

9 REHYDRATE

Apply a small amount of face cream, starting at the jaw and moving up to the forehead. Drink a large glass of water or a cold infusion to rehydrate and relax.

NEXT
Extend your pampering evening by running a bath and giving your whole body a treat (over the page)....

FULL-BODY PAMPER

Give yourself a top-to-toe pampering. This routine works just as well in the shower if you don't have a bath. Pour yourself your favourite drink and set the scene by lighting some candles in the bathroom. Run the bath and add a bath soak or your favourite bath product. Place all your products within close reach. If you have already treated yourself to a head massage (see pp160–161) and/or a spa facial (see pp162–63), skip to step 2, and get straight into the bath.

1 PREPARE

Cleanse your face. Apply a deep conditioning mask to your hair. Massage the mask into the scalp for 5 minutes, then wrap your hair in a warm towel.

2 SOAK

Get into the bath and relax for 10 minutes. If you haven't given yourself a spa facial, apply a face mask. Remove it after 10 minutes, using a flannel or muslin cloth.

3 EXFOLIATE

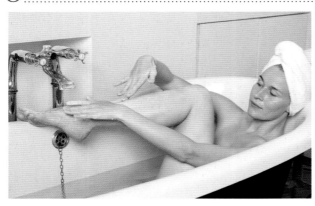

1. Apply a small amount of exfoliator to your fingertips and massage the heels. Massage your exfoliator into the skin in an upwards direction, towards the heart.

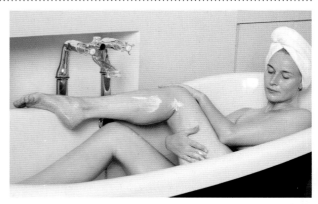

2. Move up your legs, increasing the pressure as you circulate your fingertips on the thighs and other areas prone to cellulite.

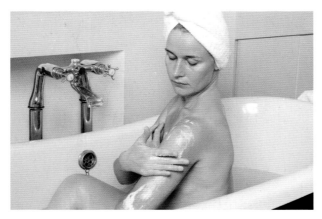

3. Exfoliate the elbows and the backs of the arms, moving up towards your shoulders.

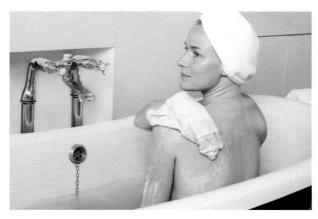

4. Using a muslin cloth wrapped around your hand, exfoliate the top of your back using large, circular movements.

4 RINSE

Rinse off the product in the bath, ensuring that all the scrub particles are rinsed off the skin. Moving slowly, step out of the bath and dry yourself using a warm towel.

5 APPLY SHAMPOO

Unless you wish to keep the hair oil or mask on for hours to give your hair even more of a treat, wash it off now. You can wash out the oil using your normal shampoo or remove your mask according to manufacturer's instructions.

6 MOISTURISE BODY

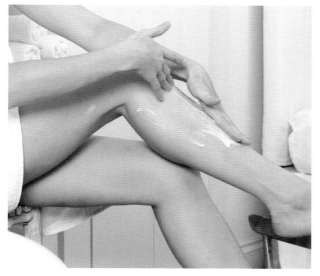

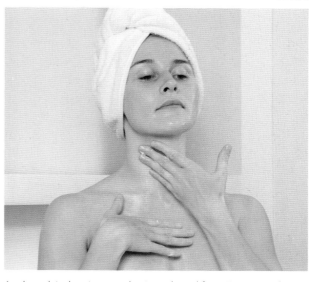

Hydrate and soften the skin by applying lotion all over your body, using strokes in an upwards direction. Put on a bathrobe and apply foot cream, paying attention to hard skin.

Apply moisturiser to your chest, neck, and face. Use upward strokes from your neck up to your forehead and pat it in with light, even pressure and gentle movements.

7 MOISTURISE HANDS

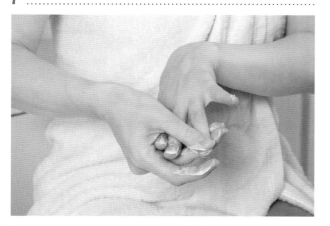

Apply hand cream to your hands, working it into the cuticles and nails. Relax for an hour. Drink plenty of water.

WHY MASSAGE?

Evidence suggests that the more massage you allow yourself to have, the better you will feel. A massage is healing, de-stressing, relaxing, and can help improve recovery from injury. The benefits of a massage include increased circulation, which enables the body to pump more oxygen and nutrients to vital organs and tissues; stimulation of the flow of lymph, the body's natural defence system; reduction of spasms and cramping; relaxation of overused and injured muscles; and increased joint flexibility and mobility. It can also help to reduce scar tissue.

Relax for at least an hour after your full-body pamper, drinking plenty of water to hydrate the skin and flush out toxins.

RECIPES FOR YOUR BODY

REVITALIZE THE WHOLE BODY WITH A WIDE RANGE OF PRODUCTS. MAKE EASY **NATURAL** SCRUBS AND MOISTURISERS THAT **REFRESH** AND **HYDRATE** YOUR SKIN. LEARN HOW TO MAKE SIMPLE BATH AND SHOWER PRODUCTS THAT NOT ONLY **CLEANSE** AND **NOURISH** THE SKIN, BUT ALSO **RELAX** AND REVIVE BOTH THE BODY AND MIND.

HONEY AND ORANGE SOAP

FOR ALL SKIN TYPES

Combine **soothing** honey and **refreshing** orange essential oil in this **moisturising** soap. Before you begin, make sure you are in a well-ventilated area. Always wear protective gloves during the making process, especially when handling sodium hydroxide. Make sure the pH of the soap is below 10, as this ensures it is safe. If you cannot find organic palm oil, you could replace it with coconut or olive oil.

MAKES A 800G (1¾LB) BATCH OF SOAP

INGREDIENTS
175g (6oz) solid palm oil
470g (1lb 1oz) solid coconut oil
150ml (5fl oz) olive oil
1 tsp honey

For the lye
115g (4oz) sodium hydroxide
20 drops orange essential oil
5 drops benzoin tincture

HOW TO MAKE

1 Heat both solid oils together in a bain-marie (see p133), until they have melted. Remove from the heat. Add the olive oil and honey, and mix well.

2 Begin the lye process, as shown in the step-by-step below.

3 Once you have poured the soap mixture into a large greased baking tray, wrap with cling film and cover with towels to insulate.

4 As the chemical reaction occurs, the soap will enter a "gel phase". The soap will become transparent and dark in the centre. The gel will spread to the edge of the soap as the chemical reaction continues to work.

5 When the gel reaches the edge of the soap, after 2–3 hours, unwrap the tray. When soft, remove the soap and cut into bars. Arrange on trays to cure, dry, and harden. This will take 4 weeks. Check the pH of the final soap before using. Store in a cool, dark place. Keeps for up to 6 months.

HOW TO APPLY

Lather on your hands or body, and rinse.

THE LYE PROCESS

Soap is the result of mixing an acid (vegetable fat/oil) with a caustic alkali (sodium hydroxide). Once the alkali is diluted with water to create a lye, it is added to the acid, and a reaction occurs. The alkali is neutralized during this reaction. After curing, the soap will no longer contain any sodium hydroxide.

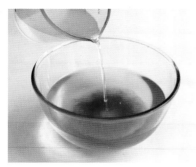

1 Mix the sodium hydroxide, 200ml (7fl oz) water, the essential oil, and tincture together. Pour into the melted oil mixture, stirring continuously.

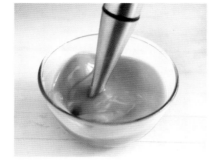

2 Mix with a stick blender. The soap mixture will thicken and become more like batter. The lye mixture begins to heat up as part of the chemical process.

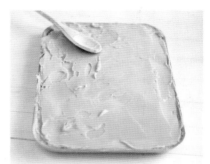

3 When the mixture reaches "trace" – or when a spoonful leaves a pattern when drizzled – slowly pour the mixture into a greased baking tray.

MELT-AND-POUR SOAP

QUICK

FOR ALL SKIN TYPES

The easiest and safest way to make soap is to use a ready-made melt-and-pour base, where the lye process has already been prepared. Go for an organic-certified base, which is usually available in 1kg (2¼lb) blocks. Use a safe dilution of essential oil to base product, following the ratio below as a guide.

MAKES 100G (3½ OZ)

INGREDIENTS

100g (3½ oz) melt-and-pour soap base
20–30 drops essential oil, if desired
pinch dried herbs, if desired

HOW TO MAKE

1 Cut the melt-and-pour soap base into cubes. Gently heat in a bain-marie (see p133), until melted.

2 Add the essential oil and dried herbs if using, and mix well.

3 Grease the soap moulds using spray oil. Pour the mixture into the moulds.

4 Leave to cool for 1–2 hours. Turn out the soaps from the moulds when cool. Store in a cool, dark place. Keeps for up to 6 months.

HOW TO APPLY

Lather on your hands or body, and rinse.

LEMON AND CORIANDER BODY BAR

MULTI-PURPOSE

FOR ALL SKIN TYPES

Make yourself a **nourishing** body bar using up any leftover pieces of bar soap. This recipe combines **moisturising** shea nut butter and glycerin with the **refreshing** scent of lemon and coriander essential oils, to **invigorate** and **energize** the skin.

MAKES ONE 85G (3OZ) BODY BAR

INGREDIENTS

1 tbsp shea nut butter
3 tbsp mineral water
1 tbsp grated bar soap
1 tsp glycerin
1 tsp honey
10 drops lemon essential oil
10 drops coriander essential oil

HOW TO MAKE

1 Melt the butter in a bain-marie (see p133).

2 Heat the mineral water in a saucepan and bring to the boil. Add the grated bar soap and continue to heat until the soap has dissolved. Add the glycerin, honey, and essential oils, and mix well.

3 Add the melted butter to the hot water mixture. Pour into a greased mould and leave to cool for 1–2 hours. Store in a cool, dark place. Keeps for up to 6 months.

HOW TO APPLY

Lather the body bar over your body in the shower or bath. It may also be used as a shaving balm.

WARMING BODY BUTTER

FOR ALL SKIN TYPES

This rich and creamy **warming** body butter contains **nourishing** cocoa butter and **skin-softening** beeswax. The combination of ginger, black pepper, and rosemary essential oils helps to increase the circulation, bringing warmth and **pain relief** to the skin. It's perfect for giving tired muscles a treat.

MAKES 100G (3½OZ)

INGREDIENTS

1 tbsp comfrey macerated oil
1 tsp cocoa butter
1 tsp beeswax
60ml (2fl oz) mineral water
1 tsp glycerin
1 tbsp emulsifying wax
2 drops ginger essential oil
2 drops black pepper essential oil
2 drops lavender essential oil
1 drop rosemary essential oil

HOW TO MAKE

1 Create an emulsion (see p109) by melting the oil, butter, and beeswax together in a bain-marie. Remove from the heat once the wax has melted.

2 Heat the mineral water in a saucepan to 80°C (175°F). Add the glycerin and emulsifying wax to the water and stir until dissolved. Add the hot oil mixture to the hot water mixture. Using a hand-held whisk or a stick blender, whisk continuously until smooth.

3 Add the essential oils and continue to stir occasionally as the mixture cools. Pour into a sterilized jar and place a lid on. Store in a cool, dry place or in the fridge. Keeps for up to 6 weeks.

HOW TO APPLY

Apply to the body with upward-sweeping movements. Pay particular attention to the areas where increased circulation is required, and if using after exercise, to the muscles and joints that have been stretched.

RICH SHEA BODY BUTTER

FOR DRY SKIN

Shea butter contains high levels of essential fatty acids and antioxidants, which lend themselves to **repairing** damaged skin. This **nourishing** body butter contains rosehip oil, which helps to even skin tone, along with hemp seed oil, which helps improve skin **elasticity**.

MAKES 100G (3½OZ)

INGREDIENTS

1 tsp rosehip oil
2 tsp hemp oil
1 tbsp shea nut butter
1 tsp beeswax
60ml (2fl oz) mineral water
1 tsp glycerin
1 tbsp emulsifying wax
6 drops jasmine essential oil
3 drops lemon essential oil
3 drops sandalwood essential oil

HOW TO MAKE

1 Create an emulsion (see p109) by melting the oils, butter, and beeswax together in a bain-marie. Remove from the heat once the wax has melted.

2 Heat the mineral water in a saucepan to 80°C (175°F). Add the glycerin and emulsifying wax to the water and stir until dissolved. Add the hot oil mixture to the hot water mixture. Using a hand-held whisk or a stick blender, whisk continuously until smooth.

3 Add the essential oils and continue to stir occasionally as the mixture cools. Pour into a sterilized jar and place a lid on. Store in a cool, dry place or in the fridge. Keeps for up to 6 weeks.

HOW TO APPLY

Apply all over the body with upward-sweeping movements. Pay particular attention to any dry patches.

5-IN-1 BODY BALM

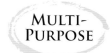

MULTI-
PURPOSE

FOR ALL SKIN TYPES

This all-purpose balm contains jojoba oil that keeps the skin moisturised, **enriching** shea butter that **softens** and **moisturises**, and cocoa butter that makes skin feel silky **smooth** and locks moisture into dry skin. Put it in your gym bag as the "one product that does all". Use as a lip balm, to tame flyaway hair, on cracked heels, knuckles, or elbows, and on cuticles. Add essential oils of your choice.

MAKES 100G (3½OZ)

INGREDIENTS

3 tbsp jojoba oil

2 tbsp solid coconut oil

1 tbsp cocoa butter

2 tsp beeswax

10 drops essential oil, such as peppermint, lavender, myrrh, neroli, or orange (optional)

HOW TO MAKE

1 Melt the oils, butter, and beeswax together in a bain-marie (see p133). Remove from the heat once the wax has melted.

2 If desired, add the essential oil of your choice to the mixture.

3 Pour into a sterilized jar and leave to cool and set before placing the lid on. Store in a cool, dry place. Keeps for up to 6 weeks.

HOW TO APPLY

Massage into the skin, all over the body, paying particular attention to any dry areas. A small amount of balm will go a long way. Use as a lip balm, an eyebrow tamer, or for cracked heels, dry elbows, or split ends.

COCOA BUTTER BODY CREAM

FOR ALL SKIN TYPES

This sweetly fragranced cream combines cocoa butter and coconut oil with vanilla and orange to leave the skin feeling **nourished**, silky **smooth**, and beautifully fragranced. Cocoa butter melts at body temperature and penetrates the skin, leaving it with a smooth and silky finish. Combined with **skin-softening** coconut oil and vitamin E-rich sunflower oil, this is a rich and creamy treat for the skin.

MAKES 100G (3½OZ)

INGREDIENTS

1 tbsp cocoa butter

1 tsp coconut oil

1 tsp sunflower oil

60ml (2fl oz) mineral water

1 tbsp emulsifying wax

1 tsp glycerin

5 drops vanilla extract

2 drops benzoin tincture

2 drops mandarin essential oil

5 drops sweet orange essential oil

HOW TO MAKE

1 Create an emulsion (see p109) by melting the butter and oils together in a bain-marie. Remove from the heat when the butter has melted.

2 Heat the mineral water in a saucepan to 80°C (175°F). Add the emulsifying wax and glycerin, and stir until the wax is fully dissolved.

3 Add the hot oil mixture to the hot water mixture. Using a hand-held whisk or a stick blender, whisk continuously until smooth.

4 Add the vanilla extract, benzoin tincture, and essential oils, and mix until smooth.

5 Pour into a sterilized jar and leave to cool before placing the lid on. Store in a cool, dry place. Keeps for up to 6 weeks.

HOW TO APPLY

Apply all over the body with upward-sweeping movements, paying particular attention to any dry patches.

TONING BODY CREAM

FOR ALL SKIN TYPES

Deeply **moisturise** the skin with this cream, restoring its **suppleness**, **tone**, and **texture**. This cream can improve lymphatic drainage – this helps to **relieve** the accumulation of water and toxic waste that can lead to cellulite. The essential oils don't just smell sweet and fruity – orange is known to **stimulate** lymph fluids, mandarin can help to **prevent stretch marks**, and cypress oil has an **astringent** effect.

MAKES 100G (3½OZ)

INGREDIENTS

1 tbsp cocoa butter
1 tsp coconut oil
1 tsp rosehip oil
1 tsp avocado oil
1 tbsp emulsifying wax
60ml (2fl oz) mineral water
1 tsp glycerin
1 tsp witch hazel water
5 drops mandarin essential oil
4 drops orange essential oil
4 drops frankincense essential oil
2 drops clary sage essential oil
2 drops cypress essential oil

HOW TO MAKE

1 Create an emulsion (see p109) by melting the butter, oils, and emulsifying wax together in a bain-marie. Remove from the heat once the wax has melted.

2 Heat the mineral water in a saucepan to 80ºC (175ºF). Add the glycerin and witch hazel water, and stir well. You may need to re-heat the water if not dissolved completely.

3 Add the hot oil mixture to the hot water mixture. Using a hand-held whisk or a stick blender, whisk continuously until smooth.

4 Add the essential oils and continue to mix until you have a smooth cream. Pour into a sterilized jar and leave to cool before placing the lid on. Store in a cool, dry place. Keeps for up to 6 weeks.

HOW TO APPLY

Apply all over the body with upward-sweeping movements, paying particular attention to any dry patches. Use in combination with dry body brushing (see pp174–75).

Combat Your Cellulite

Most women suffer from cellulite at some point in their life. It is caused by the accumulation of water and toxic waste in the connective tissue surrounding fat cells. There are many contributing factors to cellulite formation, such as poor blood circulation, hormonal imbalance, unbalanced diet, coffee, tea, cigarettes, lack of exercise, and constipation. Improving your diet and taking regular exercise should improve its appearance, as well as applying this toning, moisturising cream.

PEPPERMINT AND SEA SALT INVIGORATING BODY SCRUB

FOR ALL SKIN TYPES

This **invigorating** body scrub gives skin a very firm scrub that can remove dead skin cells, **revive** the circulation, and leave skin silky smooth. Grapefruit essential oil is a lymphatic stimulant with diuretic and **detoxifying** properties that may help with water retention and cellulite. If you want a less abrasive scrub, use table salt instead of sea salt. You could also replace the fresh mint with dried.

INGREDIENTS

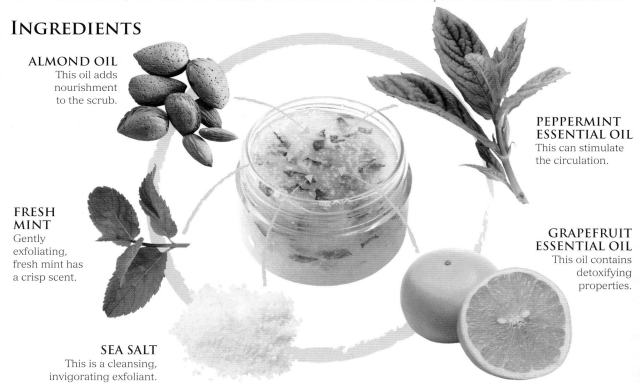

ALMOND OIL
This oil adds nourishment to the scrub.

PEPPERMINT ESSENTIAL OIL
This can stimulate the circulation.

FRESH MINT
Gently exfoliating, fresh mint has a crisp scent.

GRAPEFRUIT ESSENTIAL OIL
This oil contains detoxifying properties.

SEA SALT
This is a cleansing, invigorating exfoliant.

MAKES 100ML (3½FL OZ)

INGREDIENTS

4 tbsp sea salt
1 tsp fresh mint
4 tbsp almond oil
5 drops peppermint essential oil
2 drops grapefruit essential oil

HOW TO MAKE

1 Place the sea salt, mint, and almond oil in a bowl.
2 Add the essential oils and mix together to make the scrub. Transfer to an airtight container and store in a cool, dry place. Keeps for up to 6 months.

HOW TO APPLY

Rub into the skin, massaging into any areas of sluggish circulation. Rinse off in the shower or in the bath – as the sea salt dissolves in water, you can enjoy a relaxing mineral bath. Do not use on freshly shaved skin.

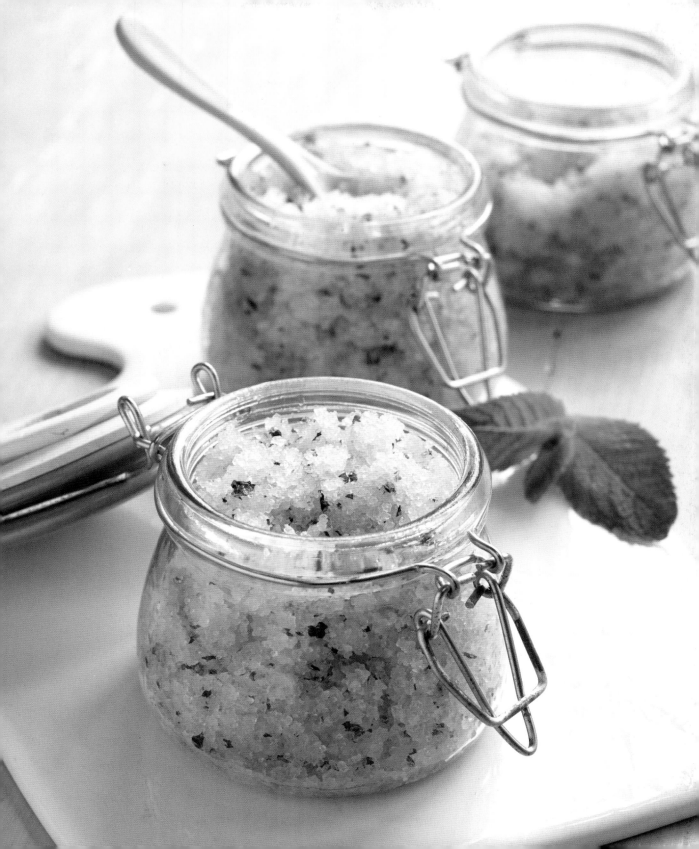

10-MINUTE DRY BODY BRUSHING

Slough off dead skin cells and boost your skin with a weekly brush. The pressure on the skin and the direction you brush in help to move lymph fluid around the body, boosting your natural elimination process and circulation at the same time. Always brush in an upwards direction, and follow each stroke with a sweep of your hand.

TOOLS

Use a firm-bristled brush. A long handle helps you to reach the whole body. If you prefer, choose one with a strap handle that helps you to control pressure.

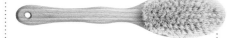

WHY BODY BRUSH?

Dry brushing stimulates and energizes the body, so it is best to do it in the morning before you shower. Regular brushing helps to deliver oxygenated blood to the skin and helps it to hydrate efficiently, contributing to a healthy skin tone. Dry brushing also helps to eliminate toxins, so can smooth unsightly lumps and bumps.

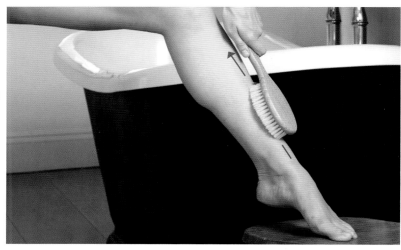

1 Holding the brush with your left hand, brush up the front of your left leg. Use long, sweeping strokes in an upward direction. Brush firmly, but not hard enough to damage the skin. Follow each stroke with a sweep of your right hand. Repeat 3 times.

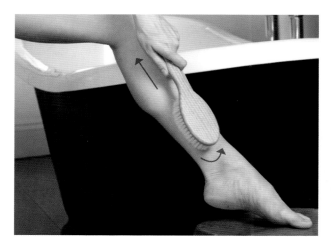

2 Using small, circular movements with your brush, travel up the inside of the same leg, starting at the ankle and moving up to the groin. Follow each stroke with a sweep of your right hand. Repeat 3 times, then switch to the outside of the leg, moving up the leg with the same small, circular movements.

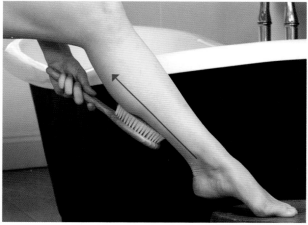

3 Move to the back of the leg, and use long sweeping strokes from the heel to the top of the thigh. Repeat twice, and on the third stroke, continue around the buttock and up towards the back. These movements accelerate the flow of lymph towards the glands where it is eliminated, stimulating your circulation.

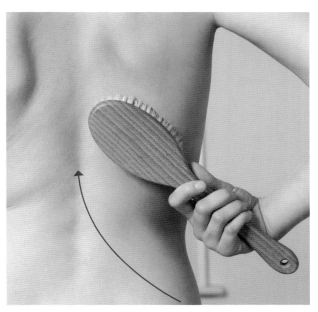

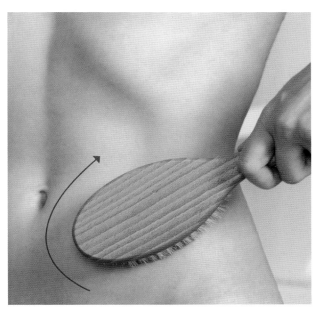

4 Move the brush across the buttocks and up onto the centre of the back, using large, sweeping, circular strokes into the centre of the body. After every stroke, put down the brush and follow the same route with your hand. Repeat 3 times.

5 Move the brush around the side of your body to your front torso, using long, circular strokes across the abdomen. After every stroke, put down the brush and follow the same route with your hand. Repeat 3 times.

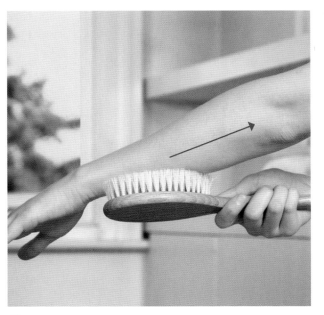

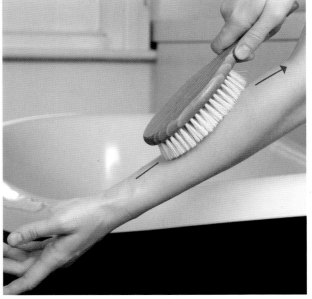

6 Passing the brush to your right hand, use long, sweeping movements to brush the outside of the left arm upwards towards the shoulder, and sweep around the outside of your left breast. After every stroke, put down the brush and sweep along the same route with your hand. Repeat 3 times.

7 To finish, brush the inside of the left arm up towards the armpit, using long, sweeping movements. After every stroke, put down the brush and sweep along the arm with your hand. Repeat 3 times. Repeat the whole sequence on the right-hand side of the body. Afterwards, your skin will feel soft and smooth.

Detox Body Oil

FOR ALL SKIN TYPES

Lymphatic problems, such as cellulite, are helped by lymphatic-drainage massage techniques using this **detoxing** oil. Juniper can treat skin conditions that lead to toxins accumulating in the body, and mandarin essential oil has a **diuretic action**, which can remove waste products and toxic materials. Using a blend of these two essential oils helps to maintain a fully functional lymphatic system.

MAKES 45ML (1½FL OZ)

INGREDIENTS

3 tbsp grapeseed oil
8 drops juniper essential oil
4 drops grapefruit essential oil
3 drops cypress essential oil
3 drops lemon essential oil
2 drops mandarin essential oil

HOW TO MAKE

1 Place all the ingredients in a bowl and mix well.
2 Pour into a sterilized bottle and place a tight-fitting lid or dropper on. Store in a cool, dark place. Keeps for up to 3 months.

HOW TO APPLY

Massage into the skin with upward-circular movements, paying particular attention to any areas of concern. Use before or after dry body brushing (see pp174–75) for optimal effect.

Rosehip Body Oil

FOR NORMAL AND DRY SKIN

This body oil contains a mixture of **nourishing** plant oils and essential oils known for their ability to increase cell turnover. This ability can promote the **healing** of wounds, burns, and stretch marks. Rosehip oil is a rich source of polyunsaturated fatty acids, and linoleic and linolenic acids. These help to **regenerate** and **repair** skin tissue, making it beneficial for treating sun-burnt, wrinkled, or scarred skin.

MAKES 45ML (1½FL OZ)

INGREDIENTS

2 tbsp rosehip oil
1 tbsp almond oil
6 drops frankincense essential oil
6 drops rose essential oil
4 drops geranium essential oil
2 drops myrrh essential oil

HOW TO MAKE

1 Place all the ingredients in a bowl and mix well.
2 Pour into a sterilized bottle and place a tight-fitting lid or dropper on. Store in a cool, dark place. Keeps for up to 3 months.

HOW TO APPLY

Massage into the skin, paying particular attention to dry areas, scars, and stretch marks.

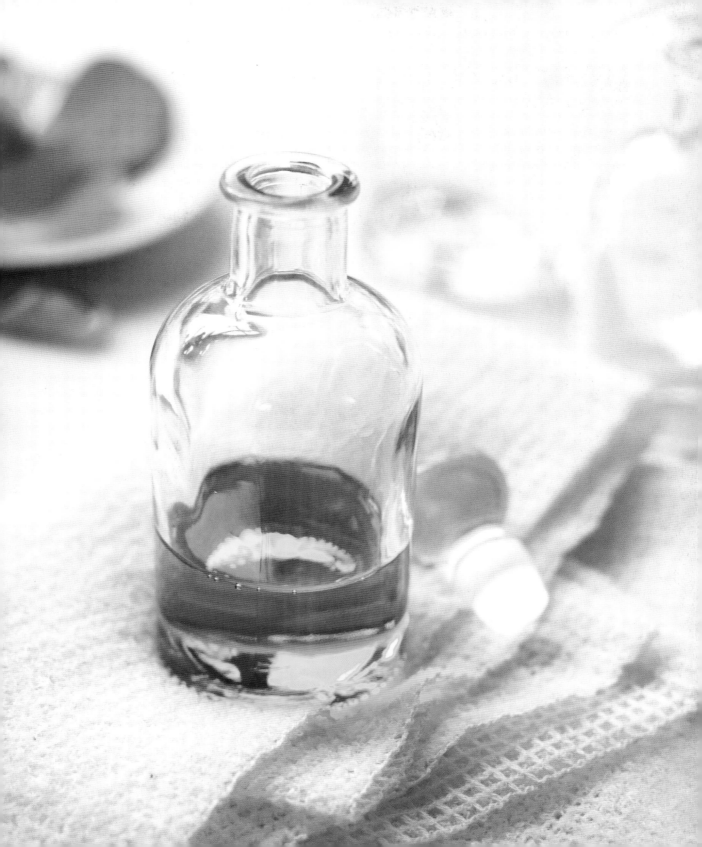

DE-STRESS MASSAGE OIL

QUICK

FOR ALL SKIN TYPES

Stress can be responsible for many illnesses. You can help to treat it with **aromatherapy**, which combines the physiological and psychological benefits of the essential oils. This de-stress massage oil blend contains fragrant and **uplifting** neroli and orange essential oils, which are combined with spiritual sandalwood and frankincense oils to help **ease anxiety** and nervous tension.

MAKES 45ML (1½FL OZ)

INGREDIENTS
1 tbsp almond oil
1 tbsp sunflower oil
1 tbsp avocado oil
6 drops neroli essential oil
4 drops frankincense essential oil
4 drops bergamot essential oil
4 drops orange essential oil
2 drops sandalwood essential oil

HOW TO MAKE

1 Place all the ingredients in a bowl and mix well.
2 Pour into a sterilized bottle and place a tight-fitting lid or dropper on. Store in a cool, dark place. Keeps for up to 3 months.

HOW TO APPLY

Massage into the skin. Use before bed to aid a restful night's sleep. Allow the oil to absorb into the skin before getting dressed.

CITRUS MASSAGE OIL

QUICK

FOR ALL SKIN TYPES

This **uplifting** massage oil helps to **tone** and **refresh** the skin and senses. Use in the mornings for a zesty, **nourishing** start to the day. Jojoba oil has a high vitamin-E content which makes it a stable oil with **antioxidant** properties. Almond oil is a light oil that **conditions** the skin, making this massage oil light but hugely **moisturising**. Cheerful citrus oils are all the excuse you need to get up and go!

MAKES 45ML (1½FL OZ)

INGREDIENTS
2 tbsp almond oil
1 tbsp jojoba oil
5 drops lemon essential oil
5 drops grapefruit essential oil
5 drops mandarin essential oil

HOW TO MAKE

1 Place all the ingredients in a bowl and mix well.
2 Pour into a sterilized bottle and place a tight-fitting lid or dropper on. Store in a cool, dark place. Keeps for up to 3 months.

HOW TO APPLY

Massage into the skin. Allow the oil to absorb into the skin before getting dressed.

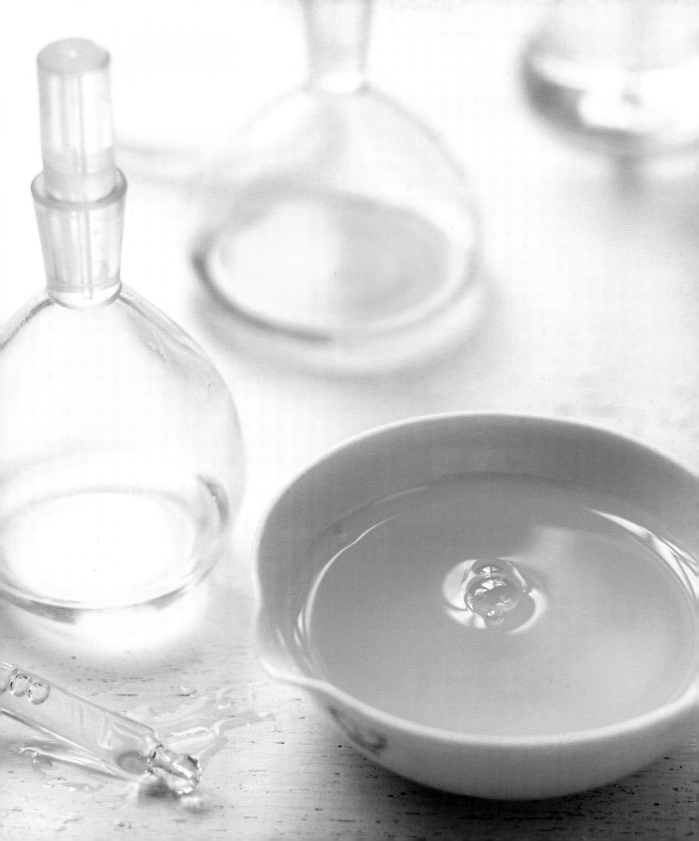

ARNICA AND COMFREY MUSCLE RUB

QUICK

FOR ALL SKIN TYPES

Use this before or after exercise to **stimulate** your circulation and encourage the body to **heal** and **protect** itself. Comfrey herb is a useful **first-aid remedy**. Arnica is not just an excellent treatment for bruising – its ability to increase circulation means it can alleviate the aches and pains of over-exertion and can treat rheumatic and neuralgic pain.

MAKES 30ML (1FL OZ)

INGREDIENTS

1 tbsp arnica macerated oil
1 tbsp comfrey macerated oil
2 drops rosemary essential oil
2 drops black pepper essential oil
2 drops lavender essential oil
2 drops sweet marjoram essential oil
2 drops lemongrass essential oil

HOW TO MAKE

1 Mix the arnica and comfrey macerated oils together in a bowl.
2 Add all the essential oils to the oil mixture.
3 Pour into a sterilized bottle and place a tight-fitting lid on. Store in a cool, dark place. Keeps for up to 3 months.

HOW TO APPLY

Rub into muscles before or after exercise. You could also create a solid muscle balm – combine the macerated oils and essential oils in this recipe with beeswax or carnauba wax (see step-by-step balm recipe, p133).

MUMMY MASSAGE OIL

FOR ALL SKIN TYPES

This is a **nourishing** massage oil for new mothers and mothers-to-be. With **moisturising** and vitamin E-rich wheatgerm oil, nourishing almond oil, and **antioxidant-rich** rosehip oil, it can help to **tone** the skin and **prevent stretchmarks**. The essential oils in this recipe have **calming** aromatherapeutic effects on the mind, **conditioning** effects on the skin, and also provide a lovely perfume.

MAKES 45ML (1½FL OZ)

INGREDIENTS

1 tbsp wheatgerm oil
1 tbsp rosehip oil
1 tbsp almond oil
8 drops neroli essential oil
4 drops frankincense essential oil
2 drops bergamot essential oil
2 drops mandarin essential oil

HOW TO MAKE

1 Mix the oils together in a bowl.
2 Add all the essential oils to the oil mixture.
3 Pour into a sterilized bottle and place a tight-fitting lid or a dropper on. Store in a cool, dark place. Keeps for up to 3 months.

HOW TO APPLY

Massage gently into the skin. Apply after a shower or bath to lock moisture into the skin.

Lemon Balm, Neroli, And Sea Salt Relaxing Bath infusion

FOR ALL SKIN TYPES

Use this mixture of **relaxing** lemon balm in combination with intoxicating neroli to **calm** the mind and body. Sea salt is rich in minerals and has **skin-healing** properties. The essential oils can encourage new cell growth, improve cell renewal, and **soften scars** as well as provide a rich, refreshing scent that is **uplifting** and can help to ease anxiety.

INGREDIENTS

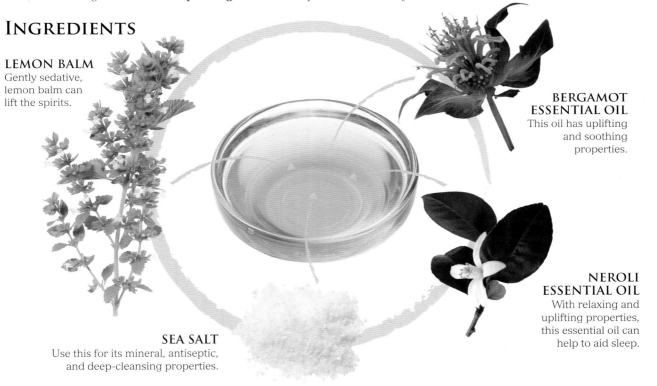

LEMON BALM
Gently sedative, lemon balm can lift the spirits.

BERGAMOT ESSENTIAL OIL
This oil has uplifting and soothing properties.

NEROLI ESSENTIAL OIL
With relaxing and uplifting properties, this essential oil can help to aid sleep.

SEA SALT
Use this for its mineral, antiseptic, and deep-cleansing properties.

MAKES ENOUGH FOR ONE BATH

INGREDIENTS
1 tbsp dried lemon balm
5 drops neroli essential oil
5 drops bergamot essential oil
1 tbsp sea salt

HOW TO MAKE

1 To make the lemon balm infusion, place the lemon balm in a teapot or glass bowl and pour 500ml (16fl oz) boiling water over the top. Leave to steep for 10 minutes, then strain.

2 Mix the essential oils and salt together to make a paste.

3 Add the paste to the infusion, and stir until dissolved.

HOW TO APPLY

Add the infusion mixture to the bath immediately and bathe as usual.

ROSE AND CHAMOMILE BATH INFUSION

FOR ALL SKIN TYPES

After a hectic day, enrich a bath with this **rejuvenating** mixture of herbs and fragrant essential oils that gently **relax** the mind and body. Rose has many therapeutic uses, and some of its key actions are **uplifting**, **revitalizing**, and **soothing**. As a fragrance it blends very well with Roman chamomile, creating a sweet yet herbal scent and a **calming**, **soothing** effect on the emotions.

MAKES ENOUGH FOR ONE BATH

INGREDIENTS

1 tbsp dried rose petals
1 tbsp chamomile flowers
5 drops rose essential oil
5 drops Roman chamomile essential oil
1 tbsp sea salt

HOW TO MAKE

1 To make the infusion, place the petals and flowers in a teapot or glass bowl and pour 500ml (16fl oz) boiling water over the top. Leave to steep for 10 minutes, then strain.
2 Mix the essential oils and sea salt together to make a paste.
3 Add the paste to the infusion and stir until dissolved.

HOW TO APPLY

Add the infusion mixture to the bath immediately and bathe as usual.

ROSEMARY AND ARNICA DETOX BATH INFUSION

FOR ALL SKIN TYPES

Use this infusion in your bath to **stimulate** the circulation and **soothe** tired muscles. This recipe contains a herbal concoction of arnica and sea salt that **relieve aches and pains**; fennel seeds that aid **digestion**, helping to relieve gas and prevent bloating; and bladderwrack that helps to **cleanse** the skin of toxins and excess fluids.

MAKES ENOUGH FOR ONE BATH

INGREDIENTS

1 tbsp dried bladderwrack (seaweed)
1 sprig rosemary
1 tbsp fennel seeds
1 tbsp dried arnica flowers
2 drops juniper essential oil
2 drops rosemary essential oil
2 drops grapefruit essential oil
1 drop black pepper essential oil
1 tbsp sea salt

HOW TO MAKE

1 To make the infusion, place the herbs, seeds, and flowers in a teapot or glass bowl and pour 500ml (16fl oz) boiling water over the top. Leave to steep for 10 minutes, then strain.
2 Mix the essential oils and sea salt together to make a paste.
3 Add the paste to the infusion and stir until dissolved.

HOW TO APPLY

Add the infusion mixture to the bath immediately and bathe as usual. Try dry body brushing (see pp174–75) to exfoliate and increase circulation before use.

LAVENDER AND ALOE VERA COOLING BATH INFUSION

FOR ALL SKIN TYPES

Cool and **soothe** the skin with this **relaxing** bath blend of aloe vera juice and lavender. The relaxing effects of lavender are well known, and a lavender bath before bed usually means a good night's sleep. Lavender also has **skin-soothing** properties, and when mixed with aloe vera juice, makes a wonderful infusion for anyone suffering with heat or redness in the skin.

MAKES ENOUGH FOR ONE BATH

INGREDIENTS

1 tbsp dried lavender flowers
10 drops lavender essential oil
1 tbsp aloe vera juice

HOW TO MAKE

1 To make the infusion, place the flowers in a teapot or glass bowl and pour 500ml (16fl oz) boiling water over the top. Leave to steep for 10 minutes, then strain.

2 Add the essential oil and aloe vera juice to the infusion, and stir.

HOW TO APPLY

Add the infusion mixture to the bath immediately and bathe as usual.

LAVENDER AND OAT BATH SOAK

FOR ALL SKIN TYPES

This soak is the ideal gift for bath lovers. The powder has a simple yet heavenly scent, made using only dried lavender flowers. Combine mineral-rich sea salts with **skin-soothing** oats to give skin a luxurious treat as you bathe. The secret ingredient is bicarbonate of soda, which **softens** and gently **exfoliates** the skin.

MAKES 450G (1LB)

INGREDIENTS

100g (3½oz) dried lavender flowers
200g (7oz) jumbo oats
50g (1¾oz) bicarbonate of soda
100g (3½oz) sea salt

HOW TO MAKE

1 Whizz all the ingredients together in an electric mixer until the mix becomes a fine powder.

2 Store in a sterilized, airtight container. Keeps for up to 3 months.

HOW TO APPLY

Add a handful of the dry mixture to a warm bath and bathe as usual. Shower the mixture off the skin if needed. If you wish to keep the bath clean, add a handful of mixture to a muslin cloth or an old pair of tights and tie into a bath float.

Pampering Bath Melt

FOR ALL SKIN TYPES

Containing deeply **nourishing** cocoa butter and shea nut butter, these bath melts **replenish** your skin. Combining the exotically scented aphrodisiac ylang ylang essential oil with **calming** clary sage and rose oils, these little pampering gems are perfect for an indulgent bath time. Pour yourself a glass of something delicious, and relax in the warm, fragrant water.

MAKES 10 SMALL MELTS

INGREDIENTS

25g (scant 1oz) cocoa butter
25g (scant 1oz) shea nut butter
1 tsp almond oil
1 tsp wheatgerm oil
1 tsp jojoba oil
4 drops ylang ylang essential oil
2 drops clary sage essential oil
2 drops rose essential oil
1 drop geranium essential oil
1 drop vanilla extract
1 tsp dried rose petals

HOW TO MAKE

1 Heat the butters together in a bain-marie (see p133), until they have melted. Remove from the heat.
2 Add the oils to the melted butters.
3 Pour in all the essential oils, the vanilla extract, and the rose petals, and mix well.
4 Pour into soap moulds or an ice-cube tray and allow to cool and set in the fridge for 1–2 hours. Remove from the fridge and press the bath melts out of the moulds. Store in a cool, dark place. Keeps for up to 3 months.

HOW TO APPLY

Add a bath melt to a warm bath and let it soften and moisturise your skin as you relax.

Nourishing Bath Melt

FOR DRY SKIN

Quick and simple to make, these **nourishing** bath melts contain deeply **moisturising** cocoa butter and almond oil and beautifully fragrant neroli essential oil. Neroli oil is steam-distilled from the blossom of the bitter orange tree and is an effective **aromatherapy remedy** for the treatment of insomnia, making a great bath time treat just before you go to bed.

MAKES 10 SMALL MELTS

INGREDIENTS

50g (1¾oz) cocoa butter
1 tbsp almond oil
10 drops neroli essential oil

HOW TO MAKE

1 Heat the butter in a bain-marie (see p133), until it turns to a golden liquid. Remove from the heat.
2 Add the oil to the melted butter. Pour in the essential oil and mix well.
3 Pour into soap moulds or an ice-cube tray and allow to cool and set in the fridge for 1 hour. Remove from the fridge and press the bath melts out of the moulds. Store in a cool, dark place. Keeps for up to 3 months.

HOW TO APPLY

Add a bath melt to a warm bath and let it soften and moisturise your skin as you relax.

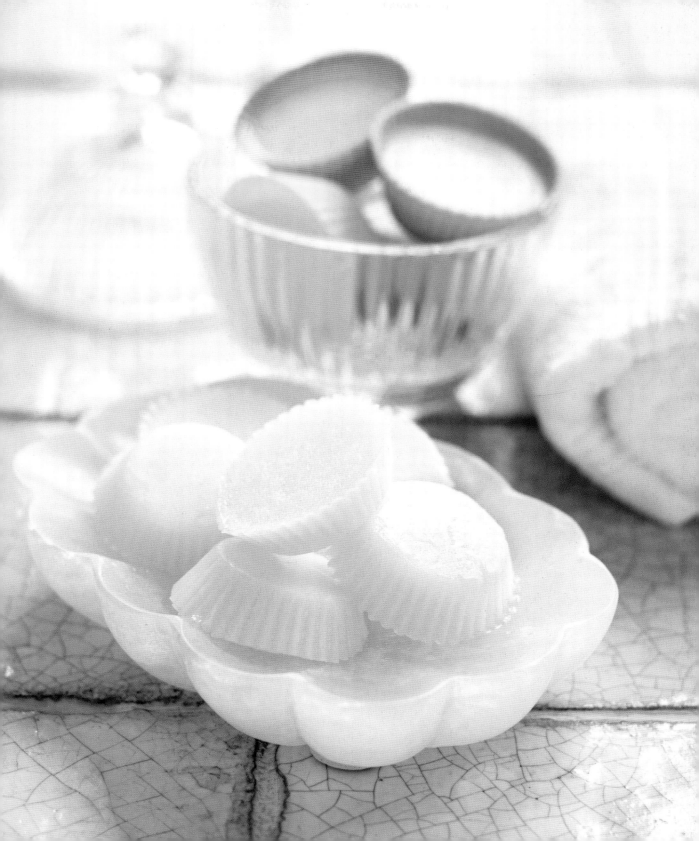

CHAMOMILE BEDTIME BOMBS

FOR ALL SKIN TYPES

Added to a warm bath, indulgent cocoa butter will help to **soften** and **moisturise** the skin. Roman chamomile and lavender essential oils are perfect bedtime partners, and have a deeply **calming** and **soothing** effect on the mind and body. This recipe is easily adaptable to include other dried flowers, such as rose petals or lavender, and essential oils, such as rosemary or jasmine.

MAKES 20 SMALL BOMBS

INGREDIENTS

400g (14oz) sodium bicarbonate
200g (7oz) citric acid
1 tsp dried chamomile flowers
1 tsp cocoa butter
10 drops Roman chamomile essential oil
5 drops lavender essential oil

HOW TO MAKE

1 Place all the dry ingredients in a bowl and, wearing protective gloves, mix them with your hands.

2 Heat the butter in a bain-marie (see p133), until melted. Remove from the heat. Add the melted butter and essential oils to the dry ingredients and mix well.

3 Pour 1 teaspoon of water into an atomizer spray. Spray the mixture with water to create the bath bomb texture, as shown in the step-by-step technique below.

4 When the bombs are set, press the bath bombs out of the moulds. Keeps for up to 3 months.

HOW TO APPLY

Add a bath bomb to a warm bath and enjoy the fizz and fragrance.

MAKING BATH BOMBS

A bath bomb is simply a mixture of citric acid, bicarbonate of soda, and water, moulded and left to dry. You can add the resulting "bomb" to a warm bath, releasing any of the herbs or fragrances that have been added to the mixture. Lightly grease the moulds before use with some spray oil.

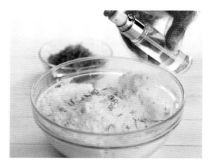

1 Using an atomizer spray, add the water to the mixture of melted butter, essential oils, and dry ingredients to bind it together.

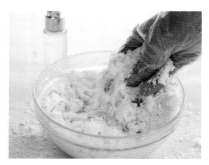

2 Continue spraying water and binding the mixture together with your hands until the mixture resembles damp sand and sticks together without fizzing. If it is dry and crumbly, add more water.

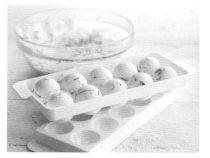

3 Firmly press the mixture into the moulds. For small, spherical bombs, press a small amount of mixture into each tray. Allow to set in the fridge for at least 1 hour. Sprinkle water on one tray, then turn out one set of halves and press them on top of the other set to form a ball.

Mandarin Bath Bombs

FOR ALL SKIN TYPES

Enjoy a **calming**, **soothing** bath with these sweet-citrus fizzing bombs. Non-toxic mandarin oil is particularly **suitable for children**. Add rose petals, marigold, borage, chamomile flowers, dried orange peel, or glitter to the mix to create beautiful-looking bath bombs. Use cosmetic glitter, which comes in a rainbow of colours, and different particle sizes. Craft glitter is not suitable for use.

MAKES 20 SMALL BOMBS

INGREDIENTS

400g (14oz) sodium bicarbonate
200g (7oz) citric acid
1 tsp dried flowers/herbs/
cosmetic glitter
15 drops mandarin essential oil

HOW TO MAKE

1 Place all the dry ingredients in a bowl and, wearing protective gloves, mix them with your hands. Add the essential oil to the dry ingredients and mix well.

2 Pour 1 teaspoon of water into an atomizer spray. Spray the mixture with water to create the bath bomb texture, as shown in the step-by-step technique (see opposite).

3 Remove from the fridge and press the bath bombs out of the moulds. Keeps for up to 3 months.

HOW TO APPLY

Add a bath bomb to a warm bath and enjoy the fizz and fragrance.

Exfoliating Bath Float

QUICK

FOR DRY SKIN

Oats are the perfect ingredient for **nourishing** and **moisturising** dry or irritated skin, yet are mild enough to be used on sensitive skin. Lavender and rose essential oils add a beautiful fragrance as well as their **calming** and **relaxing** properties. If you have sensitive skin, omit the essential oils. If you don't have a bath, you can also use this simple and effective bath float to **exfoliate** in the shower.

MAKES 1

INGREDIENTS

1 tbsp jumbo oats
1 tbsp oat bran
1 tsp lavender flowers
1 tsp rose petals
2 drops rose essential oil
2 drops lavender essential oil

HOW TO MAKE

1 Place a muslin cloth flat on a table. Place the oats, followed by the bran, in the centre of the cloth.

2 Add the lavender flowers, rose petals, and essential oils.

3 Bring the 4 corners of the cloth together and tie tightly with a ribbon or string. Use immediately.

HOW TO APPLY

Float in bath water or tie to taps and run warm water through the bag. You could also use it as an exfoliating puff in the shower. Discard contents after use and wash the cloth every time.

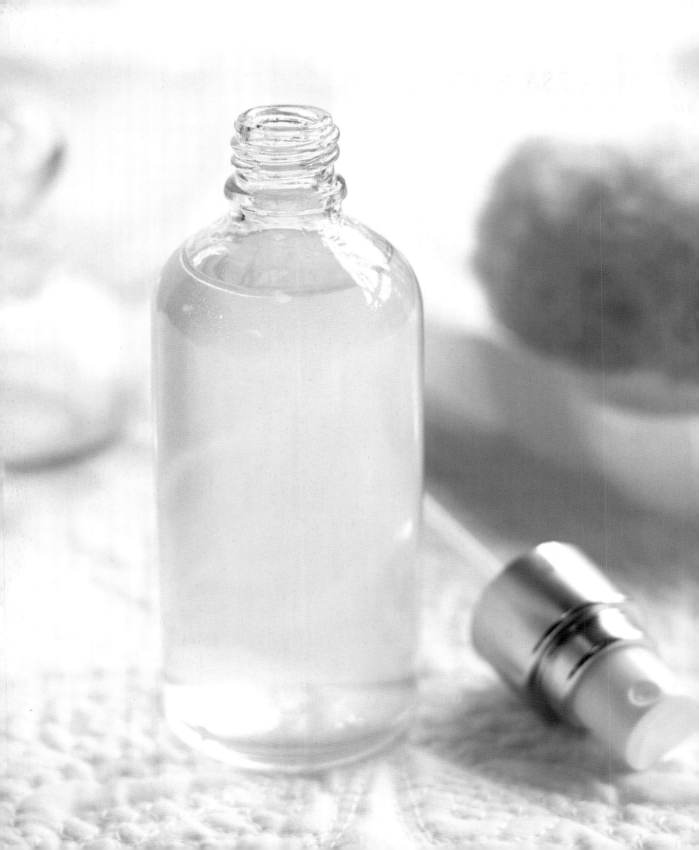

PALMAROSA AND LEMON DEODORANT

FOR ALL SKIN TYPES

Sweating is a natural function of the body that helps to regulate your body temperature and balance salt levels. Your sweat does not smell, it's the bacteria on the skin's surface that causes the odour, so preventing bacterial growth is important in a deodorant. This is a **refreshing** underarm deodorant spray containing **antibacterial** and **deodorizing** essential oils, as well as **cooling** aloe vera.

MAKES 100ML (3½FL OZ)

INGREDIENTS
90ml (3fl oz) witch hazel herbal water
1 tsp glycerin
1 tsp aloe vera juice
5 drops palmarosa essential oil
5 drops lemon essential oil
3 drops coriander essential oil
3 drops grapefruit essential oil
3 drops peppermint essential oil

HOW TO MAKE

1 Mix the witch hazel, glycerin, and aloe vera juice together in a bowl.
2 Add the essential oils and mix well. Pour into a sterilized bottle and place an atomizer on. Store in a cool, dark place. Keeps for up to 3 months.

HOW TO APPLY

Apply to clean underarms and use when required. Do not use on freshly shaved skin. Shake well before each use.

ROSE BODY POWDER

MULTI-PURPOSE

FOR ALL SKIN TYPES

This luxuriously fragranced body powder leaves your skin feeling silky **smooth** and delicately **scented** with rose, geranium, and patchouli essential oils. Body powders are primarily used to **fragrance** the skin and for **absorbing** any excess moisture. Smooth the powder into the skin after bathing, paying attention to areas where the skin folds, the underarms, and the feet.

MAKES 100G (3½OZ)

INGREDIENTS
100g (3½oz) cornflour
1 tsp rose tincture
10 drops rose essential oil
10 drops geranium essential oil
10 drops patchouli essential oil

HOW TO MAKE

1 Sift the cornflour (through a sieve) into a bowl.
2 Add the tincture and essential oils to cotton wool balls.
3 Place the cotton wool balls in an airtight container.
4 Add the cornflour, leaving some room at the top for mixing.
5 Place the lid on the container and shake vigorously to disperse the fragrance. Store in a cool, dry place. Keeps for up to 6 months.

HOW TO APPLY

Apply with a powder puff on dry skin after a shower or bath and smooth over the skin. It is great for absorbing excess moisture, so apply to areas that might get sticky during the day, like armpits and feet.

CITRUS SPLASH

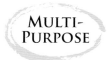

FOR ALL SKIN TYPES

Revive your skin and senses with this **refreshing** and **uplifting** blend of citrus essential oils mixed with orange floral water. Splash, pat, or atomize the lightly scented body fragrance onto pulse points or areas of the skin that need **revitalizing** or **refreshing**. The properties of these essential oils combine to make this citrus splash useful at the start and end of the day.

INGREDIENTS

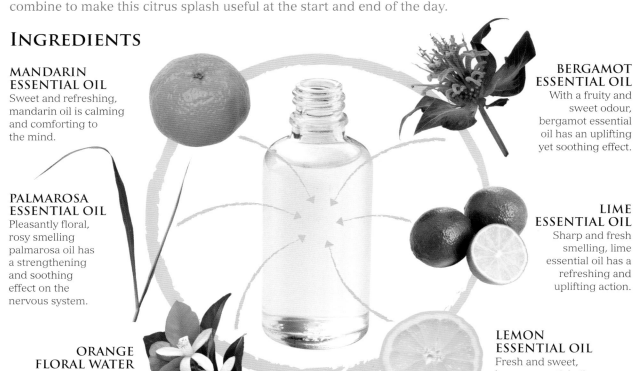

MANDARIN ESSENTIAL OIL
Sweet and refreshing, mandarin oil is calming and comforting to the mind.

PALMAROSA ESSENTIAL OIL
Pleasantly floral, rosy smelling palmarosa oil has a strengthening and soothing effect on the nervous system.

ORANGE FLORAL WATER
A beautifully fragrant by-product of the steam distillation of orange blossom.

BERGAMOT ESSENTIAL OIL
With a fruity and sweet odour, bergamot essential oil has an uplifting yet soothing effect.

LIME ESSENTIAL OIL
Sharp and fresh smelling, lime essential oil has a refreshing and uplifting action.

LEMON ESSENTIAL OIL
Fresh and sweet, lemon essential oil is truly reminiscent of the ripe fruit.

MAKES 60ML (2FL OZ)

INGREDIENTS
2 tbsp vodka
10 drops lime essential oil
5 drops lemon essential oil
5 drops bergamot essential oil
5 drops mandarin essential oil
4 drops palmarosa essential oil
1 tbsp mineral water
1 tbsp orange floral water

HOW TO MAKE

1 Mix the vodka and essential oils together in a bowl. Add the mineral water and orange floral water, and stir thoroughly.
2 Pour into a sterilized bottle and place the cap on or attach an atomizer. Store in a cool, dry place. Keeps for up to 6 months.

HOW TO APPLY

Splash, pat, or atomize the body splash onto the skin as required, when the skin is hot or needs reviving. Avoid the eyes. Men can also use it as an aftershave splash. Shake well before use.

BODY MIST

FOR ALL SKIN TYPES

This body mist is a light alternative to wearing a perfume. It contains **hydrating** rose floral water, and **skin-soothing** aloe vera, so **conditions** the skin as well as offering **fragrance**. Heavenly scented and exotic, vanilla and ylang ylang are blended with beautiful sandalwood and rose oils. The essential oils in your body mist have a therapeutic effect on the emotions, as well as the senses.

MAKES 100ML (3½FL OZ)

INGREDIENTS

75ml (2½fl oz) rose floral water
1 tbsp rose tincture
1 tsp aloe vera juice
10 drops vanilla extract
10 drops ylang ylang essential oil
6 drops sandalwood essential oil
4 drops rose absolute essential oil
2 drops clary sage essential oil
2 drops sweet orange essential oil

HOW TO MAKE

1 Mix the rose floral water with the tincture, aloe vera juice, and vanilla extract together in a bowl.
2 Add all the essential oils and mix.
3 Pour into a sterilized bottle with an atomizer. Store in a cool, dry place. Keeps for up to 6 months.

HOW TO APPLY

Apply as required for a refreshing burst of fragrance. The fragrance does not last as long as a traditional perfume, so re-apply as frequently as you like. Shake well before use. Avoid spraying on clothes, fabrics, or bed linen.

ROSE SOLID PERFUME

FOR ALL SKIN TYPES

Solid perfumes are alcohol-free as well as being very transportable. They subtly **fragrance** the skin. Create a fragrant and **therapeutic** blend of essential oils using top, middle, and base notes, and blend into a simple balm base. Look out for some attractive pots and tins to store your perfume in – you can find beautiful pill boxes that give your solid perfume an extra touch of glamour.

MAKES 30G (1OZ)

INGREDIENTS

10g (¼oz) beeswax
2 tsp sunflower oil
12 drops rose essential oil
8 drops geranium essential oil
6 drops patchouli essential oil
4 drops bergamot essential oil
3 drops cedarwood essential oil

HOW TO MAKE

1 Heat the beeswax and oil together in a bain-marie (see p133), until the wax has melted. Remove from the heat.
2 Add the essential oils and mix.
3 Pour into a sterilized jar. Once cool, apply to the skin or place the lid on. Store in a cool, dry place. Keeps for up to 6 months.

HOW TO APPLY

Rub onto pulse points when you need a fragrance boost.

NEROLI SOLID PERFUME

FOR ALL SKIN TYPES

This blend of citrus and spice works as a lovely day-to-night **fragrance**. The freshly fragrant top notes of neroli and bergamot work with a **sweet–citrus** middle note of orange and the **spicy** base notes of frankincense. Two **sweet-smelling** tinctures work as fixatives in the perfume – helping to keep the scent on your skin for as long as possible.

INGREDIENTS

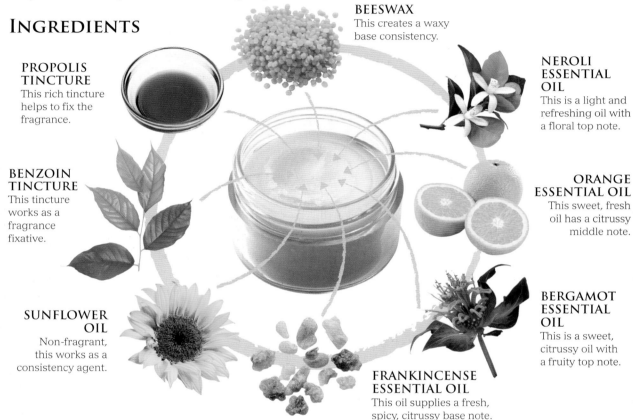

BEESWAX
This creates a waxy base consistency.

PROPOLIS TINCTURE
This rich tincture helps to fix the fragrance.

NEROLI ESSENTIAL OIL
This is a light and refreshing oil with a floral top note.

BENZOIN TINCTURE
This tincture works as a fragrance fixative.

ORANGE ESSENTIAL OIL
This sweet, fresh oil has a citrussy middle note.

SUNFLOWER OIL
Non-fragrant, this works as a consistency agent.

BERGAMOT ESSENTIAL OIL
This is a sweet, citrussy oil with a fruity top note.

FRANKINCENSE ESSENTIAL OIL
This oil supplies a fresh, spicy, citrussy base note.

MAKES 30G (1OZ)

INGREDIENTS

10g (¼oz) beeswax
2 tsp sunflower oil
1 tsp propolis tincture
1 tsp benzoin tincture
8 drops neroli essential oil
4 drops bergamot essential oil
4 drops orange essential oil
2 drops frankincense essential oil

HOW TO MAKE

1 Heat the beeswax and oil together in a bain-marie (see p133), until the wax has melted. Remove from the heat.
2 Add the tinctures and essential oils, and mix thoroughly.
3 Pour into a sterilized jar or tin. Once cool, apply to the skin and place the lid on. Store in a cool, dry place. Keeps for up to 6 months.

HOW TO APPLY

Rub onto your pulse points when you need a fragrance boost.

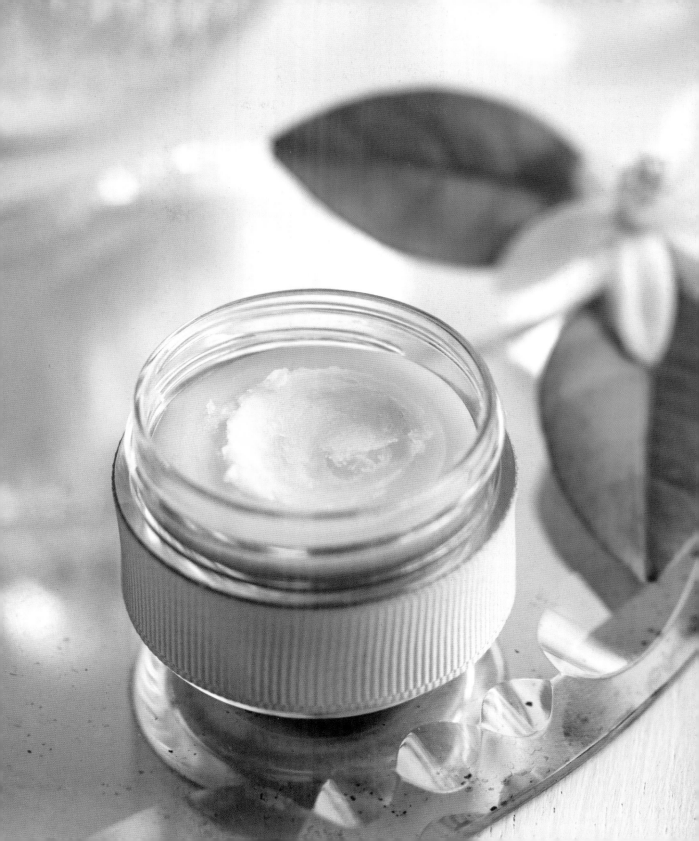

CALENDULA SOOTHING BALM

FOR ALL SKIN TYPES

Soothe and **repair** the skin with this combination of calendula, lavender, and German chamomile essential oils. Chamomile essential oil has an analgesic and **anti-inflammatory** action and can treat eczema and dry itchy skin conditions, and is also good for sensitive skin. **Antiseptic** calendula has traditionally been used to facilitate **wound healing**, due to its ability to quickly repair skin tissue.

MAKES 30G (1OZ)

INGREDIENTS

1 tsp cocoa butter
1 tsp beeswax
1 tbsp calendula macerated oil
5 drops lavender essential oil
2 drops German chamomile essential oil
1 tsp calendula tincture

HOW TO MAKE

1 Heat the cocoa butter, beeswax, and calendula macerated oil together in a bain-marie (see p133), until the wax has melted. Remove from the heat.
2 Add the essential oils and tincture, and mix thoroughly.
3 Pour into a sterilized jar. Once cool, apply to the skin or place the lid on. Store in a cool, dry place. Keeps for up to 6 months.

HOW TO APPLY

Gently massage into areas of over-exposed or irritated skin.

Soothe Irritated Skin

Your skin is the primary organ to protect you from irritants in your surroundings. As a result, most of us have suffered from a skin irritation at some point in our lives. Reactions vary from a mild tingling or red patch to more severe blisters. Irritated skin is caused by a number of factors – from allergies or sensitivities to cosmetic products, to the foods we eat. A build-up of chemicals or toxins on the skin or in the body can also contribute, as can emotional changes and anxiety. Sometimes there isn't only one source; rather, there could be a combination of irritants. Treat skin irritations with soothing balms (see above) and medicated creams. If an irritation persists or gets worse, see a practitioner.

MINTY RELIEF AID

FOR DRY SKIN

This **relieving** balm combines therapeutic essential oils with rich, emollient vegetable oils. The balm provides natural relief from minor irritation, headaches, and colds. Coconut oil is mild and **nourishing**. Combine it with peppermint oil, which has analgesic properties and is **soothing** for itchy skin, and lavender oil, which is **cooling**, **antiseptic**, and can encourage cell regeneration.

INGREDIENTS

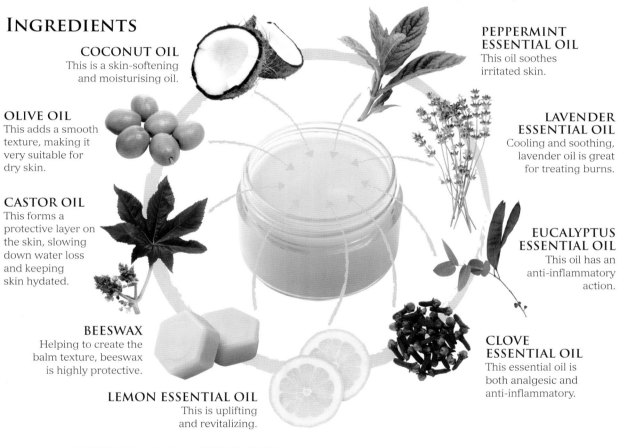

COCONUT OIL
This is a skin-softening and moisturising oil.

OLIVE OIL
This adds a smooth texture, making it very suitable for dry skin.

CASTOR OIL
This forms a protective layer on the skin, slowing down water loss and keeping skin hydrated.

BEESWAX
Helping to create the balm texture, beeswax is highly protective.

LEMON ESSENTIAL OIL
This is uplifting and revitalizing.

PEPPERMINT ESSENTIAL OIL
This oil soothes irritated skin.

LAVENDER ESSENTIAL OIL
Cooling and soothing, lavender oil is great for treating burns.

EUCALYPTUS ESSENTIAL OIL
This oil has an anti-inflammatory action.

CLOVE ESSENTIAL OIL
This essential oil is both analgesic and anti-inflammatory.

MAKES 50G (1¾OZ)

INGREDIENTS
1 tbsp coconut oil
1 tbsp olive oil
1 tbsp castor oil
1 tsp beeswax
7 drops peppermint essential oil
5 drops lavender essential oil
3 drops eucalyptus essential oil
2 drops each clove and lemon essential oil

HOW TO MAKE

1 Heat the oils and beeswax together in a bain-marie (see p133), until the wax has melted. Remove from the heat.
2 Add all the essential oils and mix thoroughly.
3 Pour into a sterilized jar. Once cool, apply to the skin or place the lid on. Store in a cool, dry place. Keeps for up to 6 months.

HOW TO APPLY

Massage into the affected areas, such as temples and forehead for headaches, the chest and neck for colds, and on insect bites.

HAIR

GREAT HAIR STARTS ON THE INSIDE. WHATEVER HAIR TYPE YOU HAVE, KEEP YOUR CROWNING GLORY LOOKING FABULOUS WITH A COMBINATION OF **NUTRITIOUS** FOODS AND LUSCIOUS **NATURAL** TREATMENTS THAT HELP TO MAKE YOUR HAIR **SHINY** AND **STRONG**.

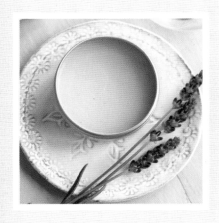
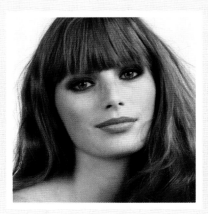
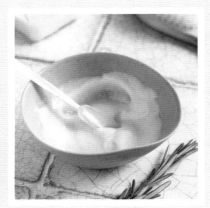

WHAT'S YOUR HAIR TYPE?

Determining your hair type is not as straightforward as you might think. Hair types are broadly defined as normal, greasy, or dry. Within these simple categories are a multitude of variations. Hair can have a fine, medium, or coarse texture, for example, and at the same time sit somewhere on a continuum that ranges from poker straight to tightly curled. However, these broad definitions can help you to care for your tresses.

IDENTIFY YOUR TYPE

This simple flowchart helps to determine your basic hair type. Work with the texture, density, and the curl of your hair to maintain healthy hair.

A STRAND OF HAIR

Whatever your type, all hair is constructed in the same basic way.

THE MEDULLA
The incredibly thin, innermost layer of the hair shaft.

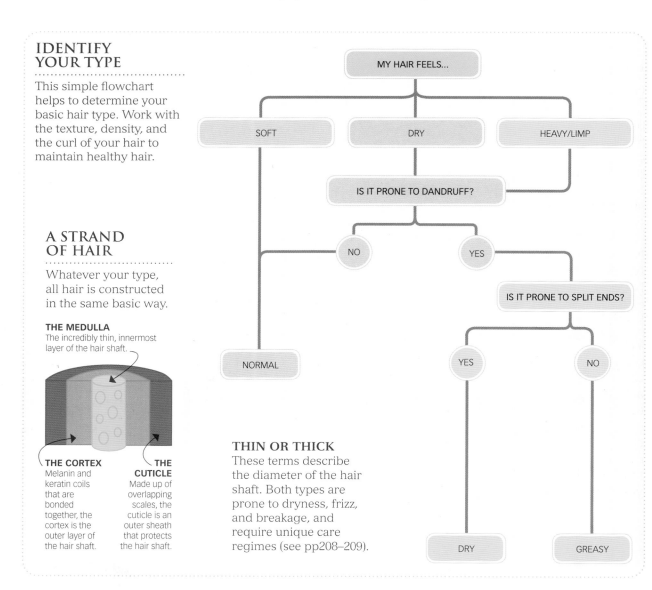

THE CORTEX
Melanin and keratin coils that are bonded together, the cortex is the outer layer of the hair shaft.

THE CUTICLE
Made up of overlapping scales, the cuticle is an outer sheath that protects the hair shaft.

THIN OR THICK
These terms describe the diameter of the hair shaft. Both types are prone to dryness, frizz, and breakage, and require unique care regimes (see pp208–209).

MY HAIR FEELS...

SOFT · DRY · HEAVY/LIMP

IS IT PRONE TO DANDRUFF?

NO · YES

IS IT PRONE TO SPLIT ENDS?

NORMAL

YES · NO

DRY · GREASY

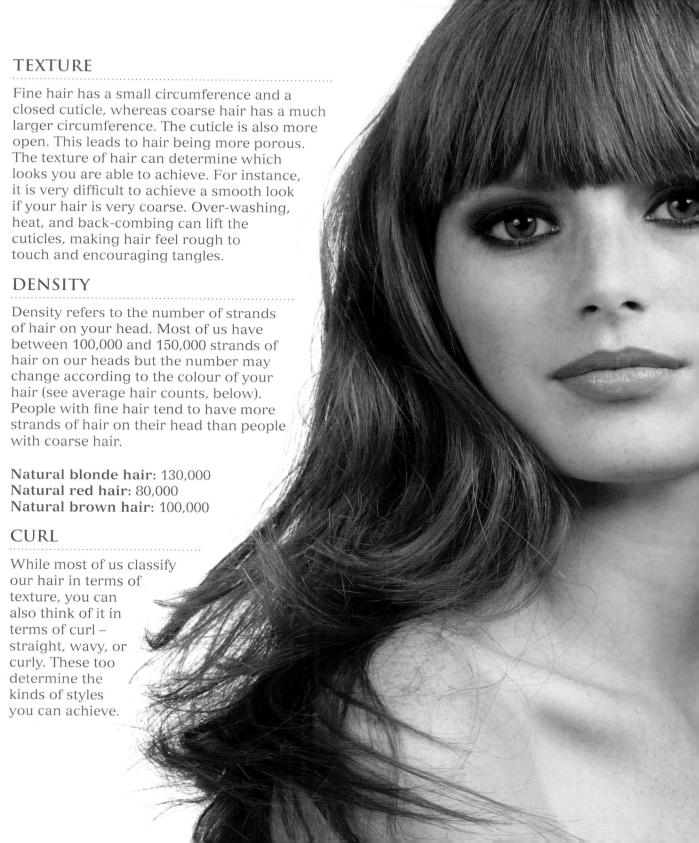

TEXTURE

Fine hair has a small circumference and a closed cuticle, whereas coarse hair has a much larger circumference. The cuticle is also more open. This leads to hair being more porous. The texture of hair can determine which looks you are able to achieve. For instance, it is very difficult to achieve a smooth look if your hair is very coarse. Over-washing, heat, and back-combing can lift the cuticles, making hair feel rough to touch and encouraging tangles.

DENSITY

Density refers to the number of strands of hair on your head. Most of us have between 100,000 and 150,000 strands of hair on our heads but the number may change according to the colour of your hair (see average hair counts, below). People with fine hair tend to have more strands of hair on their head than people with coarse hair.

Natural blonde hair: 130,000
Natural red hair: 80,000
Natural brown hair: 100,000

CURL

While most of us classify our hair in terms of texture, you can also think of it in terms of curl – straight, wavy, or curly. These too determine the kinds of styles you can achieve.

HAIR CARE: THE BASICS

Great-looking hair and a healthy scalp come from within. They are very good indicators of stress levels, diet, hormonal balance, and circulation. To achieve healthy, shiny, and strong hair, try to strike a balance between activity and rest; embrace a diet that nourishes your whole system; reduce your exposure to external factors, such as pollution and chemicals; and treat your hair with tender, loving care.

CLEANSE YOUR LIFESTYLE

Your lifestyle choices play a part in how healthy your hair is. If, like so many of us, you live in a sealed building with central heating and/or air conditioning, surrounded by electrical equipment, such as a phone, TV, and computer, this may leave your hair dry and static. A healthy diet (see box, opposite) can tackle the side effects of unavoidable factors and keep hair manageable.

TREAT STRESS AND ANXIETY, which are linked to the poor condition and thinning of hair. These do not just harm hair, but they can also lead us to indulge in habits that make the problem worse, such as smoking or excessive alcohol consumption. A good diet can also neutralize the effects of stress.

DO NOT SMOKE because it is detrimental to healthy hair. It depletes the body of nutrients, is dehydrating, puts toxic chemicals into your body, and envelopes you in fumes that leave hair looking dull. Give up smoking and not only will you be healthier, your hair will look and smell better, and will not discolour.

DRINK LESS ALCOHOL, because it is dehydrating and leeches the essential nutrients from your body.

GET ACTIVE to ensure that blood circulates to all parts of your body, including your scalp. Healthy circulation leads to strong, healthy hair.

By the time your hair reaches shoulder length, it will be at least 3 years old and will have been washed, dried, and styled hundreds of times.

ENVIRONMENTAL FACTORS

Hair changes from day to day, and week to week, responding to both internal and external environments. Your hair will not always look the same or need to be treated in the same way week in and week out.

The condition of your hair varies according to the season, most notably in winter and summer. In the winter, the scalp is tight and the hair grows at a slower rate. Central heating can also be a problem, as it dries the hair and can make it dull and more static.

In the summer, the sun has a damaging and drying effect and hair may become bleached and lose its vitality. Swimming can also damage the hair, either because of the chlorine or the salt in the water. Take care to protect your hair from damage by keeping it covered when swimming and using a balm or oil to prevent moisture loss in the hot sun.

Soft or hard water may also affect the condition of your hair, how well your shampoos clean, and how easily your conditioners rinse out.

REFRESH YOUR HAIR-CARE REGIME

The products you use regularly on your hair have a big impact on its general condition. By the time your hair reaches shoulder length, for instance, it could be at least 3 years old. It will have been shampooed, blow dried, coloured, curled, straightened, combed, sprayed, pulled back, put up, and teased into shape hundreds of times – this takes its toll on hair's condition.

SHAMPOO AND CONDITION less often – frequent shampooing can strip the natural oils from your hair and scalp. Conditioning can put some of the moisture back in, but over time causes build-up on the hair.

USE FEWER STYLING PRODUCTS, as they can dry out your hair and cause product build-up.

DO NOT BRUSH OR COMB too vigorously, especially when the hair is wet. This can damage hair, causing it to look frizzy and have split ends.

AVOID HEATED TOOLS, such as form rollers, tongs, or hairdryers that can make hair brittle and dry over time.

DO NOT USE synthetic hair dyes and bleaches – these contain an array of toxic chemicals that not only damage and weaken hair but can also cause allergic skin reactions in some individuals. The purpose of these chemicals is to damage the cuticle of the hair enough so that dye can be absorbed into the inner cortex.

GET YOUR HAIR CUT regularly to maintain healthy hair. Hair grows about 2.5cm (1in) every 6–8 weeks.

BOOST YOUR DIET

A good way to start a healthy hair regime is to eat well, as shown below.

- Enjoy a high intake of fruit and vegetables.
- Choose foods that are high in natural fibre, such as avocado, seeds, and oats.
- Eat high-quality protein, found in oily fish.
- Balance your intake of fats in favour of healthy essential fats found in foods, such as milk and hempseed oil.
- Drink plenty of water – at least 8 glasses a day.
- Find out how to eat well for shiny hair on pp226–27.

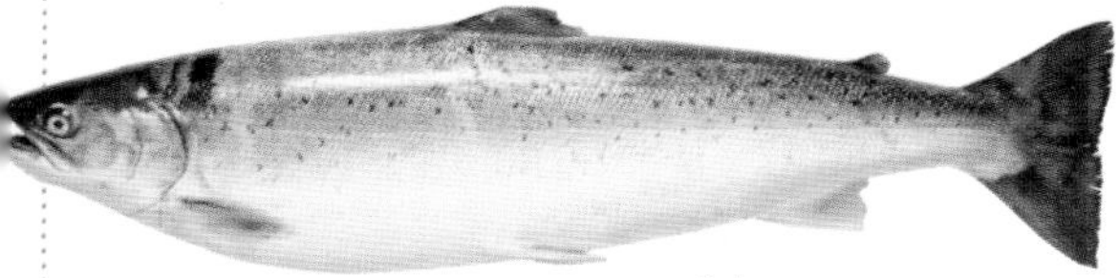

Salmon

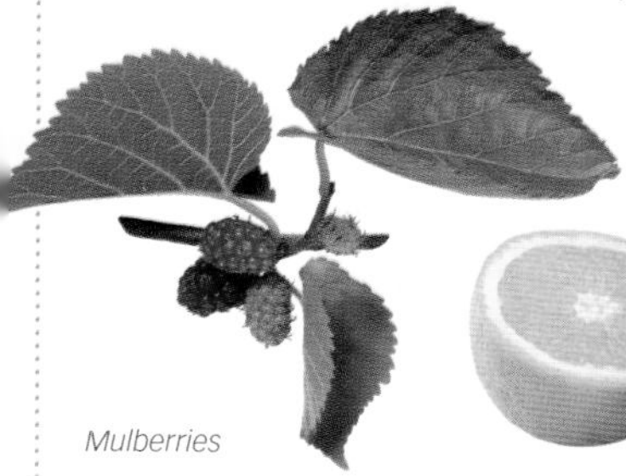

Mulberries

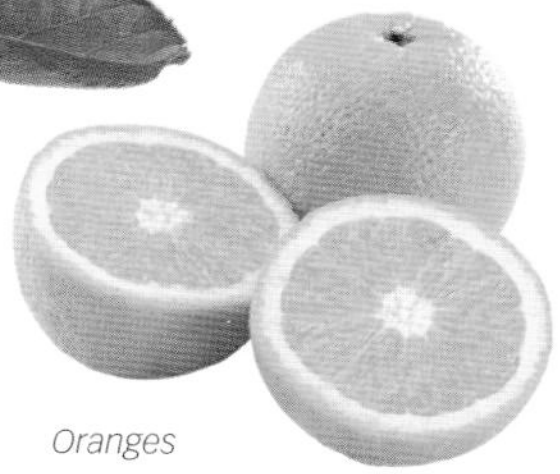

Oranges

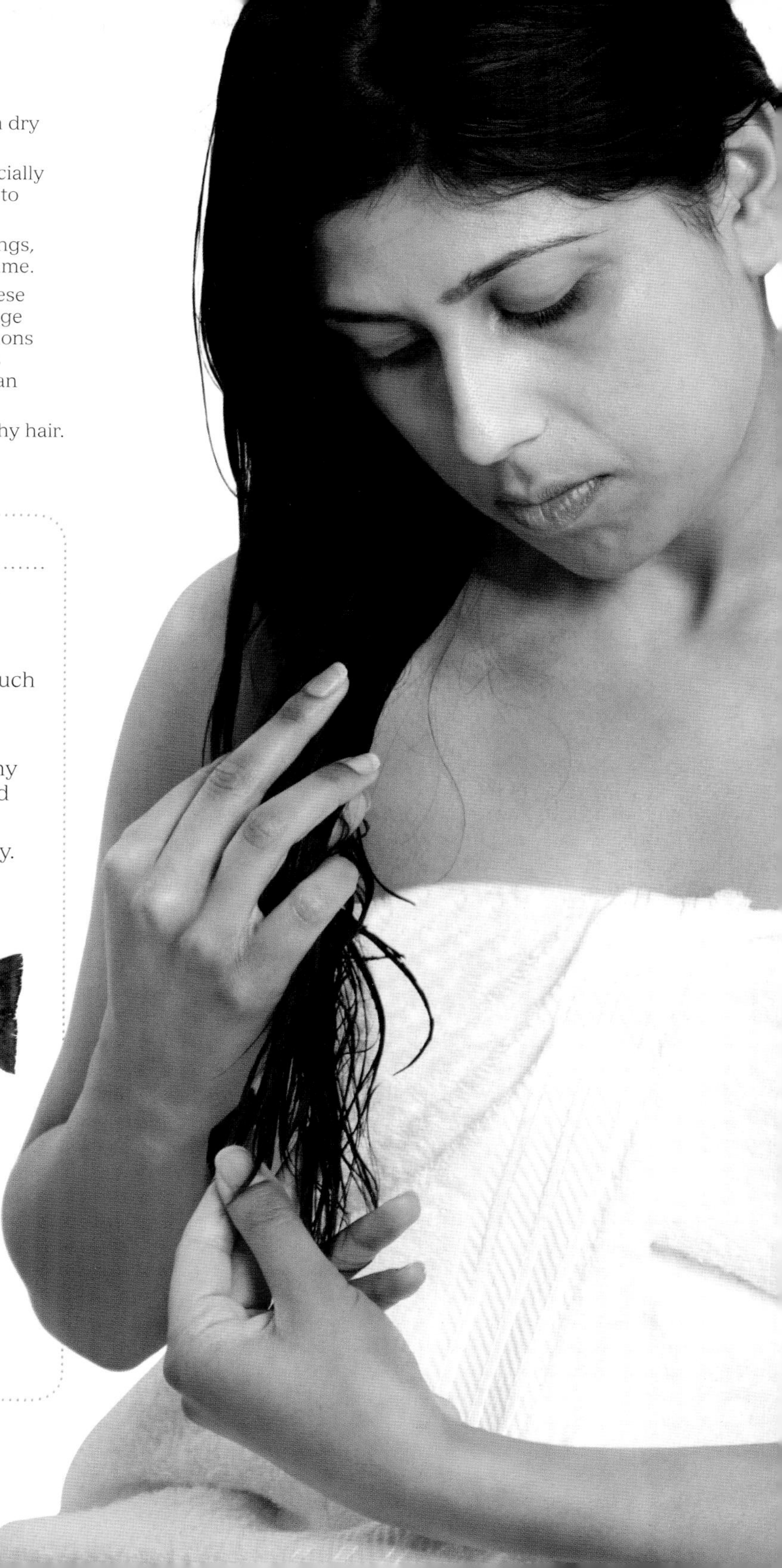

A REGIME FOR... STRONGER HAIR

Hair is made up of minerals and a type of protein called keratin. Each strand of hair lasts for about 2–5 years, and is a manifestation of our past health and habits as well as our present care. Repairing damaged hair will not happen overnight, but over time, this routine helps to make your hair glossy and strong.

TWICE A WEEK

1 SHAMPOO

Your hair type may change over time, so change your shampoo accordingly. Rotate between a clarifying shampoo and a hydrating one to keep your hair clean, shiny, and soft.

HOW TO APPLY

Apply shampoo to wet hair and massage for a few minutes. Rinse. Repeat if necessary.

2 CONDITION

Conditioners rebalance the hair and help cuticles to lie smoothly. Choose a product that suits your hair. A good conditioner nourishes, softens, and does not leave any residue.

HOW TO APPLY

Apply a generous amount to the full length of your hair, paying attention to the ends. Leave it to penetrate for 2 minutes before rinsing thoroughly.

3 RINSE

A herbal hair rinse is important, especially if you have normal–oily hair. Create your own infusion of herbs or dilute cider vinegar (see recipes p220) to add shine and balance to the natural pH of the hair and scalp.

HOW TO APPLY

Pour your home-made rinse over the hair, then rinse out thoroughly with warm water.

Hair Repair

There is a plethora of products, potions, protein, oils, and conditioners that can help to repair hair that has been damaged by exposure to the sun, hair dryers, curling tongs, flat irons, and even daily brushing. If your hair is dried out or suffers from split ends, sun damage, tangles, and brittle sections, it's time to take charge of your hair's health. It may take a bit of trial and error to find the regime that works for you, especially as our hair changes over time, so start with this regime and be responsive.

EVERY WEEK

APPLY A MASK

Rich and nourishing conditioners, masks are particularly good at repairing hair damaged by colouring or after exposure to the sea or sun. They contain nourishing oils, such as argan and jojoba, and are often combined with protein, to try to repair the keratin.

HOW TO APPLY

Apply after washing and leave on the hair – typically for 5–10 minutes – before rinsing out thoroughly with warm water.

MASSAGE SCALP

Give yourself an invigorating scalp massage, with a fruit, nut, or seed oil. Coconut, jojoba, or olive oil are all suitable as they do not clog the follicles and are extremely nourishing.

HOW TO APPLY

Rub a few drops of oil between your fingertips and massage your scalp and hair roots (see pp160–61). Then give your hair a good brushing. Rinse out if you have oily or normal hair. If you have dry hair, let the oil soak in overnight.

KEY BOTANICALS

Here are just a few of the lovely plants that can strengthen and repair your hair. Look out for them in shampoos and conditioners.

JOJOBA One of the closest botanicals to the natural oils that the scalp produces, jojoba nourishes the scalp and conditions the hair. It is an ingredient often found in good hair products.

COCONUT OIL The essential fatty acids in this oil can do wonders for dry and damaged hair. It can also be massaged into a dry scalp and the anti-fungal properties eliminate dandruff.

ROSEMARY Renowned for adding shine to dark hair, use this dried herb to make a hair rinse. Dilute the essential oil in a base oil and massage into the scalp where its stimulating properties help to promote healthy hair growth.

HONEY A classic ingredient in shampoos and conditioners because it is a humectant (capable of locking in moisture and preventing dryness and brittleness).

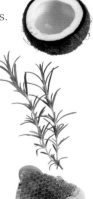

HAIR HABITS

• Try not to wash your hair every day. Once every 2–3 days, or less for some hair types, is better for the regulation of natural oils.

• Always use a conditioner after washing with shampoo. It helps to balance out any dryness or static caused by the detergents present in shampoos.

• Dry your hair gently and avoid using the hot setting on a hair dryer as it can damage the hair.

• Get your hair cut every 6 weeks or so to get rid of any split ends.

• Take a mineral supplement containing zinc, iron, and silica. They are all essential for strong, healthy hair.

Recipes to try:
Cider vinegar hair rinse, p213;
Nettle hair rinse, p213;
Rosemary conditioner, p214.

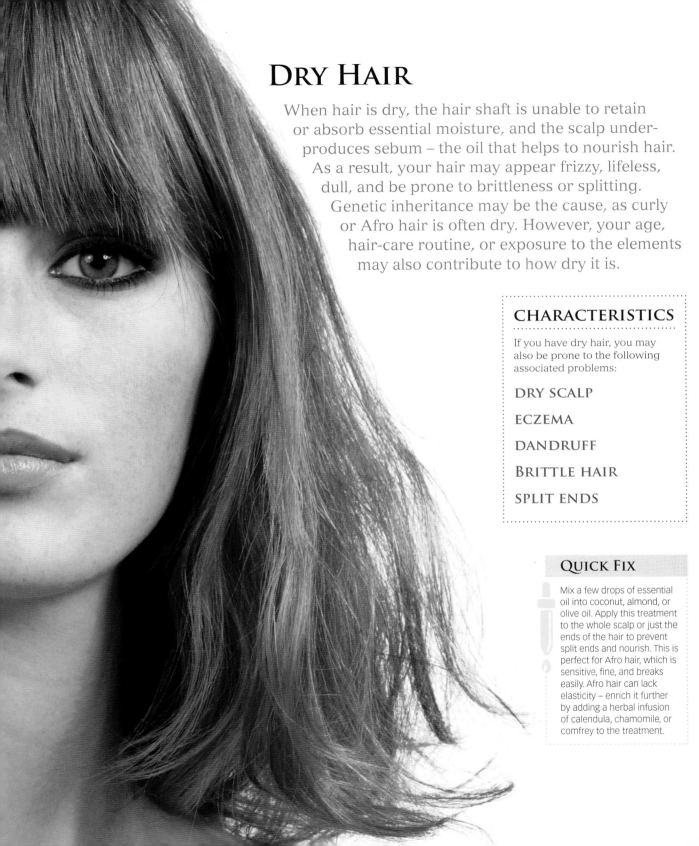

DRY HAIR

When hair is dry, the hair shaft is unable to retain or absorb essential moisture, and the scalp under-produces sebum – the oil that helps to nourish hair. As a result, your hair may appear frizzy, lifeless, dull, and be prone to brittleness or splitting. Genetic inheritance may be the cause, as curly or Afro hair is often dry. However, your age, hair-care routine, or exposure to the elements may also contribute to how dry it is.

CHARACTERISTICS

If you have dry hair, you may also be prone to the following associated problems:

DRY SCALP

ECZEMA

DANDRUFF

BRITTLE HAIR

SPLIT ENDS

QUICK FIX

Mix a few drops of essential oil into coconut, almond, or olive oil. Apply this treatment to the whole scalp or just the ends of the hair to prevent split ends and nourish. This is perfect for Afro hair, which is sensitive, fine, and breaks easily. Afro hair can lack elasticity – enrich it further by adding a herbal infusion of calendula, chamomile, or comfrey to the treatment.

TRY...

Very dry and fine hair will need to be cut regularly as the ends are brittle and easily broken. Ensure you are getting enough protein and healthy fats in your diet to support healthy hair. Many of us have dry hair due to our genetic inheritance, but there is a range of natural solutions that can help revive it.

MAKE A MASK by mixing an egg yolk and a teaspoonful of honey together. Leave it on the hair for 2 hours before washing off. Alternatively, mix 75g (2½oz) of full-fat yogurt with a generous spoonful of olive oil and 6 drops of your choice of essential oils (see Natural helpers, right). Leave on for 15–20 minutes, then rinse with warm water.

USE HOT OIL TREATMENTS once a week. Warm 60ml (2fl oz) of nourishing oil, such as jojoba or coconut oil, and massage well into the scalp and hair. If you have eczema, make sure to rub into the area behind your ears as well. Wrap your head in a towel and leave for about 20 minutes. To wash out, work a mild shampoo well into the hair.

LEAVE YOUR HAIR to dry naturally. If you need to use a hair-dryer, use it on a cool setting and keep it a good distance away from the head. After drying, apply a small amount of coconut oil or natural hair balm to the ends to add shine and protection.

BRUSH YOUR HAIR GENTLY, rotating a round barrel, natural-bristle brush downwards. This helps to close the cuticle (the outer part of the hair shaft, made up of overlapping scales) and improves shine.

USE A HAIR RINSE after washing. An infusion made with seaweed or horsetail makes a strengthening tonic. You can also use as a hairspray.

MASSAGE YOUR SCALP (see pp160–61) to relax and encourage sebum production.

AVOID...

Although our age and genetics may determine how dry our hair is, it may also be the result of washing too frequently, using harsh shampoos and styling products, or exposure to environmental factors, such as extremes in weather.

AVOID WASHING TOO MUCH – every scalp is different but if your hair is very dry you may only need to wash it every 2 or 3 days. Do not use a harsh shampoo that strips natural oils from the hair and scalp.

LIMIT YOUR USE OF HEATED TOOLS, such as curlers or straighteners, especially in conjunction with alcohol-based styling products. These dry out and damage your hair. Save these for special occasions and invest in a low-maintenance hair style for every day.

COVER YOUR HAIR if you're out in extreme weather conditions for prolonged periods of time.

AVOID HARSH CHEMICAL TREATMENTS, such as dyes, perms, and relaxers that can cause lasting damage to hair.

NATURAL HELPERS

The below natural helpers are excellent for repairing and moisturising dry hair – look out for them in shop-bought hair products and use them in your home-made treatments.

Herbal healers Calendula, chamomile, marshmallow, and comfrey

Essential oils Frankincense, palmarosa, sandalwood, geranium, chamomile, rose, patchouli, and vetiver

Moisturising oils Evening primrose, borage, avocado, sunflower, jojoba, and almond

Helpful supplements Vitamin C, biotin, iodine, selenium, and omega-3 fatty acids

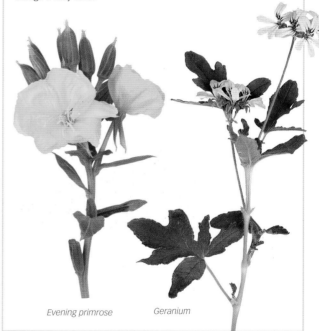

Evening primrose   *Geranium*

TREAT DANDRUFF

Dandruff is caused by yeast over-production, resulting in a flaking of skin on the scalp. To treat it, make a macerated oil (see p26) with dried peppermint, thyme, rosemary, lavender, or nettles. Alternatively, you can mix an essential oil, such as cedarwood, patchouli, sage, tea tree, thyme, or rosemary, with almond oil. Apply the macerated oil or diluted essential oil to the scalp for as long as possible, ideally overnight with hair wrapped in a turban. Wash it off with mild or diluted shampoo. If you have dry hair and dandruff, it may be a result of your diet or an allergic reaction.

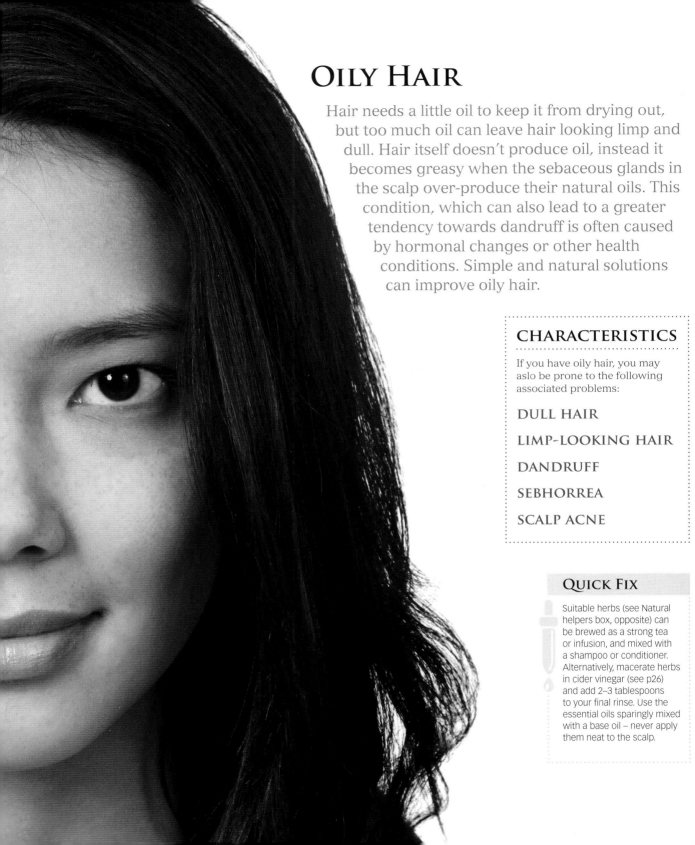

OILY HAIR

Hair needs a little oil to keep it from drying out, but too much oil can leave hair looking limp and dull. Hair itself doesn't produce oil, instead it becomes greasy when the sebaceous glands in the scalp over-produce their natural oils. This condition, which can also lead to a greater tendency towards dandruff is often caused by hormonal changes or other health conditions. Simple and natural solutions can improve oily hair.

CHARACTERISTICS

If you have oily hair, you may aslo be prone to the following associated problems:

DULL HAIR

LIMP-LOOKING HAIR

DANDRUFF

SEBHORREA

SCALP ACNE

QUICK FIX

Suitable herbs (see Natural helpers box, opposite) can be brewed as a strong tea or infusion, and mixed with a shampoo or conditioner. Alternatively, macerate herbs in cider vinegar (see p26) and add 2–3 tablespoons to your final rinse. Use the essential oils sparingly mixed with a base oil – never apply them neat to the scalp.

TRY...

People with a high density of hair – such as blondes or those with very fine hair – have more oil-producing glands in their scalp and are thus more prone to greasy hair. There are many simple and natural ways to tackle greasy hair.

DRINK LOTS OF WATER and get enough exercise to improve your circulation, which will in turn improve the condition of your hair.

TRY DUSTING A DRY POWDER into the roots in between washes. This helps to remove excess oil from your scalp. Leave for a few minutes then gently brush out. See Dry shampoo recipes (see p211).

RESTORE THE PH of your scalp by mixing a teaspoon of baking soda with clear shampoo and using it to wash your hair. Alternatively, after shampooing, rinse it with a mixture of 250ml (9fl oz) of apple cider vinegar, 250ml (9fl oz) of water, and 10 drops of either rosemary or tea tree essential oil.

RINSE THE HAIR with cold water, which will help calm overactive sebaceous glands.

TRY AN ALOE VERA RINSE to soothe a flaky and itchy scalp. Mix 500ml (16fl oz) of water with 250ml (9fl oz) of aloe vera juice. Add 20 drops of bergamot, cedarwood, cypress, geranium, grapefruit, juniper, lemon, lime, tea tree, lavender, or petitgrain essential oil, if you prefer, to make a soothing hair rinse. Use as required.

ADD SOME CURL TO YOUR HAIR – there is some evidence that this can prevent excessive oil build-up on the strands and make the oil in your hair less noticeable.

AVOID...

If your hair is greasy, you need to adjust your hair-care routine. Greasy hair can actually be made worse by frequent washing as this will affect the acid–alkaline balance of the scalp. Try to ensure that you leave at least 48 hours between each wash.

LIMIT HOW OFTEN YOU BRUSH and start your brush strokes away from your scalp. Brushing or combing your hair moves oil from the scalp to the hair. This is great if you have dry hair, but not so great if it is greasy.

AVOID HEAVY CONDITIONERS. When you do feel the need to condition, apply to the ends of the hair only. Other styling products, such as hair spray, gel, and mousse, can also make the hair oily, so avoid them too. For a novel way to set hair without too much product, try using beer. You can use warm beer, around 500ml (16fl oz), depending on how much hair you have. Add it to the final rinse, dry, and style as normal.

TURN DOWN THE HEAT. Use a hair dryer on the cool setting to ensure that you do not stimulate the sebum flow further.

STAY COOL AND DRY during warm weather, as heat and humidity accelerate oil production. Avoid exercising outside in hot and humid weather.

NATURAL HELPERS

The below natural helpers are excellent for treating and regulating oily hair – look out for them in shop-bought hair products and use them in your home-made remedies.

Herbal healers Elderflower, lemon balm, mint, rosemary, sage, yarrow, and bay

Essential oils Bergamot, cedarwood, cypress, geranium, grapefruit, juniper, lemon, lime, tea tree, lavender, and petitgrain

Moisturising oils Hazelnut, safflower, and soya

Helpful supplements Vitamins A and C, omega-3 fatty acids, and zinc

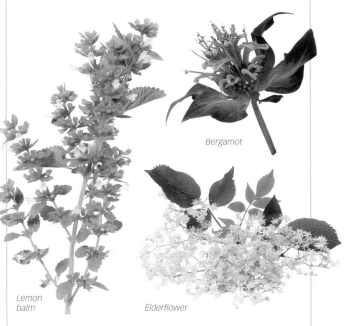

Bergamot

Lemon balm

Elderflower

KEEP CALM

Stress boosts the production of the hormone androgen and this, in turn, triggers sebum production. Take time out to relax – try meditation, gentle massage, yoga, or other nurturing and absorbing activities.

THICK HAIR

When we talk about thick hair, it refers to the diameter of the individual hair strands. Many agree that a luxurious, thick mane of hair is a blessing. However, as with all hair types, there are pros and cons. For instance, thick hair may be difficult to style, but with practice and persistence, styles can stay in place longer than other hair types. Thick hair, common in those of Asian and Latin descent, may be coarse and prone to frizz, especially when humidity is high.

CHARACTERISTICS

Thick hair may also be prone to the following problems:

FRIZZ

RIGIDITY

SURFACE DAMAGE

COARSENESS

SEBORRHEIC DERMATITIS

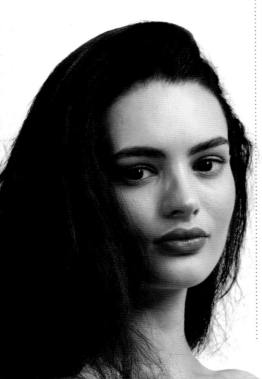

TRY...

Thick hair acts like a sponge, absorbing moisture from the environment. It absorbs up to 40 per cent more moisture than fine hair, which is why it is more prone to frizz. To keep your thick hair looking its best, keep the following suggestions in mind.

USE MILD SHAMPOOS that do not strip essential oils from the scalp and hair.

MOISTURISE YOUR HAIR to help tame the frizz. Rub a tiny bit of coconut oil on your hands and then run it through your tresses, starting a little way from the scalp.

STYLE IT – long, thick hair cries out for braiding and twisting, so experiment with a herringbone braid behind one ear or a classic French twist.

RINSE THOROUGHLY after shampooing and conditioning. Residues of product left behind can lead to an itchy, flaky scalp. Make sure the water is warm, but not hot, as hot water can remove moisture from the hair, leaving it dry and frizzy.

AVOID...

Although thick hair does not usually show dirt or greasiness as quickly as fine hair, it still needs meticulous care to keep it looking its best.

DO NOT RUSH – if you have very thick hair, your most effective styling accessory is time. For some with very long, thick hair, a wash-and-go approach to hair will just not work. It can take up to an hour to get hair completely dry after washing. Section your hair properly when drying and styling to get the best from it.

NEVER BRUSH WET HAIR – use a wide-toothed comb to gently undo tangles and leave to dry naturally if you can.

AVOID VERY HOT DRYERS as they add extra volume that you will not need. Turn down the heat while drying hair to look your best.

DO NOT USE PERMANENT COLOURS, as they can have a thickening effect. Instead, opt for semi-permanent colours.

QUICK FIX

Once a week, condition your hair with an intensive mask. Use natural conditioning ingredients such as olive oil, jojoba oil, shea nut butter, or aloe vera. Apply to wet hair and allow it to soak in for 20 minutes before washing out with a mild shampoo.

NATURAL HELPERS

Look for these natural helpers in shop-bought products and use them in your home-made remedies.

Herbal healers Rose, rosemary, thyme, nettle, and aloe vera

Essential oils Cedarwood, rosemary, orange, lavender, and geranium

Moisturising oils Coconut, almond, jojoba, and hazelnut

Helpful supplements Iron, vitamin B complex including biotin, and vitamins C and E

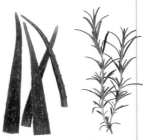

Aloe vera   *Rosemary*

FINE HAIR

The term "fine" refers to the diameter of the hair shaft, not the number of individual strands of hair on your head. In fact, people with fine hair generally have more hair on their scalp. Unless it has some natural curl, fine hair is a challenge to style – it is often flat and lifeless, and many of the products we use to style it can weigh it down, making the problem worse. However, with a little attention to detail, even very fine hair can feel lustrous.

CHARACTERISTICS

Fine hair may also be prone to the following problems:

DRYNESS

FLYAWAYS

BREAKAGE

FRIZZ

SPLIT ENDS

GETS DIRTY QUICKLY

NATURAL HELPERS

Look for these natural helpers in shop-bought products and use them in your home-made remedies.

Herbal healers Calendula, oat straw, and seaweed

Essential oils Geranium, lavender, chamomile, and lemongrass

Moisturising oils Evening primrose, borage, avocado, sunflower, jojoba, and almond

Helpful supplements Vitamin C, biotin, iodine, selenium, and omega-3 fatty acids

Sunflower

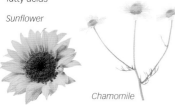

Chamomile

TRY...

Fine hair is not always a curse. Properly cared for and kept in good condition, it can be baby-soft, silky, and a joy to touch.

PRE-TREAT YOUR HAIR with jojoba or almond oil. Gently warm the oil and massage thoroughly into your hair and scalp, wrap your head in a towel, and leave it for 20 minutes. Wash the treatment out with a gentle shampoo.

EAT HEALTHILY – a diet with adequate protein is key to healthy hair. Don't forget plenty of green vegetables, fresh fruit, and wholegrains.

STAY HYDRATED by drinking at least 8 glasses of water a day.

BE WEATHER WISE and protect your hair from environmental damage – whether it's the sun, wind, or snow.

GET YOUR HAIR CUT every 6–8 weeks. Even if it is well cared for, fine hair is prone to splitting.

AVOID...

Adjusting your hair-care routine can improve the health of fine hair immediately.

AVOID HEAVY GELS and sprays that usually only make hair look more flat and dull.

BRUSH GENTLY and less frequently, especially when wet. Aggressive, frequent brushing can easily break your hair and cause split ends. Never brush wet hair.

MINIMIZE USE OF HEATED TOOLS, such as straighteners, curling irons, or hair dryers. When you do use them, make sure they are on a low setting and use a heat-protecting product.

AVOID LONG STYLES as they are more prone to damage. A short cut helps keep your hair in top condition. Blunt or one-length haircuts can make hair look fuller and thicker at the ends. If you like longer styles, try a bit of layering to give it some lift.

DO NOT USE HEAVY CONDITIONERS and apply conditioner to the ends of your hair, not the roots. This prevents your hair from being weighed down.

MINIMIZE USING ACCESSORIES, such as hairpins, clips, and rubber bands, which can cause extensive hair breakage.

QUICK FIX

Boost fine hair between washes with an infusion. In a saucepan over a medium heat, place 2 tablespoons each of dried chamomile and lemongrass in 600ml (1 pint) of boiling water. Simmer for 10 minutes, allow to cool, and strain into a bottle with an atomizer.

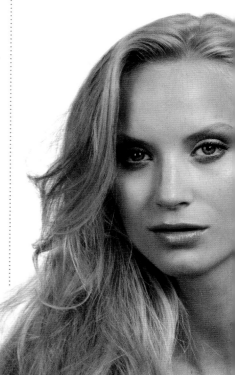

Recipes For Your Hair

REJUVENATE YOUR HAIR WITH RECIPES THAT DON'T STRIP THE HAIR OF ITS NATURAL OILS OR COAT IT. FIND CONDITIONING **TREATMENTS** THAT **MOISTURISE** WITH THE HELP OF ORGANIC OILS AND WAXES, AND RINSES THAT USE ESSENTIAL OILS TO ADD **FRAGRANCE** AND IMPROVE THE **CONDITION** OF YOUR SCALP AND HAIR.

Dry Shampoo

FOR FAIR HAIR

Dry shampoo can help **avoid oily roots,** give your hair **extra volume,** and work as a good **styling aid**, separating curls and adding a subtle hold. The arrowroot and cornflour **absorb** the excess oil. This recipe will coat your hair, leaving it dry and matt. The powders used here are light in colour, so can help to lighten the roots if your hair is dyed. Add essential oils to make your hair smell heavenly.

MAKES 30G (1OZ)

INGREDIENTS
1 tbsp cornflour
1 tbsp arrowroot
10 drops of either grapefruit, peppermint, or eucalyptus globulus essential oil (optional)

HOW TO MAKE
1 Mix the cornflour and arrowroot together in a bowl.
2 Add 10 drops of any of the essential oils, if desired, and mix well.
3 Place in a sterilized airtight container and shake well before use. Store in a cool dry place. Keeps for up to 3 months.

HOW TO APPLY
Use on dry hair. Use an old make-up brush and brush the powder into the roots or oily parts of your hair. Comb through the hair and style as usual.

Dry Shampoo with Cocoa Powder

FOR DARK HAIR

This recipe is a variation of the dry shampoo recipe shown above. The combination of **oil-absorbing** cocoa powder (to match the darker hair tones), starchy arrowroot, and cornflour, will **revive** your hair. If you do not want to use cocoa powder on your hair, you could simply use the arrowroot and cornflour mixed together before you go to bed, to allow the pale powder to absorb.

MAKES 30G (1OZ)

INGREDIENTS
4 tsp cocoa powder
1 tsp cornflour
1 tsp arrowroot
10 drops essential oil of your choice (see suggestions above)

HOW TO MAKE
1 Mix the cocoa powder, cornflour, and arrowroot together in a bowl.
2 Add the essential oil, if desired, and mix well.
3 Place in a sterilized airtight container and shake well before use. Store in a cool, dry place. Keeps for up to 3 months.

HOW TO APPLY
Use on dry hair. Use an old make-up brush and brush the powder into the roots or oily parts of your hair. Comb through the hair and style as usual.

CLEANSING HAIR PASTE

FOR ALL HAIR TYPES

This cheap, effective, chemical-free recipe **cleanses** the hair and leaves it **fresh** and soft. When you first start to use it, you may find it takes your scalp a while to adjust to the change in "washing" style. This is short-lived and is worth persevering with. You can easily personalize this hair paste to your hair type, adding essential oils that add **fragrance** and bring out the best in your hair.

MAKES 85G (3OZ)

INGREDIENTS

2 tbsp bicarbonate of soda
2 tbsp water
2 drops essential oil of your choice
(see below)

HOW TO MAKE

1 Mix the bicarbonate of soda and water together in a bowl to form a paste. Add more water if it is too stiff, or more bicarbonate of soda if it is too wet.
2 Add the essential oil of your choice and mix together thoroughly.
3 Pour into a sterilized squeezable bottle. Store in a cool, dark place. Keeps for up to a week.

HOW TO APPLY

Shake well before use. The amount required depends on the length of your hair. Apply enough of the paste to cover dry or wet hair. Work the paste into the scalp and through to the ends of the hair. Leave for 2–4 minutes and rinse with warm water. Dry and style as usual. Use 3–4 times a week in combination with the Cider vinegar hair rinse (see opposite).

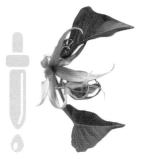

FOR NORMAL HAIR

2 DROPS
YLANG YLANG
ESSENTIAL OIL

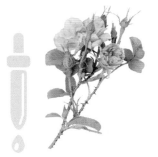

FOR DRY HAIR

2 DROPS
ROSE ABSOLUTE
ESSENTIAL OIL

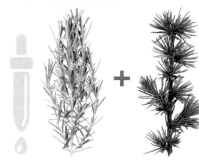

FOR OILY HAIR

1 DROP
ROSEMARY
ESSENTIAL OIL

1 DROP
CEDARWOOD
ESSENTIAL OIL

CIDER VINEGAR HAIR RINSE

FOR ALL HAIR TYPES

Cleanse and **balance** the hair with this cuticle-smoothing hair rinse. Cuticles cover the hair shaft and offer it protection. They need to be healthy and in good condition to give your hair a smooth appearance. Cider vinegar removes scaly build-up and residue from the hair shaft, giving the hair more shine, and it can balance the pH of the hair. Add essential oils for a delicious fragrance.

MAKES 120ML (4FL OZ)

INGREDIENTS

2 tbsp apple cider vinegar
8 tbsp water
8 drops rosemary essential oil
6 drops lemon essential oil
4 drops grapefruit essential oil

HOW TO MAKE

1 Mix the vinegar and water together in a bowl. Use less vinegar for dry hair and more for oily hair.
2 Add the essential oils and mix thoroughly.
3 Pour into a sterilized squeezable bottle or a bottle topped with an atomizer. Store in a cool place. Keeps for up to 3 months.

HOW TO APPLY

Shake well before use. Use on wet hair in the shower or bath. Apply the product to your hair and leave for 1–2 minues. Avoid getting it in your eyes. Rinse the hair with water until the vinegar smell is faint. Dry and style as usual. Use 3–4 times a week after the Cleansing hair paste (see opposite).

NETTLE HAIR RINSE

FOR DRY SCALP

Many of us suffer from a dry, itchy scalp at some point in our lives. This hair rinse contains a combination of English garden herbs that have wonderful properties for **scalp health**. Nettles are a fantastic **cleansing**, **detoxifying**, and **strengthening** tonic for the whole body. This combination of nettle and sage creates a very useful hair rinse for a dry and flaking, itchy, or allergic scalp.

MAKES 200ML (7FL OZ)

INGREDIENTS

200ml (7fl oz) mineral water
1 tbsp nettle dried herb
1 tbsp sage dried herb
1 tbsp rosemary dried herb
4 drops peppermint essential oil

HOW TO MAKE

1 To make the infusion, boil the mineral water in a saucepan. Place the dried herbs in a teapot or glass bowl and pour the boiling water over. Leave to steep for 10 minutes, then strain.
2 Allow to cool, then add the essential oil and mix well. Pour into a sterilized bottle and leave to cool before placing the lid on. Store in a cool, dry place. Keeps for up to 6 weeks.

HOW TO APPLY

Shake well before use. Use on wet hair before shampooing. Pour a cupful over wet hair in the shower or bath. Massage into the hair or comb through the hair, then follow with your usual shampoo. After use, dry and style as usual.

ROSEMARY CONDITIONER

FOR DRY HAIR

Invigorating rosemary is excellent for hair and scalp health, and can treat hair loss and dandruff. It is combined with three super oils for hair health – shea butter, one of the few ingredients that can help **repair** split ends; argan oil, which **conditions** and **moisturises** the hair; and coconut oil, which **softens** and **soothes** the hair and scalp.

MAKES 45ML (1½FL OZ)

INGREDIENTS

1 tbsp shea butter
1 tbsp coconut oil
1 tbsp argan oil
10 drops rosemary essential oil

HOW TO MAKE

1 Heat the butter and oils together in a bain-marie (see p133), until melted. Allow to cool for 30–40 minutes.

2 Using a hand-held whisk or a stick blender, whisk the oily mixture continuously, until you have the texture of double cream.

3 Add the essential oil and mix. Spoon the mixture into a sterilized jar and leave to cool before placing the lid on. Store in a cool, dry place. Keeps for up to 6 weeks.

HOW TO APPLY

This conditioner is very rich, so you don't need to use much. Depending on the length of your hair, a coin-sized amount of the product should be enough for one application. Massage into the hair, paying particular attention to the scalp and ends. To use as a hair mask, wrap the hair in a warm towel and leave for 30–60 minutes, or overnight. To remove the product, rub shampoo through the hair before it comes in contact with water, then rinse out the shampoo and repeat to ensure any last traces of the oils have been removed.

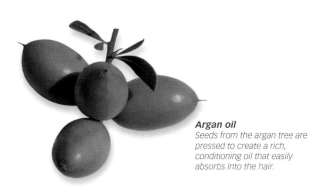

Argan oil
Seeds from the argan tree are pressed to create a rich, conditioning oil that easily absorbs into the hair.

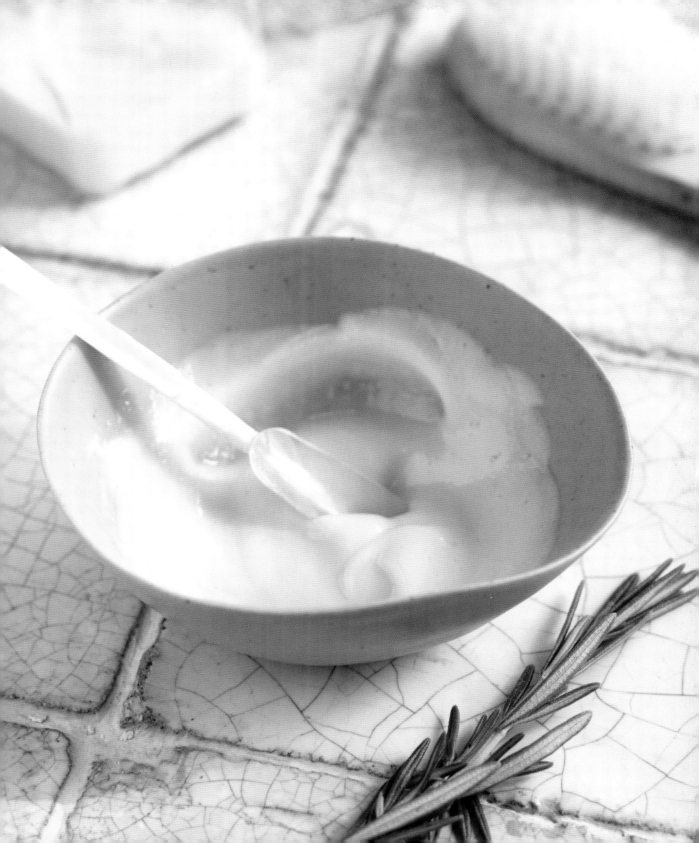

COCONUT CONDITIONER

FOR OILY HAIR

This coconut conditioner leaves the hair feeling soft and light. Coconut is often used in hair care – the oil **softens** the hair and **soothes** the scalp, and its milk has similar **conditioning** and **nourishing** effects on the hair. Egg yolk has long been used to improve the condition of hair. It can **strengthen** hair as well as **moisturise** and condition it.

MAKES ENOUGH FOR ONE APPLICATION

INGREDIENTS

1 egg yolk
1 tsp solid coconut oil
3 tbsp coconut milk

HOW TO MAKE

1 Using a hand-held whisk or stick blender, whisk the egg yolk and coconut oil together in a bowl until frothy.
2 Add the coconut milk and mix until smooth.
3 Pour into a squeezy bottle for easy application. Store in a cool, dry place. Keeps for up to 6 weeks.

HOW TO APPLY

Apply to hair and massage into the scalp. Leave for 2–5 minutes. Rinse with cool water. Dry and style hair as normal.

Massage Your Scalp

Use this simple sequence to massage the conditioner into your hair and invigorate your scalp, promoting healthy, strong hair.

- Gently massage the whole of the head with thumbs and fingers in a "shampooing motion".
- Grasp fistfuls of hair at the roots and tug from side to side, keeping the knuckles close to the scalp.
- Squeeze the temples with the heel of the hands and make slow circular movements.
- Find the occipital bone – the bone you can feel at the back of your head towards the top of your neck. Place the left thumb under the left occipital area and the right thumb on the right occipital area. Use a rubbing movement to release the muscles.

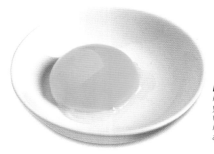

Egg yolk
Nutritionally rich, egg yolk contains protein, vitamins, and minerals. It is also perfect for treating acne and dry, flaky skin.

CHAMOMILE DETANGLER

FOR ALL HAIR TYPES

This combination of chamomile and coconut milk helps to **condition** and **smooth** the hair. Chamomile infusions have been used for years for their medicinal benefits. They can **brighten** up blonde hair and lighten darker shades, and are also very good at **soothing** irritated scalp. Coconut milk is **conditioning** and **nourishing** and acts as a natural detangler for the hair.

INGREDIENTS

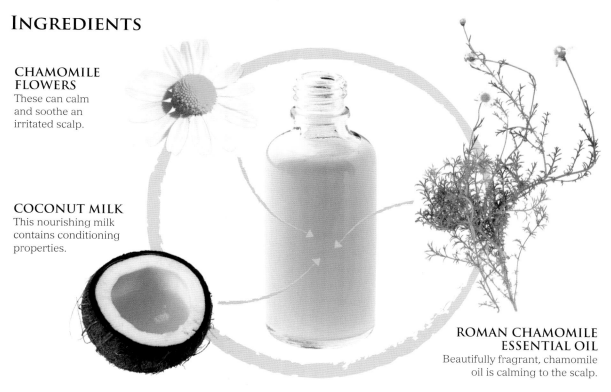

CHAMOMILE FLOWERS
These can calm and soothe an irritated scalp.

COCONUT MILK
This nourishing milk contains conditioning properties.

ROMAN CHAMOMILE ESSENTIAL OIL
Beautifully fragrant, chamomile oil is calming to the scalp.

MAKES 200ML (7FL OZ)

INGREDIENTS
200ml (7fl oz) mineral water
1 tbsp chamomile flowers
2 drops Roman chamomile essential oil
2 tbsp coconut milk

HOW TO MAKE

1 To make the chamomile flower infusion, boil the mineral water. Place the flowers in a teapot or glass bowl and pour the boiling water over. Leave to steep for 10 minutes, then strain.

2 Add the essential oil to the coconut milk and mix well.

3 Add the coconut milk mixture to the cooled infusion and mix.

4 Pour into a sterilized bottle and place an atomizer on. Store in a cool, dry place. Keeps for up to 6 weeks.

HOW TO APPLY

Shake well before use. Spray on clean wet hair, comb through, and rinse off with warm water or use as a leave-in product.

HENNA HAIR-DYE RINSE

QUICK

FOR ALL HAIR TYPES

Henna is a **natural hair dye** that has been used for thousands of years. It can dry hair, so if your hair is already dry, add a tablespoon each of any base oil and warm milk to the paste. Follow the package instructions to create your dye, and use before the Hot oil treatment (see opposite) or the Banana hair mask (see p222). You may wish to dye a cutting of your hair before you use it for the first time.

MAKES ENOUGH FOR ONE APPLICATION

INGREDIENTS

for short or cropped hair use
25g (scant 1oz) henna

for shoulder-length hair use
50g (1¾oz) henna

for long hair use
75g (2½oz) henna

HOW TO MAKE

1 Depending on your hair length, measure the henna powder you want to use and place it in a bowl. According to package instructions, heat a measured amount of water in a saucepan.

2 Pour the hot water over the powder and, wearing gloves, mix well to make a paste or "henna pack". Use immediately.

HOW TO APPLY

Wearing rubber gloves, smooth the henna paste into the hair and massage into the scalp and hair. Leave for 30–40 minutes. For a more intense colour, wrap hair in a towel and leave for 1–4 hours, or overnight. Henna may leave the hair slightly stiff but it has a long history of safe use.

Dyeing With Henna

Henna has been used by women for thousands of years to dye hair, fingernails, palms, and the soles of the feet. It comes from a small, attractive shrub with pale green leaves, which are dried and crushed into a greenish–yellow powder that is then mixed into a paste and used to colour the hair. On dark hair, henna tends to produce a brown–orange, auburn colour. Allergic reactions to it are extremely rare although it may cause irritation to very sensitive skin. Always do a patch test before use, by dabbing some of the paste onto the sensitive skin behind the ears and leaving for 24–48 hours. Wash off. Any skin irritation will show on your skin.

HOT OIL TREATMENT

FOR ALL HAIR TYPES

This hot oil hair treatment will add an extra healthy-looking **glow** to your hair and is an easy-to-make monthly **conditioning** treatment for silky tresses. Coconut is a **nourishing** hair oil, jojoba oil forms a film on the scalp and hair, making hair **silky smooth** and **soft**, while olive oil is a natural moisturiser and will **soften** and **smooth** the hair. This recipe makes enough for medium-length hair.

MAKES ENOUGH FOR ONE APPLICATION

INGREDIENTS

1 tsp soild coconut oil
1 tsp olive oil
1 tsp jojoba oil

HOW TO MAKE

1 Gently heat the oils together in a bain-marie (see p133) until the solid coconut oil has melted.
2 The mixture should be warm but not hot (you do not want to burn your scalp). It if gets too hot, allow it to cool a little before applying. Use immediately.

HOW TO APPLY

Apply to clean, damp hair. Dip fingertips into the warm oil and massage the oil into the scalp and hair, working your way from the roots to the ends. Warm up a towel on a radiator and wrap hair in the warm towel. Leave for 20 minutes. Wash hair thoroughly after use, applying shampoo to your oily hair before getting your hair wet. Dry and style as usual. Use once a month for glossy, healthy hair.

SOLID COCONUT OIL

When warm, nutritious coconut oil melts and feels luxurious in your hair and scalp.

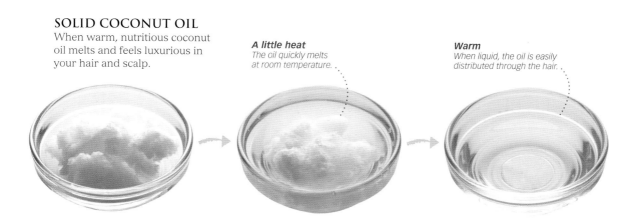

A little heat
The oil quickly melts at room temperature.

Warm
When liquid, the oil is easily distributed through the hair.

10-MINUTE LUSCIOUS LOCKS

It only takes 10 minutes to improve the condition of your hair. This conditioning, massaging, and rinsing sequence rejuvenates your hair and leaves it shiny and luscious. Herbs revive the colour in your hair, so use a herbal hair rinse after washing. Prepare your own in advance, choosing a recipe that suits your colour.

TOOLS

Choose a hairbrush made with natural bristles, not pig-hair bristles. You could use a comb instead, especially if you have short hair.

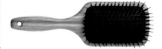

HOME-MADE HAIR RINSES

Fair hair rinse Place 1 tbsp calendula flowers, 1 tbsp chamomile flowers, and the juice of 1 lemon in a teapot. Pour over boiling water and leave to infuse for 10 minutes. Strain the infusion into a jug.

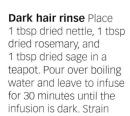

Calendula

Dark hair rinse Place 1 tbsp dried nettle, 1 tbsp dried rosemary, and 1 tbsp dried sage in a teapot. Pour over boiling water and leave to infuse for 30 minutes until the infusion is dark. Strain the infusion into a jug.

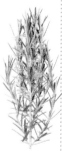

Rosemary

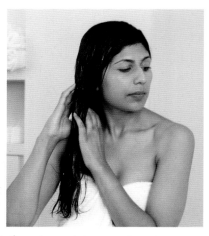

1 Wash your hair as usual. Apply a generous amount of conditioner to your wet hair, all the way to the ends.

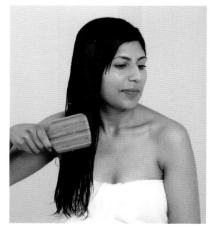

2 Using a brush or comb, spread a little conditioner through the hair, making sure it is evenly applied.

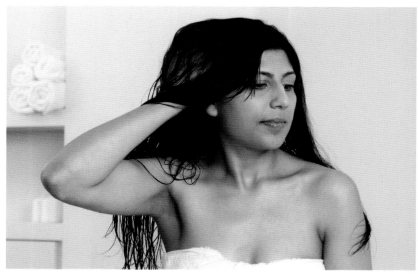

3 Massage the scalp for 3 minutes, using slow, circular movements with the fingertips as if shampooing the hair. Make sure you have covered the whole scalp.

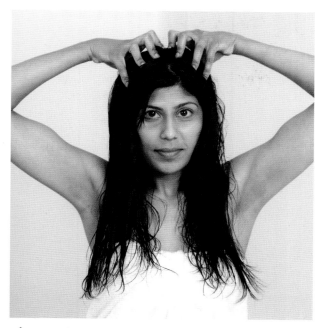

4 For another 2 minutes, invigorate the scalp by scratching it with the pads of the fingertips, being sure to cover all areas of the scalp.

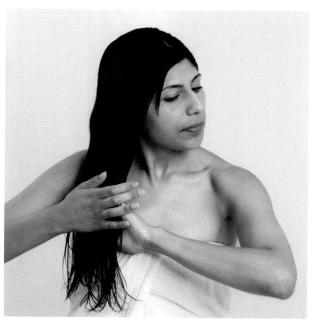

5 Using the flat palms of your hands, apply a little pressure and smooth the hair down slowly with your fingers, all the way from root to tip.

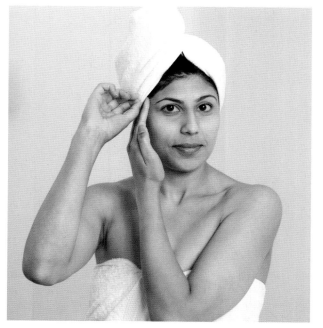

6 Wrap your hair in a warm towel, tucking in all loose strands. Sit comfortably and relax for 5 minutes, before rinsing the conditioner out of your hair using clean water.

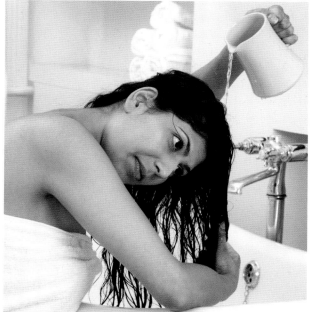

7 Pour the prepared home-made herbal rinse over your hair. Rinse it out thoroughly with clean warm water, before drying your hair and styling it as normal.

Banana Hair Mask

FOR ALL HAIR TYPES

Use overripe bananas to make a deeply **moisturising** hair mask, which can do wonders for your scalp and hair. Bananas are a rich source of potassium and vitamins A, C, and E, which are known to help hair to become **strong** and healthy. This makes them a perfect fruit for home-made hair treatments. This quick and easy recipe makes hair feel **soft** and **conditioned**.

MAKES ENOUGH FOR ONE APPLICATION

INGREDIENTS
1 medium-sized ripe banana
1 ripe avocado
3 tbsp coconut milk

HOW TO MAKE

1 Using a fork, mash the soft banana and avocado in a bowl.

2 Add the coconut milk and mix well to make a paste. If you have very dry or damaged hair, you could leave out the avocado and replace the coconut milk with 1 tablespoon almond, coconut, or olive oil.

3 Use immediately as the mask contains fresh ingredients.

HOW TO APPLY

Massage into dry hair and leave for 15 minutes. For optimal effect, wrap the hair in a towel, preferably warm, and leave for 15 minutes. Rinse the paste from the hair with warm water and wash as usual.

Cedarwood Hair Treatment

FOR OILY HAIR

The **regenerative**, **antiseptic**, and **astringent** properties of cedarwood oil can help in the treatment of oily hair, dandruff, and scalp irritation. The coconut oil in this recipe **nourishes** the hair and adds body, lustre, and shine. An excellent **antiseptic**, lavender **soothes** as well as **heals**, and has the ability to promote the formation of scar tissue.

MAKES 45G (1½OZ)

INGREDIENTS
2 tbsp solid coconut oil
3 tsp neem oil
5 drops cedarwood essential oil
5 drops lavender essential oil
5 drops rosemary essential oil

HOW TO MAKE

1 Heat the oils together in a bain-marie (see p133), until they have melted. Remove from the heat. Add the essential oils and mix well.

2 Pour into a sterilized jar and leave to cool before placing the lid on. Store in a cool, dark, and dry place. Keeps for up to 3 months.

HOW TO APPLY

Depending on the length of your hair, a coin-sized amount of the product should be enough for one application. Massage into the hair, paying particular attention to the scalp, then wrap the hair in a warm towel and leave for 30–60 minutes, or overnight. To remove the product, rub shampoo through the hair before it comes in contact with water, then rinse out the shampoo with warm water. Repeat to ensure that all traces of the oils have been removed. Leave hair to dry naturally.

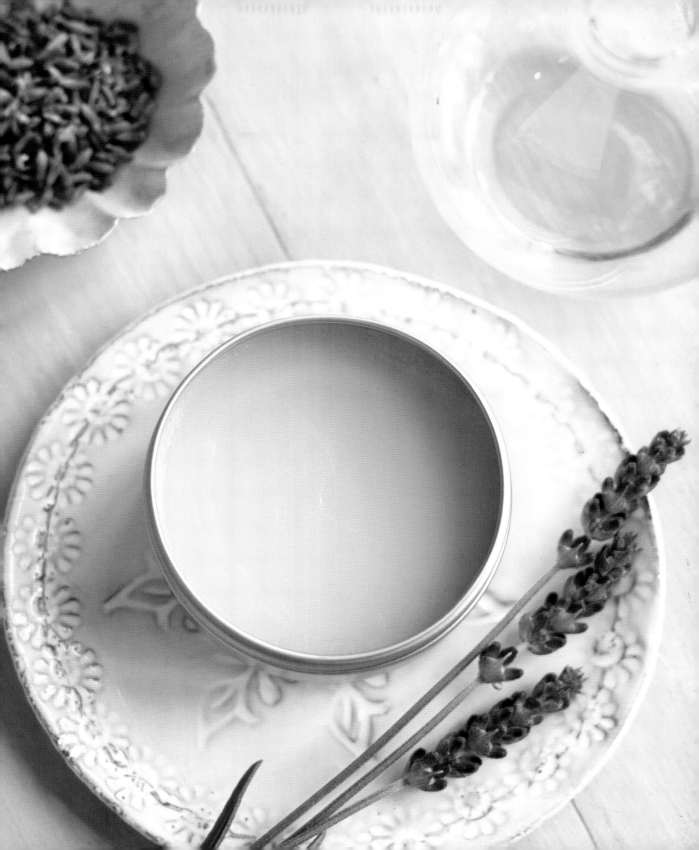

Neem And Coconut Scalp Balm

FOR DRY OR FLAKY SCALP

Neem oil is commonly used in Ayurvedic medicine, and the earliest Sanskrit writings describe its use in curing illness. The twigs of the tree are used as toothbrushes in Asia, and the leaves are commonly used for their medicinal properties. The oil is **antiseptic** and an effective insect repellent. Neem oil **treats scalp problems**, **prevents itching and dandruff**, and is an effective treatment for head lice.

MAKES 45G (1½OZ)

INGREDIENTS

1 tbsp neem oil
2 tbsp solid coconut oil
3 drops sage essential oil
3 drops tea tree essential oil
3 drops lavender essential oil

HOW TO MAKE

1 Gently heat the neem and coconut oils together in a bain-marie (see p133) until the oils have melted. Remove from the heat.
2 Add all the essential oils and mix thoroughly.
3 Pour into a sterilized jar and leave to cool for 1–2 hours. Use on the scalp or place the lid on and store in a cool, dark place. Keeps for up to 3 months.

HOW TO APPLY

Massage into the scalp once a week. Leave for 10 minutes, and wash out with shampoo, rinsing with warm water.

Rosemary And Coconut Glossy Hair Balm

FOR ALL HAIR TYPES

Hair can lose its shine and lustre, especially if you use products that leave build-up or strip the hair of its natural moisture. One of the best ways to keep hair shiny and healthy is to eat a healthy diet and take regular exercise. This simple hair gloss **enhances** natural hair as well as **protects** hair from damage. You can use it on wet or dry hair.

MAKES 20G (¾OZ)

INGREDIENTS

1 tbsp solid coconut oil
1 tsp cocoa butter
5 drops rosemary essential oil

HOW TO MAKE

1 Gently heat the coconut oil and cocoa butter in a bain-marie (see p133) until the butter has melted. Remove from the heat.
2 Add the rosemary essential oil and mix. Pour into a sterilized jar and leave to cool before placing the lid on. Store in a cool, dark place. Keeps for up to 3 months.

HOW TO APPLY

Apply to clean, damp hair. Smooth the hair gloss down the hair, concentrating on the ends, and leave on for 3–5 minutes, then rinse with warm water. Dry and style as usual. Apply sparingly to clean, dry hair, smoothing down the hair to the ends and avoiding the scalp.

SHEA BUTTER ANTI-FRIZZ BALM

FOR FRIZZY HAIR

Frizzy, messy, tangled hair is a result of the outer hair cuticle lifting up and not lying flat and smooth. To reduce frizz, avoid brushing hair when dry as it can damage the hair cuticle. Shea butter is **nourishing** and **moisturising**. Apply to the hair and work into the roots for hair that is much more manageable. It is good for split ends and **protects** the hair by coating it with a shiny layer.

MAKES 90ML (3FL OZ)

INGREDIENTS

1 tsp shea nut butter
1 tbsp argan oil
1 tsp emulsifying wax
1 tsp glycerin
4 tbsp aloe vera juice
5 drops essential oil of your choice (see below)

HOW TO MAKE

1 Create an emulsion (see p109) by melting the shea nut butter, argan oil, and emulsifying wax together in a bain-marie. Remove from the heat once the wax has melted.

2 Mix the glycerin with the aloe vera juice, and heat gently.

3 Add the warm oil mixture to the warm aloe vera mixture. Using a hand-held whisk or stick blender, whisk continuously until smooth.

4 Add the essential oil. Pour into a sterilized bottle and leave to cool before placing on a pump. Store in a cool, dark place. Keeps for up to 3 months.

HOW TO APPLY

Shake well before use. After shampooing, pump a small amount into your palm, rub your hands together, and smooth it over hair. Rinse with warm water or use as a leave-in conditioner, then dry and style as usual.

FOR DANDRUFF

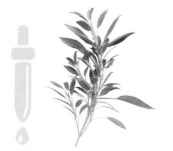

5 DROPS SAGE ESSENTIAL OIL

FOR TREATING HAIR LOSS

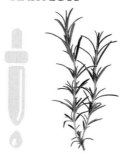

5 DROPS ROSEMARY ESSENTIAL OIL

FOR IRRITATED SCALP

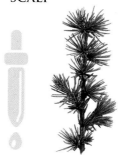

5 DROPS CEDARWOOD ESSENTIAL OIL

EAT WELL FOR... SHINY HAIR

Your diet and lifestyle reflect how healthy your hair is. In order to shine, hair requires healthy follicles and scalp, plus sufficient protein and minerals to create strong strands of hair. Improve your diet to bring shine to your hair – after about 6–8 weeks you will start to see the benefits, as nutritional deficiencies are corrected and new, healthier, and shinier hair grows.

BOOST YOUR BASICS

TRY MORE PROTEIN Hair is formed mainly of a protein called keratin. For strong hair with flat cuticles that generate shine, you need to eat lots of good-quality protein. Eat fewer refined carbohydrates and more protein with each meal. Fish, eggs, nuts and seeds, and a little organic meat, beans, and pulses are all fantastic sources of protein.

INCREASE ZINC This mineral is very important for hair health, and contributes both to the repair and growth of our hair. Many of us are zinc deficient, as intensive agriculture has depleted the soil of its normal levels. Concentrate on zinc-rich foods, such as oats, or take a zinc supplement.

GO FOR IRON Many of us are deficient in the mineral iron. One of the symptoms of iron deficiency or anaemia is thinning hair. Eat foods rich in iron, such as nuts and leafy greens, or take a supplement to improve hair growth and volume.

CHOOSE SILICA As we age, the source of silica in our bodies can become exhausted. This depletion results in lacklustre and thinning hair. Natural sources of silica include oats, brown rice, barley, green vegetables, soya beans, and apples.

TRY OMEGA-RICH OILS Keep your scalp nourished with plenty of "good" oils. Find them in fish, and nuts and seeds, such as hazelnuts or hemp.

SUPERFOODS

Supplement a balanced diet with these vitamin-rich superfoods that contain everything you need to strengthen keratin, protect the scalp, and bring shine to your hair.

OILY FISH
Salmon, mackerel, and sardines are the richest source of omega-fatty acids for scalp health, as well as containing keratin-building protein and the fat-soluble vitamins A, D, E, and K. Try to eat oily fish at least twice a week.

HAZELNUTS
A rich source of folate and the vitamin B biotin, hazelnuts are great for healthy hair. They also contain protein and omega-fatty acids. The skin contains a large amount of proanthocyanidin – an antioxidant that protects the scalp and hair-follicle cells.

HORSETAIL
This is one of the richest sources of silica, a nutrient that helps to transport other nutrients around the body. Silica can alleviate brittleness and increase shine and strength in your hair. To make a tea, add a heaped teaspoonful of horsetail to a cupful of boiling water.

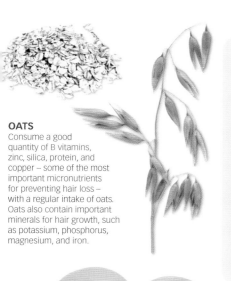

OATS
Consume a good quantity of B vitamins, zinc, silica, protein, and copper – some of the most important micronutrients for preventing hair loss – with a regular intake of oats. Oats also contain important minerals for hair growth, such as potassium, phosphorus, magnesium, and iron.

SAY NO TO...

PROCESSED AND REFINED FOODS These foods fill you up but are so poor in nutrients – including flavonoids, minerals, and vitamins – that you can actually become overweight but deficient in key nutrients.

"BAD" OILS Polyunsaturated or hydrogenated fats, found in margarine and cooking oils, such as canola, contribute to inflammation and premature ageing. They may also stimulate over-production of sebum or a flaking scalp. Replace them with "good" oils, such as those rich in omega-fatty acids like virgin coconut oil or cold-pressed olive oil.

PHYTATES (PHYTIC ACID) These are compounds found in wholegrains, legumes, nuts, and seeds. They can bind to certain dietary minerals including iron, zinc, manganese, and calcium, and inhibit their absorption. The way to avoid the potential negative effects of phytates is to break down the "anti-nutrient" properties, so make sure that cereals and legumes are cooked properly before eating. If eating cereals, such as oats, raw, then soak them in something slightly acidic, such as apple juice, yogurt, or buttermilk for several hours before eating.

EGGS
A great source of keratin-building protein, egg yolk is also a good source of omega-fatty acids for a healthy scalp, and biotin – a water-soluble vitamin B. Too little biotin can cause brittle hair and may lead to hair loss.

SPIRULINA
A blue–green algae with an incredible nutritional profile, spirulina contains 18 amino acids, making it one of the most complete sources of protein to build keratin. It also contains essential fatty acids and many antioxidants for a healthy scalp. Drink a teaspoon of spirulina mixed with apple juice daily.

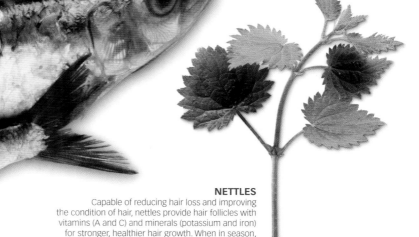

NETTLES
Capable of reducing hair loss and improving the condition of hair, nettles provide hair follicles with vitamins (A and C) and minerals (potassium and iron) for stronger, healthier hair growth. When in season, cook fresh nettles in soups and stews, or prepare a tea using a heaped teaspoonful of dried leaves.

HANDS AND FEET

WE OFTEN FORGET TO TAKE GOOD **CARE** OF OUR HARD-WORKING HANDS AND FEET. **STRENGTHEN** YOUR NAILS AND SAY GOODBYE TO ROUGH, CRACKED SKIN WITH THESE **SOOTHING** AND **PAMPERING** TECHNIQUES AND RECIPES.

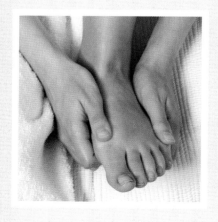
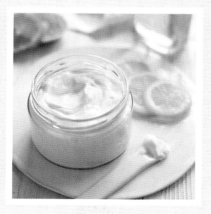
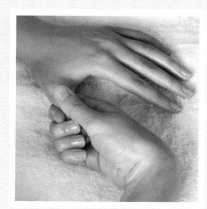

CARE FOR HANDS AND FEET

Many of our daily beauty routines focus on the face and hair, and it is easy to forget other areas of the body that need extra attention. Our hands and feet are two of the hardest-working areas of the body. Taking good care of them will pay dividends throughout your life and is an essential part of a healthy lifestyle.

BOOST YOUR DIET

Your diet has an influence on the health of your skin and nails.

- Make sure you are eating a range of healthy essential fats to nourish your skin and nails.
- Take a good multivitamin and mineral tablet – minor or trace deficiencies are often at the root of nail problems.
- For healthy nails, eat high-quality protein foods such as legumes, nuts, and seeds. Eat foods that are high in B vitamins or take a supplement.
- Drink plenty of water since a hydrated body encourages healthy skin and nails.

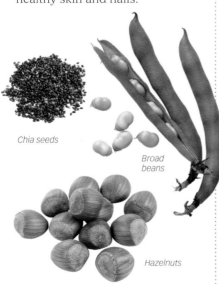

Chia seeds

Broad beans

Hazelnuts

HELP FOR YOUR HANDS

You expose your hands to sun, wind, rain, and cold every day. As we use them for washing and cleaning they are also more exposed to harsh chemicals than any other part of the body. The damage to skin and nails can build up very quickly and neglected hands in particular can show their age – and can sometimes make you look older than you are.

Healthy fingernails are generally smooth and uniform in colour. They should be free of spots, ridges, dents, or discoloration. If your nails do not look good, it could be because of a lack of regular care and attention, but it could also be an indication of an underlying condition – such as a fungal infection – that requires treatment.

WASH YOUR HANDS regularly and apply a moisturiser each time you do.

MOISTURISE YOUR NAILS because they need moisture, just like the rest of your skin does. Massage moisturiser into the nails and cuticles to encourage healthy circulation, helping oxygenated blood, full of nutrients, to reach the nails and hair.

WEAR GLOVES when washing up, gardening, or cleaning – these activities bring your hands into contact with water and harsh detergents for prolonged periods of time.

DO NOT BITE YOUR NAILS or pick at your cuticles as it damages the nail bed. Even a minor cut alongside your nail can allow bacteria or fungi to enter and cause an infection. As nails grow very slowly, an injured nail will retain signs of an injury for several months.

TRIM YOUR FINGERNAILS and clean under the nails regularly. Use sharp manicure scissors or clippers and an emery board to smooth the edges of your nails.

NEVER PULL OFF HANGNAILS – it almost always results in ripping living tissue. Instead, clip hangnails off carefully.

RETHINK NAIL POLISH because most polishes are made with toxic solvents and hormone-disrupting plastics, and the products we use to remove them are very drying for the nails and cuticles. Well-maintained, natural-looking nails are always the healthiest option.

BEST FOOT FORWARD

Most of us ignore our feet, unless they are painful. Yet taking care of your feet is a lifelong habit that can put a spring in your step. Good foot care begins with the shoes you wear, so make sure your shoes fit properly. Keep in mind that tight, poorly fitting shoes can raise the risk of fallen arches, bunions and corns, and ingrown toenails, all of which are painful and can affect your gait. Trainers can make feet sweaty, smelly, and prone to fungal infections. Research suggests that high heels can encourage poor posture and backache, and raise the risk of osteoarthritis in the knees.

WASH AND DRY your feet carefully. After washing your feet, make sure you dry thoroughly between the toes. Left damp, they are a perfect breeding ground for athlete's foot.

USE CLIPPERS to trim toenails regularly. Trim straight across only. Cutting down the sides of toenails encourages painful ingrown nails.

PUT YOUR FEET UP at the end of the day. If you are on your feet all day and you suffer from heavy or swollen legs, try to make some time daily to rest with your feet higher than your head. Slowly rotate and flex your feet from time to time to encourage circulation.

SOFTEN UP ROUGH SKIN with nourishing oils like olive, coconut, shea butter, or pure cocoa butter. Apply every night and give yourself an occasional foot massage (see p236). If your skin is particularly rough, slip on thin socks after moisturising. Leave on overnight to speed healing.

A RELAXING FOOT BATH heals and soothes aches and pains. Try adding some sea salt, Epsom salts, or refreshing essential oils such as lavender, chamomile, tea tree, or eucalyptus to the foot bath.

FIGHT INFECTION quickly to avoid it from spreading. Natural essential oils like tea tree and thyme are great for fighting infection. Seek advice from a doctor, chiropodist, or podiatrist for chronic foot problems that do not respond to simple treatments.

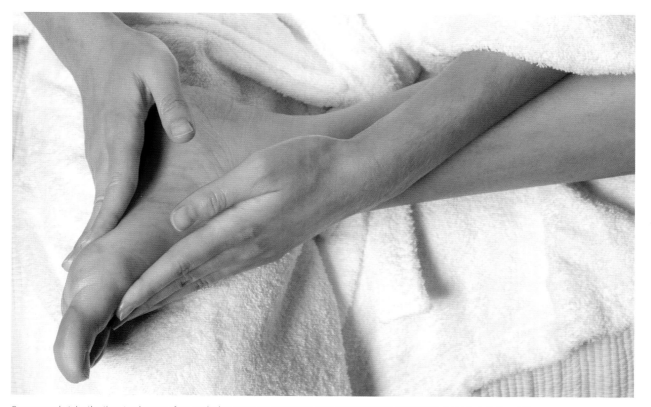

Once a week, take the time to give your feet a relaxing massage (see p236) with a moisturising oil or lotion. It can help to boost the condition of your feet and invigorates them if they are tired or achey.

GARDENERS' HAND SCRUB

FOR TIRED AND DIRTY HANDS

After a day in the garden, **soothe** and **nourish** dry hands with this easy-to-make hand scrub. It contains **exfoliating** ground rice and pumice powder, which give a firm yet gentle consistency. Almond oil is **nourishing** and mixed with olive oil, it can **soften**, **soothe**, **heal**, and **protect** the skin. The **stimulating** action of rosemary essential oil is brilliant for use on tired and overworked muscles.

INGREDIENTS

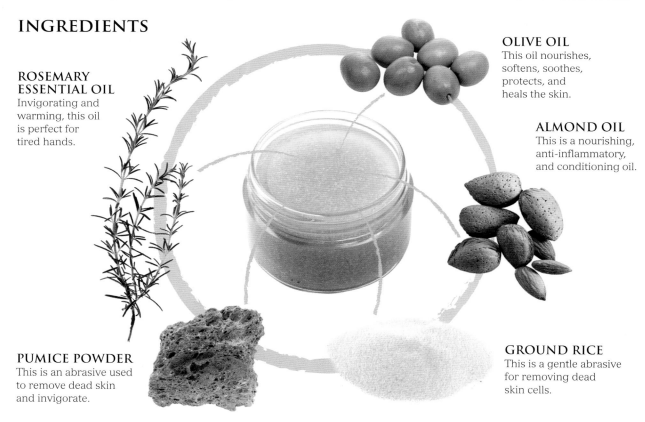

ROSEMARY ESSENTIAL OIL
Invigorating and warming, this oil is perfect for tired hands.

OLIVE OIL
This oil nourishes, softens, soothes, protects, and heals the skin.

ALMOND OIL
This is a nourishing, anti-inflammatory, and conditioning oil.

PUMICE POWDER
This is an abrasive used to remove dead skin and invigorate.

GROUND RICE
This is a gentle abrasive for removing dead skin cells.

MAKES 50G (1¾OZ)

INGREDIENTS
1 tbsp ground rice
1 tsp pumice powder
1 tbsp almond oil
1 tbsp olive oil
10 drops rosemary essential oil

HOW TO MAKE

1 Place all the ingredients in a bowl and mix well.

2 Spoon into a sterilized jar and place the lid on. Store in a cool, dark place. Keeps for up to 3 months.

HOW TO APPLY

Massage into the hands, paying attention to areas of ingrained dirt and dry skin. Rinse with warm water. Use hand cream after application, if required.

GENTLE OAT HAND SCRUB

FOR MATURE SKIN

Our hands are always working. They experience an enormous amount of wear and tear on a daily basis, and they age along with the rest of our skin. Keeping hands in good condition is often at the bottom of the priority list, but this simple scrub can help to **revitalize** dull skin, leaving hands feeling **silky smooth** and **youthful-looking.**

MAKES 45G (1½OZ)

INGREDIENTS

1 tbsp jumbo oats
1 tbsp argan oil
1 tsp sugar
1 tsp ground rice
1 tsp glycerin
4 drops geranium essential oil
4 drops orange essential oil

HOW TO MAKE

1 Place the oats, oil, and sugar in a bowl. Add the ground rice, glycerin, and essential oils and mix well.
2 Spoon into a sterilized jar and place the lid on. Store in a cool, dry place. Keeps for up to 3 months.

HOW TO APPLY

Apply to clean hands. Gently rub the scrub into your hands. Pay attention to areas of dry or rough skin. Rinse with warm water, dry carefully, and apply hand cream if required. Omit the sugar for a more gentle scrub.

ARGAN NAIL BALM

FOR WEAK NAILS

Boost nail and cuticle health with a home-made nail balm containing rich vegetable oils to help **strengthen** and **moisturise**. Intensively moisturise and **soften cuticles** with **restorative** argan oil and rich cocoa butter. Melissa and lemon essential oils help to make your nails smell deliciously clean, and zesty myrrh essential oil helps to **heal** cracked skin.

MAKES 20G (¾OZ)

INGREDIENTS

1 tsp argan oil
1 tsp evening primrose oil
1 tsp cocoa butter
½ tsp beeswax
5 drops melissa essential oil
2 drops lemon essential oil
2 drops mandarin essential oil
1 drop myrrh essential oil

HOW TO MAKE

1 Heat the oils, butter, and beeswax in a bain-marie (see p133), until the wax has melted. Remove from the heat.
2 Add the essential oils and mix well.
3 Pour into a sterilized jar and leave to cool before placing the lid on. Store in a cool, dark place. Keeps for up to 3 months.

HOW TO APPLY

Gently massage into nails and cuticles. Re-apply as required.

Hand Repair Cream

FOR DRY SKIN

Deeply **nourish**, **moisturise**, and **repair** work-worn hands with this combination of rich vegetable oils and reparative essential oils. This protective cream **enriches** the hands and nails with **soothing** and **softening** olive and jojoba oils, and vitamin and fatty acid-rich argan oil. The essential oils in this product repair the skin, **treat inflammation**, and create an **uplifting** fragrance.

Ingredients

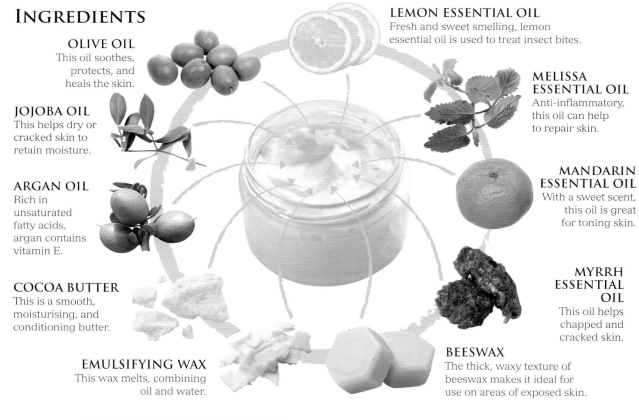

OLIVE OIL
This oil soothes, protects, and heals the skin.

JOJOBA OIL
This helps dry or cracked skin to retain moisture.

ARGAN OIL
Rich in unsaturated fatty acids, argan contains vitamin E.

COCOA BUTTER
This is a smooth, moisturising, and conditioning butter.

EMULSIFYING WAX
This wax melts, combining oil and water.

LEMON ESSENTIAL OIL
Fresh and sweet smelling, lemon essential oil is used to treat insect bites.

MELISSA ESSENTIAL OIL
Anti-inflammatory, this oil can help to repair skin.

MANDARIN ESSENTIAL OIL
With a sweet scent, this oil is great for toning skin.

MYRRH ESSENTIAL OIL
This oil helps chapped and cracked skin.

BEESWAX
The thick, waxy texture of beeswax makes it ideal for use on areas of exposed skin.

MAKES 50G (1¾OZ)

INGREDIENTS

1 tsp each argan, olive, and jojoba oils

1 tsp cocoa butter

1 tsp beeswax

60ml (2fl oz) mineral water

1 tbsp emulsifying wax

1 tsp glycerin

8 drops melissa essential oil

4 drops each lemon, mandarin, and myrrh essential oils

HOW TO MAKE

1 Create an emulsion (see p109) by melting the oils, butter, and beeswax in a bain-marie. Remove from the heat when the wax has melted.

2 Boil the mineral water to 80°C (175°F). Add the wax and glycerin, and stir.

3 Add the hot oil mixture to the hot water mixture. Using a hand-held whisk or stick blender, whisk continuously until smooth.

4 Add the essential oils and continue to mix. Pour into a sterilized jar and leave to cool before placing the lid on. Store in a cool, dark place. Keeps for up to 3 months.

HOW TO APPLY

Gently massage onto dry hands, rubbing into nails and cuticles.

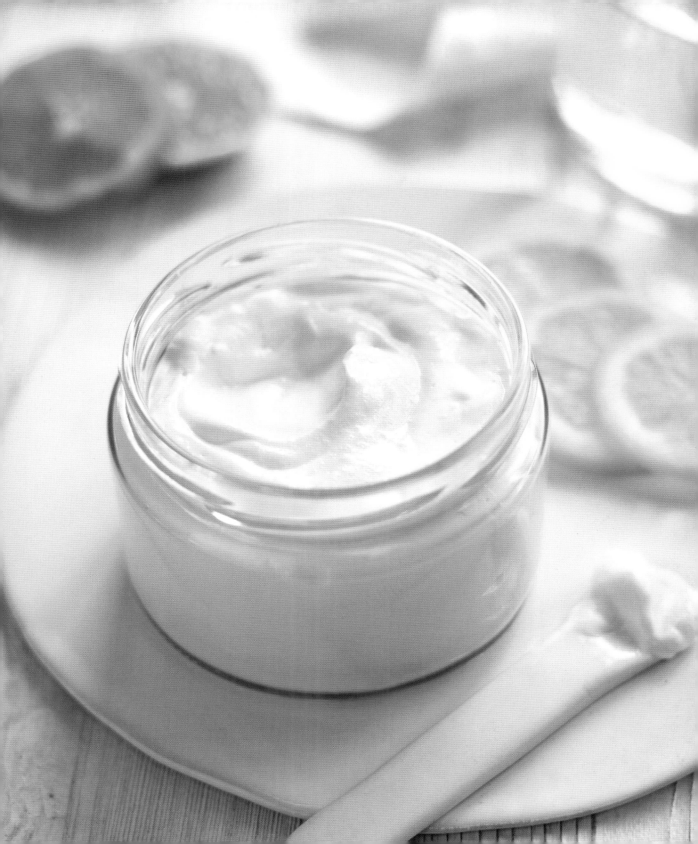

10-Minute **Foot Massage**

Relax with a weekly foot massage to keep your feet in good condition. To prepare, soak your feet in a bowl of warm water that contains 2 drops of essential oil, such as peppermint or lavender. After 5 minutes, dry your feet. Support your lower back with cushions, and rest the sole of the right foot against your left knee.

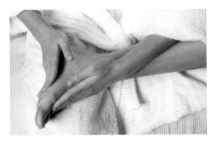

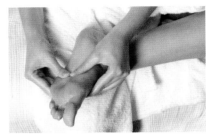

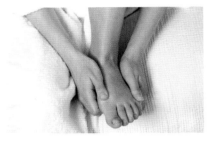

1 Rub oil or lotion between the palm of the hands. Sandwich the left foot between the hands, with fingers facing forwards. Rub the hands backwards and forwards along the foot to warm the area.

2 Using firm circular pressure, massage the sole of the foot from heel to toe with both of the thumbs. Make sure you cover the whole of the sole of the foot.

3 Hold the bottom of the foot with both of your hands and use the thumbs to gently rub the top of the foot across towards the sole. Repeat 3 times.

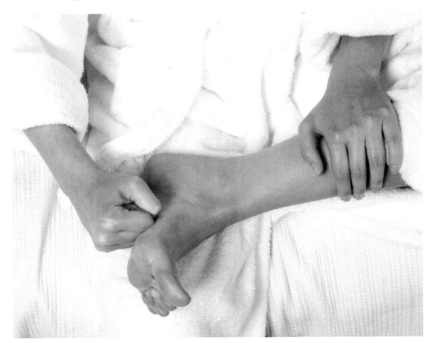

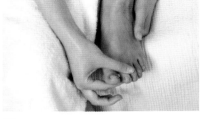

5 Support the heel of the foot with the left hand and grip the toes with the right hand. Squeeze and rotate each toe and then gently flex. Roll and squeeze each toe, one at a time.

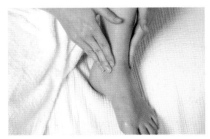

4 Arch your foot. Holding your left leg with one hand, make a closed fist with the other. Using the top part of the fingers, roll your hand backwards and forwards to gently knead the sole, working into the arch of your foot.

6 Using both hands, massage both sides of the anklebone with circular motions, gently rubbing over the top of the bone. Repeat the sequence with the right foot.

10-Minute Hand Massage

Soothe your hands and stimulate your blood flow with a weekly massage. To begin, add 2 drops of your favourite essential oil to a bowl of warm water. Leave hands to soak for 5 minutes, then dry them and sit comfortably on a chair with a towel-covered pillow on your knee. Apply lotion or oil to your hands and rub them together.

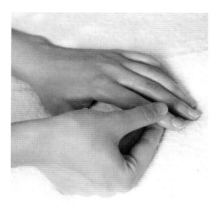

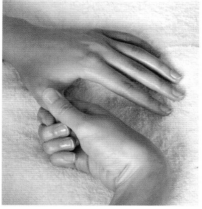

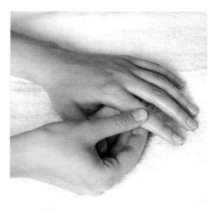

1 Place your left hand on the pillow, palm down. Starting at the base of each finger, apply firm pressure, pulling out each finger to the tip. Be careful not to pull the joints too far.

2 Grip your thumb with your right hand, and gently twist and pull towards the tip. Repeat this action with each finger of your left hand, making sure you don't pull the joints too far.

3 Gently massage each joint on your left hand with circular movements between the thumb and index finger of your right hand.

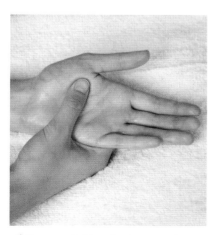

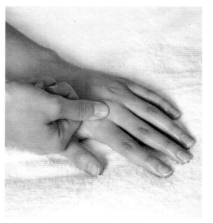

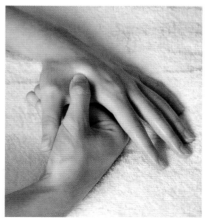

4 Turn your left hand palm up, and support it with four fingers of the right hand. Use the thumb pad to massage into the palm in clockwise and anti-clockwise circles. Concentrate on the muscles around the thumb joint.

5 Turn the hand over with the palm facing down, and make long strokes with the thumb pad from between the fingers to the wrist. Be careful to massage between the bones rather than over them. Repeat this 3 times.

6 Using the thumb pad, massage between the thumb and index finger in small clockwise and anti-clockwise circles. Gently shake the hand out. Repeat the whole sequence on the other hand, then rest for 5 minutes.

ROSE AND SHEA BUTTER HAND CREAM

FOR DRY SKIN

Care for your hard-working hands with this rich, buttery cream that **restores** and **softens**. Almond oil is well known for its **nourishing** properties and is combined with **moisturising** shea butter to create the base of this hand cream. Fragranced with a blend of **calming** rose and **balancing** geranium essential oils, this product is a handbag essential.

MAKES 100G (3½OZ)

INGREDIENTS

1 tsp almond oil
1 tsp shea nut butter
1 tbsp emulsifying wax
60ml (2fl oz) mineral water
1 tsp glycerin
5 drops rose essential oil
5 drops geranium essential oil
3 drops patchouli essential oil

HOW TO MAKE

1 Create an emulsion (see p109), by melting the oil, butter, and wax together in a bain-marie. Remove from the heat once the wax has melted.

2 Heat the mineral water in a saucepan to 80°C (175°F). Add the glycerin.

3 Add the hot oil mixture to the hot water mixture. Using a hand-held whisk or a stick blender, whisk continuously until smooth.

4 Add the essential oils and continue to mix.

5 Pour into a sterilized jar and leave to cool before placing the lid on. Store in a cool, dark place. Keeps for up to 3 months.

HOW TO APPLY

Gently massage onto dry hands rubbing into nails and cuticles. Re-apply as required.

SOOTHING HAND CREAM

FOR DRY SKIN

Our hands are exposed to the elements on a regular basis, exposed to detergents, and washed frequently, so it's no wonder that the skin on our hands gets dry. This hand cream was designed with sore, hard-worked hands in mind. The mixture of calendula macerated oil and chamomile essential oil helps to **soothe** irritated skin as well as **replenish** any moisture lost from the skin.

MAKES 100G (3½OZ)

INGREDIENTS

1 tsp jojoba oil
2 tsp calendula macerated oil
1 tsp beeswax
1 tbsp emulsifying wax
60ml (2fl oz) mineral water
6 drops lavender essential oil
5 drops Roman chamomile essential oil

HOW TO MAKE

1 Create an emulsion (see p109), by melting the oils, beeswax, and emulsifying wax together in a bain-marie. Remove from the heat once the waxes have melted.

2 Heat the mineral water in a saucepan to 80°C (175°F). Add the hot oil mixture to the hot water. Using a hand-held whisk or a stick blender, whisk continuously until smooth.

3 Add the essential oils and continue to mix.

4 Pour into a sterilized jar and leave to cool before placing the lid on. Store in a cool, dark place. Keeps for up to 3 months.

HOW TO APPLY

Gently massage onto dry hands, rubbing into nails and cuticles. Re-apply as required.

PUMICE FOOT SCRUB

FOR DRY FEET

Soften dry or hard skin on the feet with this **cleansing** foot scrub. Pumice powder and ground rice can **exfoliate** the dead skin cells from feet, and purifying kaolin draws out impurities and helps with foot perspiration problems. The combination of essential oils works alongside a foot massage to **stimulate** the circulation and leave feet warm, **smooth**, and cleansed.

MAKES 45G (1½OZ)

INGREDIENTS

1 tsp pumice powder
1 tsp ground rice
1 tsp kaolin
5 drops lemongrass essential oil
2 drops ginger essential oil
2 drops grapefruit essential oil

HOW TO MAKE

1 Place the pumice powder, ground rice, and kaolin in a bowl and mix together.

2 Add 1–2 tablespoons of water gradually and mix to make a paste. Add the essential oils and continue to mix.

3 Spoon into a sterilized jar and place the lid on. Store in a cool place. Keeps for up to a month.

HOW TO APPLY

Massage the scrub into the skin on the feet in circular movements, paying particular attention to areas of dry skin and the heels. Leave the scrub on the feet for 5 minutes for extra cleansing. Rinse feet well with clean, warm water. Pat skin dry with a clean towel.

SEA SALT AND TEA TREE FOOT SCRUB

FOR DRY FEET

Give dry, hard skin on the feet a treat by combining this quick and easy-to-make foot scrub with a **soothing** foot soak. Sea salts are **relaxing** and **soothing** and make a great **exfoliating** particle. Mixed with **nourishing** jojoba oil and **cleansing** tea tree oil, use this scrub every day to **revive** tired feet and remove dry skin.

MAKES 45G (1½OZ)

INGREDIENTS

1 tbsp sea salt
3 tbsp jojoba oil
10 drops tea tree essential oil

HOW TO MAKE

1 Place all the ingredients in a bowl and mix together to make a spreadable paste. Add more oil if required.

2 Spoon into a sterilized jar and place the lid on. Store in a cool place. Keeps for up to 3 months.

HOW TO APPLY

Soak feet first in a warm-water foot bath for 5 minutes. Remove from the water and massage the scrub into the skin on the feet in circular movements, paying particular attention to areas of dry skin and the heels. Return the feet to the foot bath and leave to soak for a further 5 minutes. Rinse feet well with clean, warm water. Pat skin dry with a clean towel. Avoid use on broken skin.

HEEL REPAIR OINTMENT

FOR DRY, CRACKED HEELS

Keep the skin on the heels **moisturised** and avoid cracks with this intensive oil-based ointment. The ointment contains **restorative** essential oils to encourage **healing**, and **skin-softening** and **hydrating** base oils with protective waxes that address dryness. It is best to apply after washing and, if possible, exfoliating the feet.

MAKES 50G (1¾OZ)

INGREDIENTS

1 tsp beeswax
1 tsp carnauba wax
1 tsp castor oil
1 tsp hemp seed oil
1 tbsp sunflower oil
1 tbsp jojoba oil
5 drops myrrh essential oil
4 drops lavender essential oil

HOW TO MAKE

1 Heat the waxes and oils in a bain-marie (see p133). Remove from the heat when the wax has melted.

2 Add the essential oils, mix, and allow to cool for about an hour, stirring occasionally.

3 Scoop into a sterilized jar and use immediately, or store in a cool, dry place. Keeps for up to 6 weeks.

HOW TO APPLY

First exfoliate the area with a pumice stone, then wash the feet thoroughly and dry. Massage into the skin, paying particular attention to dry, chapped areas.

Nourish Broken Heels

Dry, broken heels can be painful. The cracks can deepen and start bleeding if they are neglected for too long. To prevent them, soften up rough skin on your feet with nourishing oils, such as olive, coconut, shea butter, or pure cocoa butter on a regular basis. To treat broken heels, nourish them with a rich ointment (see above) or medicated creams that get into the root of the cracks, fast. Apply generously at night, slip on some thin socks, and in the morning your heels will be visibly smoother and softer.

SEA SALT FOOT SOAK

FOR ALL SKIN TYPES

Use this at the end of a busy day. Sea salt has long been known for its **deep-cleansing** and **antiseptic** properties. This foot soak contains a combination of dead sea salt and **skin-softening** and **soothing** oats, mixed with muscle-soothing arnica macerated oil. Lavender essential oil relaxes the muscles and lends its **fragrance** to the product.

INGREDIENTS

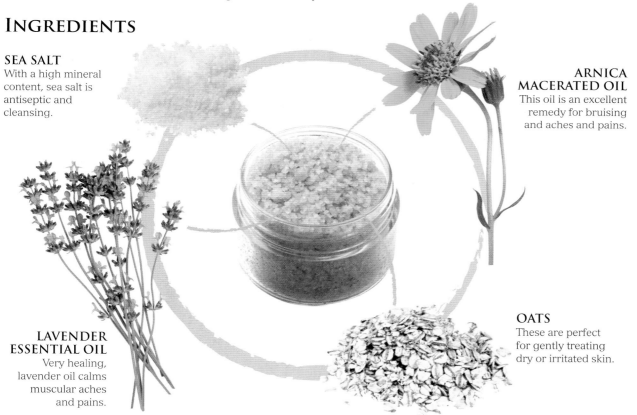

SEA SALT
With a high mineral content, sea salt is antiseptic and cleansing.

ARNICA MACERATED OIL
This oil is an excellent remedy for bruising and aches and pains.

LAVENDER ESSENTIAL OIL
Very healing, lavender oil calms muscular aches and pains.

OATS
These are perfect for gently treating dry or irritated skin.

MAKES 45G (1½ OZ)

INGREDIENTS
2 tbsp sea salt
1 tbsp jumbo oats
1 tsp arnica macerated oil
10 drops lavender essential oil

HOW TO MAKE

1 Blitz the sea salt and oats together in an electric blender until they form a fine powder.

2 Add the arnica macerated oil and the essential oil, and mix together.

3 Transfer to a sterilized jar. Store in a cool, dark place. Keeps for up to 6 months.

HOW TO APPLY

Add a tablespoon of the mixture to a foot bath and leave feet to soak for 10 minutes. Remove from the water, pat dry, and apply foot cream.

TEA TREE FOOT CREAM

FOR ALL SKIN TYPES

Our feet need looking after – so many of us wear ill-fitting shoes, and neglect our feet until the warmer months. This rich, **refreshing** foot cream contains luxurious cocoa butter and **nourishing** jojoba oil, along with **antiseptic** tea tree and myrrh essential oils, which will give your feet a well-deserved, **moisturising** treat.

MAKES 100G (3½OZ)

INGREDIENTS

1 tsp jojoba oil
1 tsp cocoa butter
1 tsp beeswax
1 tbsp emulsifying wax
60ml (2fl oz) mineral water
6 drops tea tree essential oil
5 drops lemon essential oil
2 drops myrrh essential oil

HOW TO MAKE

1 Create an emulsion (see p109) by melting the oil, butter, beeswax, and emulsifying wax together in a bain-marie. Remove from the heat once the wax has melted.

2 Heat the mineral water in a saucepan to 80ºC (175ºF). Add the hot oil mixture to the hot water. Using a hand-held whisk or a stick blender, whisk continuously until smooth.

3 Add the essential oils and continue to stir occasionally as the mixture cools. Pour into a sterilized jar and place the lid on. Store in a cool, dry place. Keeps for up to 6 weeks.

HOW TO APPLY

Gently massage into dry feet, concentrating on dry areas such as the heels. Re-apply as required.

TEA TREE FOOT POWDER

FOR ACTIVE FEET

This is an ideal product for helping to control sweat. It contains a blend of **antiseptic** essential oils and absorbent cornflour, which work to absorb moisture and prevent odour. Tea tree essential oil is an antifungal that can treat athlete's foot, while lavender essential oil has an **antibacterial** action, which is perfect for combatting any odour-causing bacteria.

MAKES 50G (1¾OZ)

INGREDIENTS

50g (1¾oz) organic cornflour
1 tsp propolis tincture
10 drops tea tree essential oil
10 drops lavender essential oil

HOW TO MAKE

1 Place the cornflour in a salt or sugar shaker, leaving some room at the top for mixing.

2 Add the tincture and essential oils to cotton wool balls and add to the shaker.

3 Leave for 2 hours, regularly shaking the mixture to disperse the fragrance and propolis tincture.

4 Shake well before applying to feet. Store in a cool, dry place for up to 6 months.

HOW TO APPLY

Apply to clean, dry feet.

BANANA FOOT TREATMENT

QUICK

FOR DRY FEET

Dry feet not only look unattractive, but can also cause more serious issues. If the skin on your feet becomes too dry, it can crack under daily stresses and strains. Bananas have a high moisture content, and when you apply them to skin, they can provide an instant **moisture boost**, leaving you with **softer**, **smoother**, and more **supple** skin on your feet.

MAKES ENOUGH FOR ONE APPLICATION

INGREDIENTS

2 medium-sized ripe bananas

HOW TO MAKE

Using a fork, mash the bananas in a bowl into lump-free, smooth paste.

HOW TO APPLY

Apply to clean, dry feet 1–2 times a week. Massage into cracked heels. Leave for 10 minutes and rinse with warm water. Pat skin dry with a clean towel.

Try a Natural Pedicure

Give your feet a natural, organic pedicure every few weeks to improve their health and appearance.

- Soften your feet in a foot soak, such as Sea salt foot soak (see p241) for 10 minutes.

- Apply an exfoliator to your feet, such as Pumice foot scrub (see p239), gently massaging the product all over using small, circular movements. Remove with warm water and cotton wool. Gently pat your feet dry using a warm towel.

- Moisturise your feet using a generous amount of cream, such as Tea tree foot cream (see p242). Massage the product in, paying close attention to the joints of the toes and the heel area.

- Cut your nails carefully using nail scissors or clippers. Always cut straight across, to prevent ingrowing toenails. Buff them with a nail file to even the shape. Avoid painting your nails with polish, as it contains harmful, synthetic ingredients. Instead, rub a drop of almond or evening primrose oil into each toenail and cuticle.

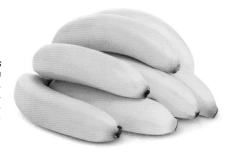

Bananas
Nutritionally rich, bananas contain vitamins, minerals, and antioxidants. They also have a high water content, making them excellent for moisturising, nourishing, and brightening dull skin.

Vitamins, Minerals, And Nutrients

Essential to the healthy functioning of our body systems, vitamins, minerals, and nutrients help to strengthen hair and nails, build collagen, and keep skin healthy. We should get all the nutrients we need from a good diet, but modern farming and food-processing methods have had a negative impact on nutritional levels in our food. Boost these levels with particular foods or regular supplements.

Vitamin or Nutrient	Functions for Skin, Hair, and Nails	Rich Food Sources	Notes	Average Daily Intake/ Supplemental Range
Vitamin A (Retinol) and Carotenoids	**Vitamin A:** This is a rich antioxidant and is anti-ageing. It helps to produce collagen. **Carotenoids:** Precursors to vitamin A, carotenoids have antioxidant properties and help to protect skin from sun damage.	**Vitamin A:** Fish-liver oils, animal liver, oily fish, egg yolks, whole milk, and butter. **Carotenoids:** Green and yellow fruits and vegetables, green leafy vegetables, peppers, sweet potato, and broccoli.	Animal sources of vitamin A may be much better absorbed than vegetable sources.	**Vitamin A:** ADI: 5,000–9,000IU SR: 10,000+ **Beta-carotene:** ADI: 5–8mg SR: 10–40mg
B-complex Vitamins	These are required for healthy skin, hair, and eyes, as well as a healthy liver and nervous system.	Yeast, animal liver, kidneys, almonds, wheatgerm, brown rice, mushrooms, egg yolk, red meat, and mackerel.	These may be destroyed by refining and processing.	Variable, check individual vitamin B.
Vitamin C (Ascorbic Acid)	This is necessary for antioxidant function. Vitamin C encourages healthier bones, teeth, gums, cartilage, capillaries, immune system, and connective tissue. Important for healing and anti-ageing. Anti-inflammatory.	Acerola cherry, sweet peppers, kale, parsley, green leafy vegetables, broccoli, watercress, strawberries, papaya, oranges, grapefruit, cabbage, lemon juice, elderberries, liver, and mangoes.	This vitamin is unstable to heat and light. Cooking may lead to a 10–90 per cent loss of vitamin C content.	ADI: 75–125mg SR: 250–2,000mg
Vitamin D (Calciferol)	Cancer-protective vitamin D regulates calcium absorption for healthy bones, teeth, hair, and nail growth. It balances hormones and boosts a healthy immune system.	**Vitamin D3:** Fish-liver oils, sardines (tinned and fresh), salmon, tuna, shrimps, butter, liver, egg yolk, milk, and cheese. **Vitamin D2:** Sunflower seeds, spirulina, mushroom, flaxseed, and sprouted seeds.	Vitamin D is synthesized by sunlight on the skin. Vitamin D3 is easier to absorb than vitamin D2.	ADI: 200–400IU SR: 400–3,000IU
Vitamin E (Tocopherol)	This is necessary for antioxidant function, healthy immune system, heart, circulation, and lipid balance. A sex hormone regulator, it has an anti-ageing effect on the skin.	Sunflower seeds, sunflower oil, safflower oil, almonds, sesame oil, peanut oil, corn oil, wheatgerm, peanuts, olive oil, butter, spinach, oatmeal, salmon, and brown rice.	Losses caused by heat and light. Milling/refining flour causes up to 80 per cent loss of vitamin E content.	ADI: 30mg SR: 100–800mg
Bioflavonoids, such as Citrin, Hesperidin, Rutin, and Quercetin	Anti-inflammatory bioflavonoids are necessary for antioxidant function and a healthy immune system. They are good for healthy blood vessels and may help to prevent broken capillaries. Rutin can combat skin redness.	Apples, black and red berries, blackcurrants, buckwheat, citrus fruit, apricots, garlic, green-growing shoots of plants, onions, rosehips, and cherries.	Cooking and processing foods causes a loss in levels of bioflavoid.	ADI: N/A SR: 500–3,000mg
Essential Fatty Acids (Omega Oils)	These acids help to regulate inflammation and hormones. Good for lipid balance, growth, the nervous system, eyes, skin, joints, and metabolism.	Fish-liver oils, oily fish, milk, cheese, flaxseed (linseed) oil, hempseed oil, canola, and walnut oil.	Loss of content is caused by hydrogenation, light, and heat.	3–8 per cent of calories.

Vitamin or Nutrient	Functions for Skin, Hair, and Nails	Rich Food Sources	Notes	Average Daily Intake/ Supplemental Range
Hyaluronic Acid	This acid is necessary for wound healing, cartilage and joint functioning, tissue repair, and skin regeneration.	Offal, fish oil, fruits (cherries, guavas), and parsley.	Foods rich in vitamin A (retinol) are also likely to be high in hyaluronic acid.	40–200mg daily
Methyl Sulfonyl Methane (MSM)	MSM improves collagen and keratin production, reduces signs of ageing, and has detoxifying and anti-inflammatory benefits. It strengthens the skin's support matrix and may help eczema, acne, and psoriasis.	Onions, garlic, cruciferous vegetables, and protein-containing foods, such as nuts, seeds, milk, and eggs.	Lost during cooking and processing, methyl sulfonyl is present in raw and rain-watered (outdoor-grown) foods.	500–6,000mg daily

Mineral	Functions	Rich Food Sources	Notes	Average Daily Intake/ Supplemental Range
Calcium	This mineral aids bone, teeth, and nail formation, regulates nerve and muscle function, and boosts hormones.	Kelp, seaweed, cheese, molasses, carob, almonds, yeast, parsley, corn, watercress, goat's milk, cow's milk, tofu, figs, sunflower seeds, yogurt, beet greens, green leafy vegetables, wheat bran, buckwheat, and sesame seeds.	Water softeners remove calcium from your water supply.	ADI: 800–1400mg SR: 1000–2500mg
Copper	Copper helps the synthesis of enzymes required for iron absorption. It builds collagen and red blood cells and maintains skin, bone, and nerve formation.	Oysters, shellfish, nuts, brazil nuts, almonds, hazelnuts, walnuts, pecans, legumes, split peas, liver, buckwheat, peanuts, lamb, sunflower oil, and crab.	High levels of zinc and calcium prevent the absorption of copper.	ADI: 1–3mg SR: 2–10mg
Iron	Necessary for red blood cell function, energy release, growth, and bone regulation, iron is great for hair, skin, and nails.	Kelp, yeast, molasses, wheat bran, dried apricots, liver, sunflower seeds, millet, parsley, clams, almonds, prunes, cashews, red meat, eggs, and nuts.	Vitamin C enhances iron absorption.	ADI: 10–20mg SR: 15–50mg
Magnesium	This aids the synthesis of proteins, carbohydrates, and lipids. It helps DNA repair, energy production, and healthy hair and nails.	Kelp, seaweed, wheat bran, wheatgerm, almonds, cashews, molasses, brewer's yeast, buckwheat, Brazil nuts, and nuts.	Milling/refining of grains and cereals can cause a loss of up to 90 per cent.	ADI: 350mg SR: 300–800mg
Selenium	This aids antioxidant function, the detox of chemicals, and fertility. It aids DNA repair and sperm, reproductive system, and thyroid health and is anti-carcinogenic.	Butter, wheatgerm, Brazil nuts, cider vinegar, barley, prawns, oats, chard, shellfish, milk, fish, red meat, molasses, garlic, barley, eggs, mushrooms, and alfalfa sprouts.	Milling/refining of cereals causes a 40–50 per cent loss in selenium content.	ADI: 50–200ug SR: 200–800ug
Silica (Silicon)	This is an essential mineral for healthy and strong skin, hair, and nails. Required for collagen production. It balances calcium/ magnesium levels and hormones.	Apples, leeks, green beans, bamboo shoots, cucumber, mango, celery, asparagus, rhubarb, cabbage, cereals, horsetail, and certain mineral waters.	As we age, silica levels decline, so taking supplements becomes more important.	10–30mg daily
Zinc	This is an antioxidant-rich enzyme activator. It aids DNA and RNA synthesis, fertility and reproductive health, wound healing, and skin, hair, muscle, and respiratory health.	Oysters, ginger, red meat, nuts, dried beans, liver, milk, egg yolk, whole wheat, rye, oats, brazil nuts, peanuts, chicken, sardines, buckwheat, oily fish, prawns, and white fish.	Milling/refining of cereals causes an 80 per cent loss of zinc content. Freezing vegetables causes a loss of 25–50 per cent.	ADI: 15mg SR: 10–70mg

Note An Average Daily Intake (ADI) is set by public health officials to meet the requirements of most healthy people. Supplemental Range (SR) is the range of intake considered safe – it is used when taking nutritional supplements. ADIs are not set for every nutrient, so for some only an SR is given.

SUPERFOODS

Nourishing and nutritious, superfoods can give your inner health and outer beauty a real boost. They are becoming more popular as a way to enhance an everyday diet. Some of them are delicious as food ingredients – simply add them to your daily recipes. Others are better taken in supplement form. If you are pregnant or on any medication, check with your doctor before taking any supplements.

Superfood	Main Constituents	Properties	Notes	Daily Intake
Acerola Cherry	This cherry is one of the richest sources of vitamin C and flavonoids, such as hesperidin and rutin.	Vitamin C boosts collagen formation and skin healing, and is anti-inflammatory. Rutin is good for broken capillaries and acne rosacea.	The cherries are often used in supplements for a natural source of vitamin C.	Eat a few fresh cherries when they are in season, or make a jam. Try also as a powder or capsule.
Avocado	Avocado contains omega-fatty acids; vitamins A, B complex, E, and K; fibre; potassium; magnesium; sterolin; and lecithin.	It is an excellent source of healthy oils with anti-inflammatory, skin-nourishing, and skin-softening properties.	Sterolin may help to reduce the apperance of age spots.	Eat fresh avocado daily or try a tablespoon of cold-pressed oil in salad dressings.
Bee Pollen	Pollen contains 40 per cent protein, free amino acids, and vitamins including B complex.	Bee pollen stimulates cell renewal and rejuvenates the skin.	Each bee pollen pellet contains over two million flower pollen grains.	Take up to one teaspoon a day.
Blueberries	These berries offer an excellent source of antioxidants, anthocyanins, flavonoids (quercetin), and resveratrol.	Providing whole-body benefits, especially to circulation, eyes, and skin, blueberries have antioxidant, anti-ageing, and regenerative properties.	Eat organic – there are higher levels of antioxidants, and pesticide residues are a problem in non-organic.	Eat a handful a day of fresh blueberries, when in season.
Boswellia (Indian Frankincense)	Boswellia contains essential oils and boswellic acids.	This contains highly effective anti-inflammatory properties and provides anti-ageing and regenerative actions.	This is used as a traditional Ayurvedic remedy for any inflammatory condition.	Capsules 300–1200mg (at 37.5–65 per cent boswellic acid content) daily.
Chia Seeds	These seeds contain omega-3 fatty acids, fibre, protein, calcium, and manganese.	They are good for clear skin and strong teeth, nails, and hair.	One of the best conversions of omega-3 usable by the body.	Add a tablespoon daily to juice or cereal.
Chlorella	Chlorella algae contains protein; chlorophyll; vitamins A, B12, and D; minerals (iron); and nucleic acids.	Chlorella is a highly effective blood cleanser that helps to clear the skin and has a regenerative action.	The "chlorella growth factor" is thought to provide excellent cell-protective effects.	Maintenance dose 3–10g daily.
Goji Berries	These berries contain vitamins A and C, carotenoids, beta carotene, iron, selenium, essential fatty acids, and dietary fibre.	Goji berries help to build collagen that nourishes and plumps the skin and have an anti-ageing action.	The berries have been used for over 6,000 years in Traditional Chinese medicine due to their nourishing properties.	Eat 4 tablespoons of dried goji berries daily.
Grapeseed Extract	Grapeseed extract contains proanthocyanidin complexes (OPCs).	A powerful antioxidant, grapeseed extract has anti-ageing, wound-healing, and anti-inflammatory properties.	Grape skin extract (containing resveratrol) is also a powerful antioxidant.	Capsules 50–300mg daily.

Superfood	Main Constituents	Properties	Notes	Daily Intake
Green Tea and White Tea	Green tea and white tea are excellent sources of antioxidants, especially catechins (ECGC).	These tea aid healthy cells in all stages of growth and provide anti-ageing properties. They may aid weight loss.	Do not add tea to boiling water; heat water to 80–90°C (160–170°F) to preserve antioxidant levels.	Drink 2–3 cups a day or take a supplement of 100–750mg every day.
Tree Nuts, such as Hazelnuts, and Cobnuts	These are high in essential fatty acids (oleic and linoleic), vitamins B complex and E, iron, copper, and manganese. Nuts also help to produce the antioxidant enzyme superoxide dismutase (SOD).	SOD enzymes have anti-ageing properties – they repair cellular damage and are anti-inflammatory, neutralizing damage that can lead to wrinkles.	Choose nuts with a brown outer coating on, as it contains many of the nutrients and helps nuts keep for longer. The oil is also an excellent source of essential fatty acids.	Eat several nuts daily or drizzle cold-pressed oil on salads.
Hemp	Hemp contains proteins, essential fats (omega 3 and 6), gamma linoleic acid, vitamins (B, D, and E), and enzymes, as well as calcium, iron, magnesium, copper, phospholipids, and phytosterols.	Hemp provides digestible protein for healthy hair and nails. The essential fatty acids in hemp promote healthy skin by reducing inflammation. Properties can treat acne, eczema, and dry skin.	Hemp oil has the best balance of omega 3:6 of any plant oil.	Add seeds or powder to cooking, baking, cereals, and smoothies. You could also add a tablespoon of oil to juice and salad dressings.
Flaxseed (Linseed)	Flax contains omega fatty acids, alpha linoleic acid, fibre, lignans, minerals (calcium, iron, zinc, magnesium, and selenium), and vitamins (B complex and E).	Flax improves digestion (works as a bulk laxative) and is good for acne, eczema, and dry skin. Essential fatty acids promote healthy skin by reducing inflammation.	Flaxseed oil has an excellent omega-3 fatty acid content.	Add a tablespoon of seeds to cereals, or use them in baking. You could also soak them in water. Add a tablespoon of flaxseed oil to juice and salad dressings.
Mulberries	These berries contain antioxidants, anthocyanins, resveratrol, vitamin C, fibre, iron, magnesium, potassium, and zinc.	With anti-ageing and collagen-boosting properties, mulberries can balance blood-sugar levels and are good for hair growth and skin health.	The berries were traditionally used to prevent prematurely grey hair.	Eat a handful of fresh or dried berries a day.
Oats	Oats contain fibre, protein, minerals (manganese, copper, biotin, magnesium, selenium, silica, and zinc), antioxidants, and beta glucan.	They can stabilize blood sugar and therefore are good for weight management. Silica and other minerals help keep hair and nails healthy and strong.	Soak or cook oats before eating them to break down the phytates they contain.	Eat a bowl of porridge, daily.
Rosehips	Rosehips contain vitamins A, C, and K, bioflavonoids, and carotenoids.	They are incredibly rich sources of vitamin C to boost collagen and reduce inflammation. Good for inflammatory skin conditions, such as acne rosacea.	Rosehip is often combined with vitamin C in supplements to boost absorption.	Drink 2–3 cups of rosehip tea a day or take 2–10g rosehip powder.
Oily Fish, such as Salmon	Oily fish contains protein, omega-3 fatty acids (DHA and EPA), vitamins (B complex and D), minerals (selenium, iodine, and potassium).	Boosting collagen and acting as an anti-inflammatory, oily fish helps to reduce wrinkles and signs of ageing.	Eat a variety of oily fish and wild salmon if possible to avoid the pesticide residues from farmed fish.	Eat a portion of oily fish at least 3 times a week.
Spirulina	Contains high-value protein, minerals (magnesium, calcium, potassium, iron, and zinc), vitamins (B complex, E, beta carotene), and chlorophyll.	Purifying spirulina algae has antioxidant and anti-ageing properties. It can aid weight management and promotes healthy skin, hair, and nails.	This combines well with other algae, such as chlorella.	Try 1–8g daily – add the powder to smoothies, soups, and juices, or take in tablet form.

INDEX BY BEAUTY AREA

INDEX

Index entries in italic are full recipes for products. Bold type indicates ingredients with their own directory entry.

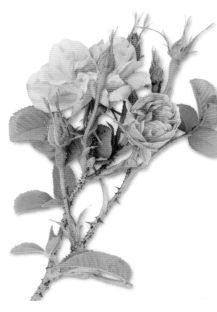

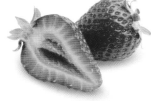

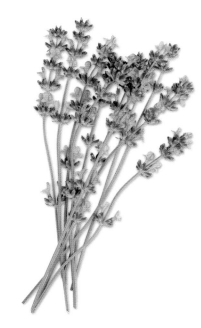

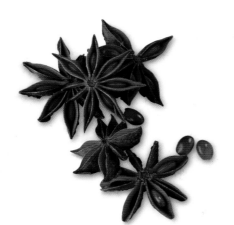

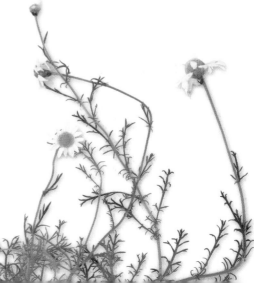

ACKNOWLEDGMENTS

The authors would like to thank the following people for their valuable contribution to making this book happen: Peter Kindersley for his tireless support for the principles of natural health and beauty; NYR's formulation and technical team, past and present; Kristina Koestler for advice on beauty regimes; Justine Jenkins for her natural make-up expertise, and Billie Scheepers for her photographic skills; and all at Dorling Kindersley for their enthusiasm and support in seeing this volume through to completion.

Dorling Kindersley would like to thank the great team at Neal's Yard Remedies.

Recipe and ingredient photography William Reavell
Recipe styling Jane Lawrie and Kat Mead
Prop styling and art direction Isabel de Cordova
Beauty photography Billie Scheepers
Make-up artist Justine Jenkins
Assistant make-up artist Jo Hamilton
Hair stylist Lisa Eastwood
Models Chloe Blanchard, Olivia Burchell, Tatiana Chechetova, Sarah Edwards, Jessi M'Bengue, Kasimira Mosich Miller, Marie Sander, Poonam Vasani, Alea Wiles, and Sarah Willey
Beauty therapists Margherita De-Cristofano and Kristina Koestler
Proofreading Corinne Masciocchi, Dorothy Kikon, Nidhilekha Mathur, Neha Samuel, and Arani Sinha
Indexing Marie Lorimer
Recipe testing Francesca Dennis
Editorial assistance Claire Gell
Design assistance Mandy Earey